theclinics.com

# SURGICAL CLINICS OF NORTH AMERICA

## Obstetrics and Gynecology for the General Surgeon

GUEST EDITOR
Charles S. Dietrich III, MD

CONSULTING EDITOR
Ronald F. Martin, MD

April  2008  •  Volume 88  •  Number 2

**SAUNDERS**

An Imprint of Elsevier, Inc.
PHILADELPHIA   LONDON   TORONTO   MONTREAL   SYDNEY   TOKYO

**W.B. SAUNDERS COMPANY**
*A Division of Elsevier Inc.*

1600 John F. Kennedy Blvd., Suite 1800, Philadelphia, PA 19103-2899

http://www.theclinics.com

SURGICAL CLINICS OF NORTH AMERICA
April 2008
Editor: Catherine Bewick

Volume 88, Number 2
ISSN 0039–6109
ISBN-10: 1-4160-5804-4
ISBN-13: 978-1-4160-5804-5

The ideas and opinions expressed in *The Surgical Clinics of North America* do not necessarily reflect those of the Publisher. The Publisher does not assume any responsibility for any injury and/or damage to persons or property arising out of or related to any use of the material contained in this periodical. The reader is advised to check the appropriate medical literature and the product information currently provided by the manufacturer of each drug to be administered to verify the dosage, the method and duration of administration, or contraindications. It is the responsibility of the treating physician or other health care professional, relying on independent experience and knowledge of the patient, to determine drug dosages and the best treatment for the patient. Mention of any product in this issue should not be construed as endorsement by the contributors, editors, or the Publisher of the product or manufacturers' claims.

*Surgical Clinics of North America* (ISSN 0039–6109) is published bimonthly by Elsevier Inc., 360 Park Avenue South, New York, NY 10010-1710. Months of publication are February, April, June, August, October, and December. Business and Editorial Offices: 1600 John F. Kennedy Blvd., Suite 1800, Philadelphia, PA 19103-2899. Customer Service Office: 6277 Sea Harbor Drive, Orlando, FL 32887-4800. Periodicals postage paid at New York, NY and additional mailing offices. Subscription prices are $238.00 per year for US individuals, $382.00 per year for US institutions, $119.00 per year for US students and residents, $292.00 per year for Canadian individuals, $466.00 per year for Canadian institutions, $309.00 for international individuals, $466.00 per year for international institutions and $154.00 per year for Canadian and foreign students/residents. To receive student/resident rate, orders must be accompanied by name of affiliated institution, date of term, and the *signature* of program/residency coordinator on institution letterhead. Orders will be billed at individual rate until proof of status is received. Foreign air speed delivery is included in all *Clinics* subscription prices. All prices are subject to change without notice. POSTMASTER: Send address changes to *Surgical Clinics*, Elsevier Journals Customer Service, 6277 Sea Harbor Drive, Orlando, FL 32887-4800. **Customer Service: 1-800-654-2452 (US). From outside of the United States, call 1-407-563-6020. Fax: 1-407-363-9661.** E-mail: JournalsCustomerService-usa@elsevier.com.

*The Surgical Clinics of North America* is also published in Spanish by McGraw-Hill Interamericana Editores S.A., P.O. Box 5-237 06500 Mexico D.F. Mexico; and in Portuguese by Interlivros Edicoes Ltda., Rua Comandante Coelho 1085, CEP 21250, Rio de Janeiro, Brazil; and in Greek by Paschalidis Medical Publications, Athens Greece.

*The Surgical Clinics of North America* is covered in *Index Medicus, EMBASE/Excerpta Medica, Current Contents/Clinical Medicine, Current Contents/Life Sciences, Science Citation Index*, and *ISI/BIOMED*.

Printed in the United States of America.

# CONSULTING EDITOR

**RONALD F. MARTIN, MD,** Staff Surgeon, Marshfield Clinic, Marshfield; and Clinical Associate Professor, University of Wisconsin School of Medicine and Public Health, Madison, Wisconsin; Lieutenant Colonel, Medical Corps, United States Army Reserve

# GUEST EDITOR

**CHARLES S. DIETRICH III, MD,** Chief, Gynecologic Oncology Service, Department of Obstetrics and Gynecology, Tripler Army Medical Center, Honolulu, Hawaii

# CONTRIBUTORS

**SONAL BAKAYA, MD,** Resident, Department of Obstetrics and Gynecology, Tripler Army Medical Center, Honolulu, Hawaii

**BRYAN D. BERKEY, MD,** Chief, Ultrasound Imaging, Department of Radiology, Tripler Army Medical Center, Honolulu, Hawaii; Assistant Professor, Department of Radiology and Radiologic Sciences, Uniformed Services University of the Health Sciences, F. Edward Hébert School of Medicine, Bethesda, Maryland

**KEVIN J. BOYLE, MD,** Teaching Staff Obstetrician and Gynecologist, Department of Obstetrics and Gynecology, Tripler Army Medical Center, Honolulu, Hawaii

**BRIAN H. CHING, DO,** Staff, Interventional and Diagnostic Radiology, Department of Radiology, Tripler Army Medical Center, Honolulu, Hawaii

**NISHAN CHOBANIAN, MD,** Director, Gynecologic Oncology, Saint John's Mercy Medical Center, Saint Louis, Missouri

**CHRISTOPHER P. DESIMONE, MD,** Assistant Professor, Division of Gynecologic Oncology, Department of Obstetrics and Gynecology, University of Kentucky Markey Cancer Center, Lexington, Kentucky

**CHARLES S. DIETRICH III, MD,** Chief, Gynecologic Oncology Service, Department of Obstetrics and Gynecology, Tripler Army Medical Center, Honolulu, Hawaii

**JOHN H. FARLEY, MD,** Department of Obstetrics and Gynecology, Uniformed Services University of the Health Sciences, Bethesda, Maryland

**ALAN GEHRICH, MD,** Chief, Urogynecology Service, Department of Obstetrics and Gynecology, Tripler Army Medical Center, Honolulu, Hawaii

ANDREW C. GJELSTEEN, MD, Chief, Emergency Radiology, Department of Radiology, Tripler Army Medical Center, Honolulu, Hawaii

CHRISTINA C. HILL, MD, Residency Program Director, Gynecologic Oncology Service and Maternal Fetal Medicine, Department of Obstetrics and Gynecology, Tripler Army Medical Center, Honolulu, Hawaii

MICAH J. HILL, DO, Obstetrician and Gynecologist, Department of Obstetrics and Gynecology, Blanchfield Army Community Hospital, Fort Campbell, Kentucky

MATTHEW HUEMAN, MD, Fellow, Surgical Oncology, and Instructor, General Surgery, Department of Surgery, The Johns Hopkins Hospital, Baltimore, Maryland

GRANT D.E. MCWILLIAMS, DO, Obstetrician and Gynecologist, Department of Obstetrics and Gynecology, Tripler Army Medical Center, Honolulu, Hawaii

MARK W. MEYERMANN, DO, Chief, Interventional Radiology, Department of Radiology, Tripler Army Medical Center, Honolulu, Hawaii

LEX A. MITCHELL, MD, Diagnostic Radiology Resident, Department of Radiology, Tripler Army Medical Center, Honolulu, Hawaii

THOMAS F. MURPHY, MD, Chief, Abdominal Imaging, Department of Radiology, Tripler Army Medical Center, Honolulu, Hawaii

JENNIFER PICKINPAUGH, DO, Resident Physician, Department of Obstetrics and Gynecology, Tripler Army Medical Center, Honolulu, Hawaii

DOUGLAS A. PRAGER, MD, Chief, Nuclear Medicine, Department of Radiology, Tripler Army Medical Center, Honolulu, Hawaii

MICHAEL P. STANY, MD, Division of Gynecologic Oncology, Walter Reed Army Medical Center, Washington, District of Columbia

SAIOA TORREALDAY, MD, Resident in Obstetrics and Gynecology, Department of Obstetrics and Gynecology, Tripler Army Medical Center, Honolulu, Hawaii

FREDERICK R. UELAND, MD, Associate Professor, Division of Gynecologic Oncology, Department of Obstetrics and Gynecology, University of Kentucky Markey Cancer Center; Department of Obstetrics and Gynecology, University of Kentucky, Lexington, Kentucky

BRADFORD P. WHITCOMB, MD, Gynecologic Oncologist, Associate Residency Program Director, Department of Obstetrics and Gynecology, Tripler Army Medical Center, Honolulu, Hawaii; Assistant Professor, Obstetrics and Gynecology, Uniformed Services University of the Health Sciences, Bethesda, Maryland

# CONTENTS

Female pelvic anatomy encompasses the reproductive, urologic, and gastrointestinal systems. Knowledge of the inherent relations between these organ systems, as well as the ability to develop pelvic spaces, will enable the surgeon to approach pelvic pathology confidently. This article highlights basic anatomy of the female pelvis and emphasizes points of caution during pelvic surgery, as well as reviews the essential principles of pelvic support.

Benign gynecologic conditions constitute the majority of the general gynecologist's practice. Along with health maintenance examinations, contraceptive management, family planning issues, and concerns about incontinence, the gynecologic conditions for which patients commonly present include adnexal masses, leiomyomata, endometriosis, and pelvic inflammatory disease. This article addresses each of these last four entities and incorporates a discussion of their etiologies, clinical presentations, keys to diagnosis, and the various treatment options available.

for the nonpregnant patient, but pregnancy may mask some of the typical presenting symptoms, leading to delayed diagnosis. This article highlights some of the more common surgical diseases that may present during pregnancy, including appendicitis, biliary diseases, bowel obstruction, hemorrhoids, inflammatory bowel disease, and malignancies.

Pregnancy always must be considered when evaluating a female trauma victim of reproductive age. When managing the pregnant trauma victim, one must optimize the well-being of two patients, but the health of the mother is of paramount importance. Rapid assessment, treatment, and transport are critical to optimizing maternal and fetal outcome. Evaluation must be performed with an understanding of the physiologic changes that occur in pregnancy. These changes alter maternal response to trauma and require adaptations to care.

## FORTHCOMING ISSUES

## RECENT ISSUES

---

## The Clinics are now available online!

### www.theclinics.com

**ELSEVIER SAUNDERS**

Surg Clin N Am 88 (2008) xi–xii

**SURGICAL CLINICS OF NORTH AMERICA**

# Foreword

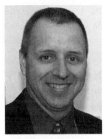

Ronald F. Martin, MD
*Consulting Editor*

Dr. Ephraim McDowell is credited with performing the first ovariotomy in 1809, well before the time of general anesthesia, antibiotics, decades before Lister, and nearly half a century before the first American textbook of surgery, Gross' *System of Surgery* (1859), was published. The practices of general surgery and gynecology have a long history of being linked and still are in some communities. Those who have been around the practice of surgery for a little while can probably remember when the *Journal of the American College of Surgeons* was called *Surgery, Gynecology and Obstetrics*.

In much of general surgery, there has been a continued trend of hyper-fractionation of scope of practice that has probably been a benefit to patients in the aggregate. However, all changes that yield benefits usually come at a cost. With the development of gynecology as a very distinct specialty and gynecologic oncology as an even more distinct subspecialty, there has been a trend for many general surgeons to be less comfortable with complex pelvic dissections. Furthermore, this trend is probably not limited to dissection in the female pelvis only.

Independent of the scope of practice of a general surgery in the current era, or even independent of how many "specialty" colleagues one has to turn to, those of us in this discipline shall all encounter situations in which a better than fair knowledge of gynecology and obstetrics is highly desirable. Patients who develop any general surgical problem while gravid pose an obvious example. And certainly the group of patients with gynecologic malignancies is highly likely to have intestinal complications or associated

doi:10.1016/j.suc.2008.02.001                    *surgical.theclinics.com* enteric involvement, either before, during, or after some oncologic therapy has been provided.

Gynecologists were well ahead of the curve in performing laparoscopic procedures, compared to general surgeons. Some of us general surgery residents received our initial training in laparoscopy or pelviscopy before laparoscopic cholecystectomy was even performed in the United States (or elsewhere), though the equipment was considerably more primitive than it is today. Many of our current trainees would find it hard to believe that in early laparoscopic procedures, the operating surgeon looked through the lens itself and no one else could see anything but the operating surgeon's head—yet, this is true. The advent of the laparoscopic cholecystectomy and the boom in videoscopic surgery volume of the late 1980s and early 1990s provided a tremendous economic incentive for surgeons and industry alike to spend substantially on research and development of the newer products that we currently enjoy along with our gynecologic colleagues.

Perhaps a less obvious reason for a general surgeon to wish to enjoy a better knowledge of pelvic anatomy is penetrating trauma—especially the kind seen in current warfare. The individual body armor worn by United States military personnel at present is highly effective at preventing thoracic and upper abdominal injuries (depending, of course, on the nature of the ballistic element and the direction of impact), but it is not as effective at reducing pelvic trauma. Other than the obvious problem of balancing mobility with protection for the combatant in a war environment, this presents a clinical problem of increased penetrating pelvic trauma as a percentage of trauma victims for the medical responders. Fortunately for me, our Guest Editor, Dr. Dietrich, was assigned to the 8th Forward Surgical Team, which was co-located with our unit in Iraq. Having a person with skills such as his is extremely helpful under those conditions, even if we performed very, very few elective gynecologic oncology procedures.

Whether you practice as a general surgeon with high levels of gynecologic support in a large center or you are the de facto gynecologist in a small community (or just plain have an interest in this topic), this issue and its contents, which Dr. Dietrich and his colleagues have prepared, should be of value to you. We are deeply indebted for his work on this project, as well as his service for our country.

Ronald F. Martin, MD
*Department of Surgery*
*Marshfield Clinic*
*1000 North Oak Avenue*
*Marshfield, WI 54449, USA*

*E-mail address:* martin.ronald@marshfieldclinic.org

ELSEVIER
SAUNDERS

Surg Clin N Am 88 (2008) xiii–xiv

SURGICAL
CLINICS OF
NORTH AMERICA

# Preface

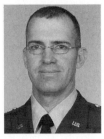

Charles S. Dietrich III, MD
*Guest Editor*

This issue of the *Surgical Clinics of North America* is dedicated to the general surgeon who, at some point in his or her career, is likely to encounter a gynecologic surgical condition, be asked to operate on an obstetrical patient, or be urgently consulted for intraoperative assistance with a gynecologic procedure. In these scenarios, the general surgeon can play a critical role in the treatment team and will often be relied upon for surgical expertise. To provide the best support, however, basic knowledge in pelvic anatomy and gynecologic disease processes should be well understood.

The origins of surgery, gynecology, and obstetrics can be traced to antiquity. During the last two centuries, these fields have been intimately intertwined, with pioneers practicing in both arenas simultaneously. Discoveries and improved surgical techniques were mutually beneficial, as they had applications in both fields. As techniques and anesthesia were further developed, some surgeons began operating exclusively in the pelvis. By the turn of the twentieth century, Johns Hopkins Hospital started training physicians dedicated solely to practicing gynecology. Since then, the two fields have had divergent courses, and on a day-to-day basis general surgeons and obstetricians or gynecologists have limited interactions.

In reality, many patient symptoms often overlap and the differential diagnosis usually includes both general surgery as well as gynecologic conditions. Furthermore, the obstetrical patient can manifest a multitude of surgical problems. Knowledge in both areas is critical for appropriate patient triage and management. Collegial interactions between surgeons and obstetricians or gynecologists can also be invaluable, as techniques in one

0039-6109/08/$ - see front matter © 2008 Elsevier Inc. All rights reserved.
doi:10.1016/j.suc.2008.02.002
*surgical.theclinics.com*

field are adapted to the other. The mutual benefit of close associations became acutely clear for me during a recent deployment with a forward surgical team. As a gynecologic oncologist working side-by-side with general surgeons and an orthopedic surgeon, we quickly learned our colleagues' strengths and capitalized on these to care for a multitude of problems in an austere environment. In the process, I think we all learned something.

The purpose of this issue is to briefly outline common gynecologic and obstetrical issues that may arise in the operative patient undergoing an abdominal surgery. The first few articles will focus on pelvic anatomy and benign and malignant gynecologic diseases. Next, pelvic imaging, managing surgical complications, and gynecologic laparoscopy will be discussed. The final articles will review obstetrical implications in trauma patients and in those with surgical problems.

I would like to thank all of the contributing authors for their endless hours of hard work and dedication. Without their efforts, this issue would still be an idea. I would also like to thank Ron Martin for his mentorship over the past year. Finally, Catherine Bewick deserves praises for her editorial guidance and patience.

Charles S. Dietrich III, MD
*Gynecologic Oncology Service*
*Department of Obstetrics and Gynecology*
*Tripler Army Medical Center*
*1 Jarrett White Road*
*Honolulu, HI 96859-5000, USA*

*E-mail address:* chuck.dietrich@us.army.mil

ELSEVIER
SAUNDERS

Surg Clin N Am 88 (2008) 223–243

SURGICAL
CLINICS OF
NORTH AMERICA

# Surgical Exposure and Anatomy of the Female Pelvis

## Charles S. Dietrich III, MD[a],*, Alan Gehrich, MD[b], Sonal Bakaya, MD[c]

[a]Gynecologic Oncology Service, Department of Obstetrics and Gynecology,
1 Jarrett White Road, Honolulu, HI 96859-5000, USA
[b]Urogynecology Service, Department of Obstetrics and Gynecology,
1 Jarrett White Road, Honolulu, HI 96859-5000, USA
[c]Department of Obstetrics and Gynecology, 1 Jarrett White Road,
Honolulu, HI 96859-5000, USA

The female pelvis is a complex three-dimensional anatomic space where the reproductive, urologic, and gastrointestinal systems converge. These systems are supported by an extensive array of bone, muscles, and ligaments, as well as extensive vascular and neurologic networks. Understanding the inherent relations between different structures will help ensure a successful operation.

The purpose of this article is to introduce the general surgeon to common approaches to the female pelvis, its essential anatomy, and a brief overview of pelvic support. While an exhaustive review of pelvic anatomy is beyond the scope of this article, the authors' intent is to familiarize readers with key pelvic landmarks and to emphasize points of caution.

## Surgical approach and abdominal incisions

Surgical pelvic problems can be approached via laparotomy, laparoscopy, and vaginally. The ultimate decision is based upon many factors, including surgeon preference and skill, ovarian and uterine size, pelvic organ mobility, prior surgeries, the risk of adhesions, the risk of encountering malignancies, and patient preference. This article focuses primarily on

The views expressed in this manuscript are those of the authors and do not reflect the official policy or position of the Department of the Army, Department of Defense, or the United States Government.

* Corresponding author.

E-mail address: chuck.dietrich@us.army.mil (C.S. Dietrich III).

0039-6109/08/$ - see front matter. Published by Elsevier Inc.
doi:10.1016/j.suc.2008.01.003

surgical.theclinics.com

abdominal approaches, as this is the most likely scenario to be encountered by surgeons.

There are several abdominal incisions typically used to approach female pelvic pathology, which can be grouped into vertical or transverse groups. Midline vertical incisions are the most versatile type and allow flexibility in incision length while maximizing lateral and vertical exposures. They are best for patients with known or suspected malignancies where upper abdominal exposure may be required, for the hemodynamically unstable patient where rapid entry is needed, for obese patients, or for patients with large benign pelvic masses or extensive adhesions. Optimal pelvic exposure can be obtained by ensuring that the fascial incision extends to the pubic symphysis, being careful to protect the bladder in the process. Vertical incisions are weaker than their transverse counterparts; therefore, meticulous attention to closure is required to prevent postoperative dehiscence and hernia formation. Patients with vertical incisions also tend to have more pulmonary complications postoperatively, usually resulting from shallow breathing and increased atelectasis.

Transverse incisions include Pfannenstiel, Cherney, and Maylard incisions. They are associated with improved cosmetic results, lower postoperative pain, fewer eviscerations, and lower pulmonary morbidity [1]. Despite their apparent benefits, however, the surgeon must remember that transverse incisions are more time consuming, offer limited exposure, and have a higher neurovascular injury rate.

Pfannenstiel's incision was first described by Hans Pfannenstiel in 1900 and is perhaps the most commonly used transverse incision today in obstetrics and gynecology [2]. The incision is usually made two finger-breaths above the pubic symphysis, in a curvilinear fashion following the lines of Langerhans. The length of the incision can vary from a 4-cm minilaparotomy to 12 cm to 14 cm, depending on the operative indications. Incisions larger than this are rarely beneficial, as further lateral exposure is limited by the rectus muscles. Of note, the superficial epigastric vessels are often encountered, especially with larger incisions. The rectus fascia is incised in a similar curvilinear transverse manner, 2-cm to 3-cm superior to the pubic symphysis. The lateral fascia has two layers formed from the external oblique aponeurosis and the fused aponeuroses of the internal oblique and transversus abdominis muscles [2]. Once the fascia is incised, the underlying rectus muscles are separated from the anterior sheath. Exposure is controlled by the extent of this dissection, which can proceed from the pubic symphysis to the umbilicus. Separating the rectus raphe and pyramidalis muscles in the midline exposes the posterior sheath and peritoneum, which are opened vertically. Meticulous hemostasis must be achieved before closure, as multiple perforating vessels to the fascia and the potential spaces created place the patient at risk for subfascial hematoma.

Cherney's [3] incision, first described in 1941, while similar to a Pfannenstiel incision, differs in that the rectus muscles are detached from their tendonous insertion on the pubic symphysis. The muscles are isolated by perforating the transversalis fascia at the lateral muscle border and by bluntly dissecting them free from the underlying bladder. It is helpful to leave a 0.5-cm to 1-cm segment of the tendon on the symphysis if possible [2]. The inferior epigastric vessels can either be ligated or left intact, depending on exposure needs. Once detached, the rectus muscles are retracted cranially, offering excellent visualization of the retropubic space and lateral pelvis. The aponeuroses can be opened laterally to the iliac crests. The operative field is often 1.5 to 2 times that of an infraumbilical midline vertical incision. Upper abdominal exposure, however, may still be limited [4]. At closure, the rectus muscles can be reattached to either the remaining tendon on the pubis or to the anterior sheath using permanent suture.

Maylard's [5] incision, reported in 1907, is a transverse incision that can be made at any level on the abdomen. Once the anterior sheath is identified, it is also cut transversely. Unlike Pfannenstiel or Cherney incisions, the underlying rectus muscles are minimally dissected from the anterior sheath. Instead, they are bluntly isolated and transected at the level of the incision with electrocautery. The inferior epigastric vessels, lateral and inferior to the rectus muscles, are most often isolated and ligated. The peritoneum is then opened transversely, offering exposure rivaling that of a vertical incision [6]. The rectus muscle stumps do not need to be reapproximated when closing a Maylard incision. A simple running suture of the anterior sheath is all that is required [7]. Occasionally, oozing from the muscles will require closed suction drainage that can be positioned underneath the fascia. Maylard incisions may be contra-indicated in patients with extensive lower extremity vascular disease as collateral flow via the epigastric vessels develops [4]. It should also probably be avoided in patients planning to undergo future procedures involving rectus abdominus flaps, so as not to compromise blood supply.

In addition to the superior and inferior epigastric vessels commonly encountered during transverse lower abdominal incisions, the ilioinguinal and iliohypogastric nerves can be injured and are the second most common neuropathy following gynecologic surgery. The reported incidence may be as high at 3.7% after a Pfannenstiel incision [8]. The ilioinguinal and iliohypogastric nerves have only sensory function, supplying innervations to the groin and gluteal regions, respectively. In a study by Whiteside and colleagues [9], the course of the ilioinguinal and iliohypogastric nerves were mapped in female cadavers. The ilioinguinal nerve terminated 2.7-cm lateral to the midline and 1.7-cm superior to the pubic symphysis. The iliohypogastric nerve terminated 3.7-cm lateral to midline and 5.2-cm superior to the pubic symphysis. When the typical Pfannenstiel incision was overlaid, almost all of the nerves crossed its path. The investigators concluded that most injuries are likely under recognized and underreported. Injury generally causes local parathesia that in most cases resolves overtime. In rare cases, severe neuropathic pain can develop, requiring local injections or surgery for treatment.

## Gynecologic viscera

When viewing the female pelvis, looking caudally from an open abdominal incision, the pelvic viscera can be easily identified, including the uterus, fallopian tubes, and ovaries. These gynecologic structures are closely associated with the bladder anteriorly, and rectosigmoid colon posteriorly (Fig. 1).

Centrally located, the uterus is a thick muscular organ. Embryologically, it is derived from the fusion of the paramesonephric (müllerian) ducts. These paired ducts form during the seventh week of gestation adjacent to the

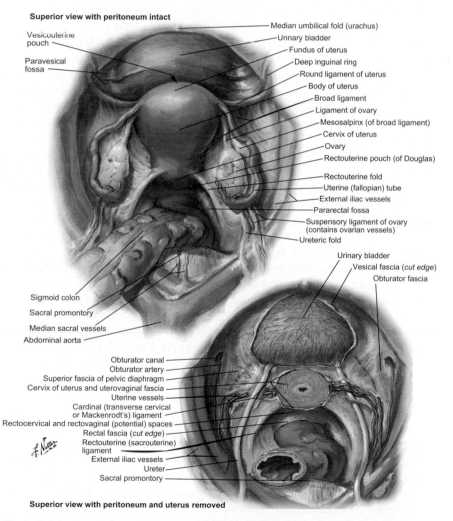

**Superior view with peritoneum intact**

Vesicouterine pouch

Paravesical fossa

Median umbilical fold (urachus)
Urinary bladder
Fundus of uterus
Deep inguinal ring
Round ligament of uterus
Body of uterus
Broad ligament
Ligament of ovary
Mesosalpinx (of broad ligament)
Cervix of uterus
Ovary
Rectouterine pouch (of Douglas)
Rectouterine fold
Uterine (fallopian) tube
External iliac vessels
Pararectal fossa
Suspensory ligament of ovary (contains ovarian vessels)
Ureteric fold

Sigmoid colon
Sacral promontory
Median sacral vessels
Abdominal aorta

Urinary bladder
Vesical fascia (*cut edge*)
Obturator fascia

Obturator canal
Obturator artery
Superior fascia of pelvic diaphragm
Cervix of uterus and uterovaginal fascia
Uterine vessels
Cardinal (transverse cervical or Mackenrodt's) ligament
Rectocervical and rectovaginal (potential) spaces
Rectal fascia (*cut edge*)
Rectouterine (sacrouterine) ligament
External iliac vessels
Ureter
Sacral promontory

**Superior view with peritoneum and uterus removed**

Fig. 1. Pelvic viscera. (*Reprinted* with permission from Netter Anatomy Illustration Collection, © Elsevier Inc. All rights reserved.)

mesonephric (wolffian) ducts. They also form the upper two-thirds of the vagina and the fallopian tubes. Without the Y chromosome, a lack of müllerian-inhibiting factor permits the paramesonephric system to develop. Furthermore, without testosterone, the male mesonephric ducts regress. Incomplete unification of the müllerian ducts results in multiple anomalies of the uterus and vagina, ranging from minor changes—such as an arcuate uterus—to completely separate genital tracts, as in uterine didelphys. Müllerian anomalies mandate evaluation of the urinary tract, as concurrent anomalies are frequently found. Mesonephric remnants are relatively common and can be found lateral to the entire female genital tract. Clinical examples include paraovarian cysts within the broad ligament, hydatids of Morgagni near the fimbria of the fallopian tubes, and Gartner's duct cysts in the lateral upper vagina [10].

The uterus can be divided into three segments: the fundus, lower segment, and cervix. The organ resembles an upside down pear and usually weighs less than 110 grams. During a term pregnancy, the uterus increases up to 20-fold in both size and weight, and following menopause, it usually atrophies. The uterus has three layers. The outer peritoneum (serosa) is densely attached in all areas except anteriorly near the internal cervical os. Incising the peritoneum in this region allows creation of a bladder flap during hysterectomies and cesarean sections. The middle muscular layer (myometrium) is relatively thick and can be subdivided into three groups of alternating longitudinal and oblique smooth muscle groups. The outer most muscular layer is contiguous with the vagina and the fallopian tubes. The third uterine layer (endometrium) ranges from a few millimeters to over a centimeter in thickness, depending on the hormonal status. It can be divided into the stratum basale and the stratum functionale. Only the stratum functionale is hormonally responsive. The endometrium lines the flattened triangular uterine cavity. Most women have an anteverted and anteflexed uterus in relation to the vaginal axis and cervical axis, respectively. Approximately 25% of women can be found to have a retroflexed uterus, a normal variant [11]. The uterine axis is important to note when invasive transcervical uterine procedures are performed to prevent inadvertent perforation and subsequent injury to adjacent vital structures or viscera.

The cervix is the dense fibromuscular lower portion of the uterus that extends into the vagina. The vagina obliquely attaches around the middle of the cervix, dividing it into the supravaginal section and the portio vaginalis. The endocervical canal is approximately 3 cm in length and leads into the uterine cavity. It is lined with a single layer of columnar epithelium, which abruptly changes to nonkeratinized stratified squamous cells on the portio vaginalis. This transition zone is termed the "squamo-columnar junction." The transformation zone, where metaplastic changes from columnar to squamous epithelium occur, is the site of most dysplastic cervical changes. The cervical stroma is composed primarily of collagenous connective tissue, 15% smooth muscle cells, and a small amount of elastic tissue [11].

The fallopian tubes extend from the superiolateral portion of the uterus bilaterally and are approximately 10 cm to 14 cm in length. They generally are less than 1 cm in external diameter, but can become markedly swollen if the tubes become blocked, leading to a condition known as a hydrosalpinx. The fallopian tube can be divided into four different segments. The intramural segment travels from the cornua of the uterine cavity through the myometrium for 1 cm to 2 cm to connect to the isthmic portion. The isthmus is relatively narrow, with an internal diameter of only 1 mm, therefore making it the preferred site for tubal sterilization procedures. Traveling distally, the inner diameter begins to enlarge in the ampulla to approximately 6 mm. Fertilization usually occurs in this segment and the ampulla is also the site of most ectopic pregnancies. The most distal portion of the fallopian tube is called the infundibulum. It contains multiple fingerlike projections called fimbria, which line the tubal opening into the peritoneal cavity. The highest concentration of ciliated epithelium is also found here, which assist in oocyte transport to the uterine cavity.

Several ligamentous structures emanate from the uterus (see Fig. 1). Anterior to the fallopian tubes, the round ligaments can be readily identified. They are composed of fibrous and muscle tissue and correlate with the male gubernaculums. They extend laterally, cross the external iliac vessels, enter the internal inguinal ring, and insert into the labia majora. Sampson's artery, a branch off of the uterine artery, usually runs along the length of the round ligament. The broad ligament is a double reflection of the peritoneum, which is draped over the round ligaments bilaterally. Ligating the round ligament is usually the first step in performing an abdominal hysterectomy as it provides safe access to the retroperitoneum. Neither the round ligament nor the broad ligament provides much support to the uterus. Occasionally the round ligament is attached to the anterior abdominal fascia to correct symptomatic retroverted uteri. Found within the peritoneal leaves at the base of the broad ligament, the cardinal ligament provides the main support for the uterus and cervix. It attaches to the cervix and extends laterally, connecting to the endopelvic fascia, which in turn is affixed to the pelvic bone [11]. The uterosacral ligaments provide minor cervical support. They originate from the upper posterior cervix, travel around the rectum bilaterally, and fan out to attach to the first through the fifth sacral vertebrae. The course of the uterosacral ligaments can be highlighted by placing the uterus on traction. Uterine and pelvic support will be discussed more later in this article.

The ovaries are paired whitish-gray organs that are supported along the lateral pelvic sidewalls by the ovarian ligaments (short fibrous bands attaching to the posteriolateral aspect of the uterus), the mesovarium (containing anastomotic regions of the uterine and ovarian vessels), and the infundibulo-pelvic ligaments (reflections of the broad ligament attaching the ovaries to the lateral pelvis). They rest in an indentation of the peritoneum called the ovarian fossa, immediately adjacent to the iliac vessels and ureters. Ovaries contain three distinct cell populations: germ cells, stromal cells, and epithelium. Around the sixth week of gestation, primordial germ cells migrate from the yolk sac to the genital ridges. Failure to complete migration can lead to extra-ovarian teratomas, most commonly found in the retroperitoneum [10]. At birth, 1 to 2 million oocytes are present. The number of oocytes steadily declines thereafter, so that at the onset of puberty only 500,000 are present. In a reproductive span of 35 to 40 years, multiple follicles can be found at any given time in varying stages of development, but only 400 to 500 oocytes will be selected to ovulate [12]. Stroma cells are tightly packed around developing follicles and secrete hormones. The outer cortex of the ovary is composed of a single layer of cuboidal epithelium, derived from coelomic mesothelium, and is essentially the same as other peritoneal surfaces within the abdomen. Multiple ovulations cause significant injury and repair cycles in a relatively small area, increasing the risk of malignant transformation when compared with other peritoneal surfaces.

## The urinary system and rectum

Thorough understanding of the urinary system and its anatomy is critical for safe gynecologic procedures. The bladder can be found anterior to the uterus. Embryologically, it is formed from the cloaca/urogenital sinus and mesonephric ducts. It is a distendable hollow organ with three sections: the mucosa, detrusor muscles, and serosa. The serosa is only present on the superior surface. Inferiorly, the bladder directly rests on the uterus and cervix, and in most cases a bladder reflection can be clearly seen on the anterior peritoneum. Opening the peritoneum 1-cm distal to this reflection allows formation of a bladder flap during a hysterectomy or other uterine procedure. The base of the bladder is adjacent to the endopelvic fascia and anterior vagina. The trigone is a triangular region at the bladder base, outlined by the two ureteral orifices and the urethra. This region lacks mucosal folds and is slightly raised when compared with the remainder of the bladder. Anteriorly, the bladder is connected to the pubic symphysis by fibrous ligaments. The urachus, a remnant of the allantois, extends from the bladder dome to the umbilicus. Occasionally its proximal portion is still patent, therefore secure ligation is necessary when dividing it to prevent urinomas from developing.

The ureters are paired retroperitoneal muscular tubes approximately 34 cm in length, originating from the renal calyxes, which insert into the inferior bladder at the trigone. They are often within 1 cm of key ligation points during a hysterectomy, therefore knowledge of their course and relationship to landmarks is necessary to prevent injuries (see Fig. 1). After leaving the kidneys, the ureter rests on the anterior psoas muscle lateral to the ovarian vessels and vena cava. Prior to reaching the iliac vessels, the ovarian vessels cross the ureters to assume a more anterior and lateral position. At the pelvic brim the ureters cross over the common iliac arteries, then dive deeply into the pelvis along the lateral pelvic sidewall. Identification of the ureters during gynecologic procedures is often first accomplished at this point after opening the retroperitoneal spaces. This site is also a common place for ureteral injuries during ligation of the infundibulo-pelvic ligament. In the pelvis, the ureter runs medial to and parallel with the internal iliac artery. The uterine artery crosses over the ureter (water under the bridge) as the obturator fossa is approached at the level of the cardinal ligament. The remaining 2 cm to 3 cm of the ureter passes through a dense fibrous tunnel within the cardinal ligament. Rich venous plexuses exist in this region and the vaginal artery lies posteriorly, making exposure challenging. Ninety percent of ureteral injuries occur here [13].

The rectum lies posterior to the uterus following the curvature of the sacrum. It begins where the sigmoid mesentery ends. Embryologically, it forms when the cloaca is divided by the urorectal septum into the urogenital sinus and rectum. Anteriorly, the proximal rectum is covered with peritoneum. The posterior cul-de-sac is a deep pouch demarcated by the most inferior extent of the peritoneum between the uterus and rectum. Not infrequently, this space is completely obliterated by pathology, such as cancer, endometriosis, or pelvic adhesions. Rectal injuries can occur during dissection of obliterated planes or during entry into the posterior cul-de-sac during vaginal hysterectomies. The distal third of the rectum parallels the posterior vagina beneath the peritoneal reflection and empties into the anus.

## Retroperitoneal spaces

Appreciation of the retroperitoneal spaces is paramount to solving complex surgical pelvic problems. These spaces are typically avascular and exist because the pelvic viscera are derived from different embryologic structures. Developing these spaces early during an operation exposes vital structures and allows access to pelvic vasculature. In the midline, the pelvic spaces include the retropubic space, the vesicovaginal space, the rectovaginal space, and the retrorectal space. Laterally, two spaces are present that are separated by the cardinal ligament and include the paravesical space and pararectal space (Fig. 2).

The retropubic space is a potential extraperitoneal space located between the bladder and the pubic symphysis. This space is commonly entered during anti-incontinence and anterior vaginal suspension procedures. The floor of the retropubic space is formed by a sheet of endopelvic fascia. A large plexus of veins, known as the veins of Santorini, run within the vaginal wall and are commonly encountered during retropubic surgery. The obturator neurovascular bundle exits the pelvis in the lateral aspects of this space. These structures can be injured with any retropubic procedure and lead to significant blood loss or neuropathy. Fortunately, the space is contained and generally tamponades itself.

The vesicovaginal space exists between the lower uterine segment, cervix, vagina, and bladder. Development of this space is critical when performing

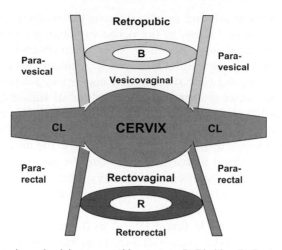

Fig. 2. The retroperitoneal pelvic spaces. *Abbreviations:* B, Bladder; R, Rectum; CL, Cardinal Ligament.

any type of hysterectomy or procedure on the lower uterus, for obvious reasons. Sharp dissection of loose areolar tissue is performed overlying the cervix until the pubocervical fascia is identified. At this point, blunt dissection can further expose this space. Inadequate dissections increase the risk for postoperative vesicovaginal fistula formation. In patients with prior procedures, significant scarring can make this dissection challenging. Dissection is limited laterally by the bladder pillars, and the space can be extended to the origin of the urethra at the bladder neck [14]. The rectovaginal space can be entered by excising the peritoneum in the posterior cul-de-sac at the level of the uterosacral ligament insertions on the cervix. The uterosacral ligaments demarcate the lateral extent of this space, and dissection can extend to the pelvic floor. When posterior anatomy is distorted and during radical pelvic surgery, this space must be developed to prevent rectal injuries.

The retrorectal space is occasionally entered during benign gynecologic operations, most commonly for pelvic suspension procedures, and is also developed during exenterative surgery. It can be entered by retracting the sigmoid colon to the left and identifying the sacral promontory. The peritoneum over the second sacral vertebrae between the common iliac vessels is opened. Caution should be exercised during dissection, as presacral vasculature arises directly from the aorta and inferior vena cava. Furthermore, bleeding can be difficult to control because the veins often retract into bony crevices. The anterior longitudinal ligament is the usual site for suspension sutures. Identification of the middle sacral artery and ureters are important before suture placement. The presacral nerve plexus supplying visceral innervation to the pelvis can also be injured during dissection in this space.

The paravesical and pararectal spaces are most often fully developed during oncology operations. These spaces exist lateral to the pelvic viscera along the pelvic sidewalls and are separated by the cardinal ligament. Transperitoneal entry allows access to the pelvic vasculature and ureters. Exposure of the pararectal space begins by opening the broad ligament lateral to and parallel with the infundibulo-pelvic ligament. Blunt dissection of loose areolar tissue between the external iliac artery (overlying the psoas muscle) and the ureter (found deeply on the medial leaf of the broad ligament) exposes the space. The medial border is limited by the uterosacral ligaments, and the pelvic sidewall defines its lateral extent. Structures that can be readily identified following exposure include the ureter, the common iliac artery, the external iliac artery and vein, the internal iliac artery, the uterine artery, and the superior vesical artery. Once the pararectal space is fully developed, the obturator space can be entered allowing visualization of the obturator nerve and vessels.

The paravesical space is found lateral to the bladder. Once the lateral peritoneum is opened, the space is developed by blunt dissection, mobilizing the bladder medially away from the bony pelvis. The space can be extended into the retropubic space. The superior vesical artery borders the medial side. Laterally and posteriorly, the obturator neurovascular bundle travels through the obturator foramen.

## Pelvic vasculature

The blood supply to the pelvis is complex, contains several anastomotic regions, and is able to extensively expand flow during certain physiologic or pathologic states. For example, during pregnancy, the uterine arteries channel 500 mL per minute of blood to the uterus, and in malignant states, rich neovascularization commonly occurs [15]. Further complicating matters, numerous variations in the course of specific vessels are possible. Despite all of these potential issues, certain characteristics of the pelvic vasculature are constant and understanding the basic layout will benefit any surgeon entering the pelvis.

The majority of the blood supply to the pelvis originates from the internal iliac artery (also known as the hypogastric artery). Additional supply comes from the ovarian arteries, the inferior mesenteric artery, and the external iliac artery. Numerous branches supply the pelvic viscera, the abdominal wall, the pelvic floor, the external genitalia, the buttocks, and the upper thighs (Fig. 3).

The common iliac artery divides into the external and internal iliac arteries. This bifurcation is easily identified following development of the pararectal space. The external iliac artery eventually becomes the femoral artery and is the primary blood supply to the lower extremity. It is also the only vessel in the pelvis without adequate collateral circulation and if ligated will cause significant sequellae. The internal iliac artery divides into an anterior and posterior division approximately 3 cm to 4 cm from the bifurcation. The posterior division, rarely seen during pelvic surgery,

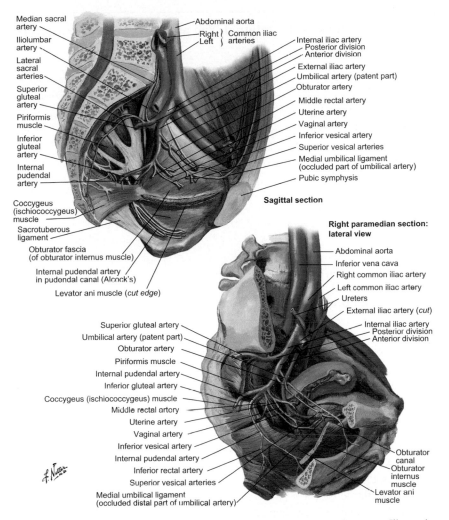

Median sacral artery
Iliolumbar artery
Lateral sacral arteries
Superior gluteal artery
Piriformis muscle
Inferior gluteal artery
Internal pudendal artery
Coccygeus (ischiococcygeus) muscle
Sacrotuberous ligament
Obturator fascia (of obturator internus muscle)
Internal pudendal artery in pudendal canal (Alcock's)
Levator ani muscle (*cut edge*)

Abdominal aorta
Right ) Common iliac
Left  ) arteries
Internal iliac artery
Posterior division
Anterior division
External iliac artery
Umbilical artery (patent part)
Obturator artery
Middle rectal artery
Uterine artery
Vaginal artery
Inferior vesical artery
Superior vesical arteries
Medial umbilical ligament (occluded part of umbilical artery)
Pubic symphysis

**Sagittal section**

**Right paramedian section: lateral view**

Abdominal aorta
Inferior vena cava
Right common iliac artery
Left common iliac artery
Ureters
External iliac artery (*cut*)
Internal iliac artery
Posterior division
Anterior division

Superior gluteal artery
Umbilical artery (patent part)
Obturator artery
Piriformis muscle
Internal pudendal artery
Inferior gluteal artery
Coccygeus (ischiococcygeus) muscle
Middle rectal artery
Uterine artery
Vaginal artery
Inferior vesical artery
Internal pudendal artery
Inferior rectal artery
Superior vesical arteries
Medial umbilical ligament (occluded distal part of umbilical artery)

Obturator canal
Obturator internus muscle
Levator ani muscle

Fig. 3. Pelvic vasculature. (*Reprinted* with permission from Netter Anatomy Illustration Collection, © Elsevier Inc. All rights reserved.)

supplies the gluteal region with three branches: the superior gluteal, iliolumbar, and lateral sacral arteries. The anterior division has many branches, including the uterine, vaginal, superior/middle/inferior vesicals, middle and inferior rectal, obturator, inferior gluteal, internal pudendal, and obliterated umbilical arteries (Box 1). During retroperitoneal surgery, the primary branches identified include the superior vesical artery, the uterine artery, and occasionally the obturator artery. The superior vesical artery is the most prominent branch of the internal iliac artery and in most cases appears to be a continuation of it. Identification is possible with development of the paravesical space and during dissection of the obturator space. The uterine

---

**Box 1. Branches of the internal iliac artery (hypogastric artery)**

*Posterior division*
Superior gluteal
Iliolumbar
Lateral sacral

*Anterior division*
Uterine
Vaginal
Superior vesical
Middle vesical
Inferior vesical
Middle rectal
Inferior rectal
Obturator
Internal pudendal
Inferior gluteal
Obliterated umbilical

---

artery often branches off of the superior vesical artery, crosses over the ureter, and enters the lateral uterus at the level of the internal cervical os. The obturator artery can be identified in the obturator fossa during lymphadenectomy, usually resting just inferior to the obturator nerve. It can also be identified laterally in the paravesical and retropubic spaces as it leaves the pelvis through the obturator foramen. The terminal branch of the internal iliac artery is the internal pudendal artery. It exits the pelvis through the greater sciatic foramen and courses around the ischial spine, providing the main blood supply to the perineum and external genitalia. The ovarian arteries originate directly from the aorta inferior to the renal arteries and are most frequently identified at the infundibulo-pelvic ligament.

The venous supply of the pelvis closely approximates the arterial supply. The primary exception is the ovarian veins. The left ovarian vein drains into the left renal vein, while the right ovarian vein drains directly into the inferior vena cava. Most pelvic veins are not visualized unless deep retroperitoneal dissection occurs, with the exception of the external iliac vein.

Multiple anastomotic regions exist in the pelvic vasculature, ensuring adequate blood flow should compromise to one region occur. Unfortunately, this can also make control of hemorrhage more challenging. The ovarian arteries freely anastomose with the uterine artery. The superior rectal artery, originating from the inferior mesenteric artery, anastomoses with the middle and inferior rectal arteries. Furthermore, lumbar and vertebral arteries anastomose with branches of the posterior division of the internal iliac artery. Other collaterals are found involving the external iliac and femoral arteries to the posterior division and obturator artery [15]. These anastomotic regions are rarely directly visualized.

The risks of bleeding associated with pelvic surgery are real. Most gynecologic surgery involves the creation of pedicles, without direct ligation of specific vessels. Surgery for pelvic pathology often leaves extensive regions devoid of peritoneum, increasing the risk for venous oozing. Additionally, bulky tumors can limit lateral exposure to the blood supply, furthering the risk of increased blood loss. Careful attention to controlling the blood supply early in an operation, meticulous surgical technique, and development of the retroperitoneal spaces can minimize these risks. Should hemorrhage occur, options exist. As previously mentioned, with the exception of the external iliac artery, any vessel in the pelvis can be ligated. Bilateral hypogastric artery ligation has long been relied on to decrease the pulse pressure in the pelvis [15]. More selective ligation of the uterine arteries is also possible but may take more time for identification. For diffuse venous bleeding, a number of hemostatic matrix products, such as FloSeal (Baxter), can be invaluable. In other cases, switching to damage-control mode with pelvic packing can allow for resuscitation and correction of coagulopathies.

## Pelvic lymphatics

Understanding the lymphatic drainage of pelvic organs and external female genitalia is very important when faced with malignant pathology. It is conceivable for a generalist obstetrician and gynecologist to call the general surgeon or urologist into a case for assistance with staging biopsies and pelvic lymph node dissections for an unsuspected cancer. Knowledge of essential anatomy and the extent of lymphatic sampling could prevent the morbidity of restaging operations and improve patient survival.

The lymphatic drainage of the pelvic viscera typically follows the venous blood supply in a stepwise fashion, with only a few exceptions. Regional lymphatic sites include the obturator nodes, internal and external pelvic nodes, common iliac nodes, and para-aortic nodes. Cervical lesions drain first to the parametrial nodes (which are removed during a radical hysterectomy during parametrectomy), then to the obturator nodes, pelvic nodes, and finally to the para-aortic region. Most uterine cancers drain first to the pelvic nodes; however, some fundal tumors can metastasize directly to the para-aortic region via the ovarian and presacral lymphatics. Ovarian neoplasms can metastasize to either the pelvic or para-aortic nodes. Inguinal metastases can also occur with advanced gynecologic malignancies via lymphatics following the round ligament.

Pelvic lymph node dissection begins by opening the retroperitoneum and developing the pararectal and paravesical spaces. Optimal exposure is critical and may require extension of the peritoneal incision into the white line of Toldt. The external iliac artery is then identified and the ureter is retracted away medially. The safest point to begin dissection is along the external iliac artery. Lymphatic tissue overlying the iliac vessels is removed from the point where the circumflex iliac vein crosses over the external iliac artery to the bifurcation of the common iliacs. The genitofemoral nerve overlying the psoas muscle defines the lateral extent of dissection. This nerve has only sensory function supplying the upper vulva and medial thigh. Occasionally, the genitofemoral nerve must be sacrificed if bulky nodes are present. Caution should be taken at the bifurcation of the internal and external iliac arteries, as bleeding can be difficult to control here. Dissection can proceed cephalically to remove low para-aortic nodes overlying the inferior vena cava. This typically is easier to perform on the patient's right side. Careful protection of the ureter is essential at this point of the dissection. The Fellow's vein (a perforating vein into the inferior vena cava, so named as it is often inadvertently transected by fellows-in-training) should be ligated with clips when identified. The upper extent of the para-aortic dissection typically ends at the level of the renal veins. These high para-aortic nodes can also be accessed through a separate transperitoneal incision. The obturator space is exposed by placing a vein retractor under the external iliac vein and gently lifting anteriorly. Lymphatic tissue resting between the obturator nerve and superior vesical artery is then removed. Initial identification of the obturator nerve makes the dissection easier. If tissue below the nerve must be removed, ligation of the obturator artery and vein may be required. Extreme care must be exercised in this region as a rich plexus of fine veins rests of the pelvic floor.

Lymphatic drainage of the external female genitalia also follows a stepwise progression. The lymphatic channels run anteriorly through the labia majora, then turn laterally at the mons to drain into the superficial inguinal nodes. In general, lymphatic channels do not extend beyond the labiocrural folds. Eight to ten superficial inguinal nodes are found in the femoral triangle between Camper's fascia and the cribiform plate surrounding the saphenous vein and adductor longus muscle. Beneath the cribiform plate, additional three to five deep inguinal lymph nodes can be found medial to the femoral vein. Cloquet's node is the most superior node in this group. The deep inguinal lymph nodes drain into the pelvic lymph node chain overlying the external iliac vessels. Lateral vulvar lesions typically drain to ipsilateral superficial inguinal nodes first, with only rare exceptions. Midline lesions on the clitoris or on the perineal body require bilateral lymph node dissections. Clitoral lesions can also directly metastasize under the pubic symphysis to the pelvic and obturator node groups.

## The anatomy of pelvic support

Pelvic support relies on a complex combination of muscles and ligaments, with their accompanying vasculature and innervation, which act dynamically to provide support for the visceral organs of the pelvis. The bladder, uterus, and rectum have a direct external connection via the urethra, vagina, and anus, respectively. A coordinated functioning of these anatomic regions is critical in maintaining continence of urine and feces and yet at the same time allowing for appropriate, socially acceptable, defecation and urination. Pelvic support must maintain its integrity in the face of severe stressors, the most acute of which is labor and vaginal delivery. These structures are not visualized during conventional gynecologic procedures and their function can generally only be gauged with physiologic or radiographic testing. The general surgeon is not often called to evaluate this anatomy in the acute setting. Nevertheless, a well-grounded understanding of this anatomy can be helpful in evaluating pelvic organ dysfunction and pain in the perioperative period. This section will cover the bony pelvis, pelvic diaphragm, perineal anatomy, and external genitalia.

## The bony pelvis

The bony pelvis is a basin shaped ring formed by four bones: two hip bones (consisting of the ilium, ischium, and pubis) and the sacrum and coccyx (Fig. 4). The pelvis is divided by the ileopectineal line into the false pelvis above and the true pelvis below. In a normally developed nonpregnant female, all pelvic organs are found within the confines of the true pelvis. The bony pelvic inlet is bounded posteriorly by the sacral promontory, laterally by the ileopectineal line, and anteriorly by the superior aspect of the pubic symphysis. The bony pelvic outlet is bounded posteriorly by the

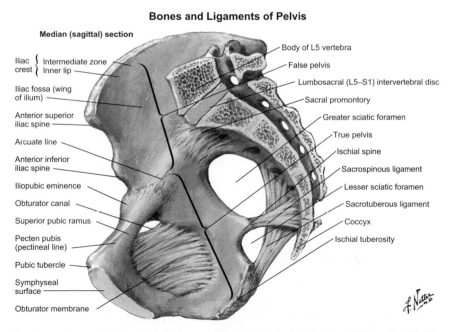

**Bones and Ligaments of Pelvis**

Median (sagittal) section

Iliac { Intermediate zone
crest { Inner lip

Iliac fossa (wing of ilium)

Anterior superior iliac spine

Arcuate line

Anterior inferior iliac spine

Iliopubic eminence

Obturator canal

Superior pubic ramus

Pecten pubis (pectineal line)

Pubic tubercle

Symphyseal surface

Obturator membrane

Body of L5 vertebra

False pelvis

Lumbosacral (L5–S1) intervertebral disc

Sacral promontory

Greater sciatic foramen

True pelvis

Ischial spine

Sacrospinous ligament

Lesser sciatic foramen

Sacrotuberous ligament

Coccyx

Ischial tuberosity

Fig. 4. The bony pelvis. (*Reprinted* with permission from Netter Anatomy Illustration Collection, © Elsevier Inc. All rights reserved.)

caudal sacrum and coccyx, laterally by the ischial tuberosities and sacrotuberous ligaments, and anteriorly by the inferior aspect of the pubic symphysis and ischiopubic rami. The obturator foramen is covered by the internal
obturator muscle and the pelvic outlet is closed by the pelvic and urogenital
diaphragm.

The sacrospinous and sacrotuberous ligaments create the greater and
lesser sciatic foramen. The greater sciatic foramen allows for the exit of
major neurovascular structures, such as the sciatic nerve, the nerve to the
quadratis femoris, and the major vasculature to the gluteum and posterior
thigh. The pudendal neurovascular bundle exits out of the greater sciatic
foramen and reenters the pelvis through the lesser sciatic foramen.

## Pelvic diaphragm

The pelvic diaphragm is the central component of pelvic support. It lies
retroperitoneal and provides support for all viscera. It is formed by the
levator ani muscle group and the coccygeus muscles with their fascial cover-
ings (Fig. 5). The levator ani is composed of three muscles: the puborectalis,
pubococcygeus, and ileococcygeus. These muscles extend from the lateral
pelvic walls downward and medially to fuse with each other posteriorly.
The levator hiatus lies anteriorly and accommodates the urethra, vagina,
and anus. The gap left by the levator hiatus is closed caudally by the urogenital diaphragm. The superior fascial layer of the levator ani muscle group
projects cranially to envelop the bladder, superior vagina, and uterus, as
well as the rectum to provide support. The inferior fascial layer extends
caudally along the urethra, distal vagina, and anus to provide distal support,
and fuses with the urogenital diaphragm. This fascia is often referred to as
the endopelvic fascia. The cardinal and uterosacral ligaments previously
described also arise from this fascia.

The pelvic diaphragm has multiple functions that require tonic activity. It
must maintain constant tone to provide support. Upon contraction, it raises
the entire pelvic floor and flexes the anorectal canal to provide continence of
stool and augments voluntary control of micturition. It must relax effectively
to allow for straightening of the anorectal canal, resulting in the passage of
stool. It must effectively relax during urination, and it helps direct the fetal
head toward the birth canal at parturition. The ability of the pelvic diaphragm to perform these functions arises from the fact that they have a unique
histology. They are hybrid muscles composed of both smooth and striated
elements and have somatic innervation from S2-4 nerve roots [16].

## Female perineum

The female perineum is the subcutaneous tissue bound deeply by the
levator ani muscles and superficially by skin (Fig. 6). It is circumscribed
by the bony pelvic outlet, which includes the pubis and ischiopubic rami
anteriorly, the ischial spines laterally, and the coccyx posteriorly. The

**Superior view**

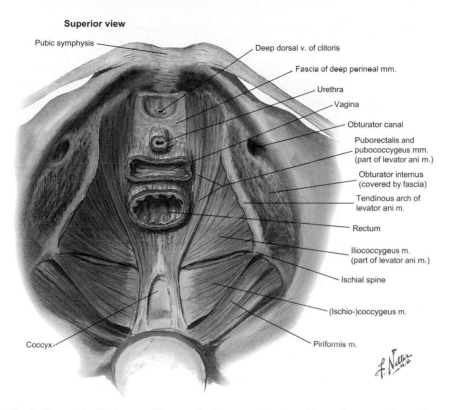

Fig. 5. The pelvic diaphragm. (*Reprinted* with permission from Netter Anatomy Illustration Collection, © Elsevier Inc. All rights reserved.)

perineum is generally divided into two triangles: the urogenital triangle anteriorly and the anal triangle posteriorly. The urogenital diaphragm is a strong musculomembranous partition stretched across the anterior half of the pelvic outlet between the ischiopubic rami. It contains the deep perineal muscles and the urethral sphincter musculature. The anal triangle is delineated anteriorly by the superficial transverse perineal muscles, laterally by the sacrotuberous ligament and gluteus maximus muscles, and posteriorly by the coccyx. It contains the anal sphincter musculature.

The perineal compartment contains the muscles which help close the genital hiatus, including the bulbocavernosus, transverse perinei muscles, and the urethral and anal sphincter musculature. The perineal body is also an important component of the perineum. It lies at the base of the urogenital diaphragm between the vaginal and anal orifices. It is the common fibrous point of attachment for the bulbocavernosus, the transverse perineal, the levator ani, and external anal sphincter muscles. In a healthy female it is pyramidal in shape.

Important anatomic reference points for the pelvic surgeon in the perineum include access to the ischiorectal fossa, a space found between the

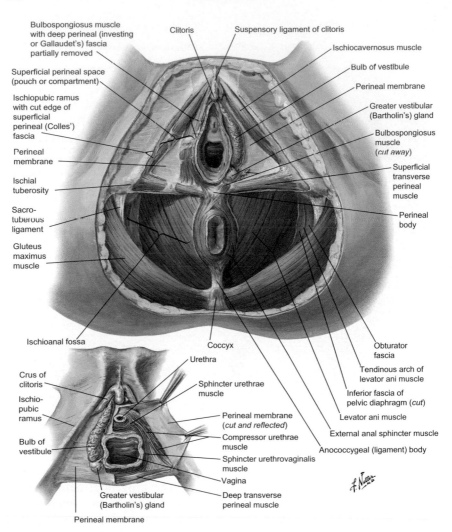

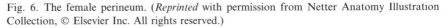

Fig. 6. The female perineum. (*Reprinted* with permission from Netter Anatomy Illustration Collection, © Elsevier Inc. All rights reserved.)

rectum medially, the levator ani superiorly, and bordered laterally by the obturator internus fascia. This space can become a site of severe ascending perineal infections and necrotizing fasciitis, requiring aggressive debridement [17]. Large vulvar hematomas can complicate vaginal deliveries or trauma. These can be of vital significance if they extend into the ischiorectal fossa, or paravaginally as the bleeding is not contained and extends into the large potential retroperitoneal space. This can be difficult to diagnose early but in the face of shock, the space must be explored and the bleeding tamponaded.

*Female external genitalia*

The female external genitalia are comprised of the mons, labia majora, labia minora, clitoris, and vestibule of the vagina. The mons is a fatty prominence overlying the pubic bone. The labia majora are two longitudinal skin folds that run inferiorly from the mons pubis. They are joined anteriorly by the anterior commisure, and with pubertal development are covered with terminal hairs. They are homologous to the scrotum of the male and contain the terminations of the round ligaments of the uterus. Also contained within this sac is a vestigial remnant of peritoneum. This may persist in the child as the canal of Nuck and may give rise to inguinal hernias.

The labia minora lie medial to the labia majora, contain no fat, and are hairless. Superiorly they fuse to form the prepuce and frenulum of the clitoris. Lying beneath the labia minora anteriorly is the clitoris. The clitoris is homologous to the penis in the male and consists of erectile tissue that is enlarged during engorgement with blood. It consists of two crura, two corpora cavernosa, and a glans, and is covered by sensitive epithelium. Innervation to the clitoris arises anteriorly from the ilioinguinal nerve as well as posteriorly from the pudendal nerve. As previously mentioned, clitoral innervation can be compromised by injury to the ilioinguinal nerve with transverse lower abdominal incisions.

The vestibule of the vagina is space between the labia minora, which has the openings of the urethra and vagina. It is bordered internally and separated from the vagina by the hymen, a thin vascularized membrane that is generally perforated in adults. Skene's ducts open in the posteriolateral aspect of the urinary orifice. Bartholin's gland ducts are visible near the hymenal ring at 4 and 8 o'clock. These structures can become clinically significant as they become infected and require incision and drainage. On visual inspection of the female external genitalia, it is also important to evaluate the perineal body and anus. The perineal body is defined as the structure between the posterior vestibule of the vaginal opening and the anus. Clinically significant findings along the external genitalia may include benign or malignant epithelial or dermal growths, such as condyloma accuminata, lipoma, fibroma, squamous cell carcinoma, melanoma or hydrandenitis suppurativa, which in general require excision.

## Functional innervation of the pelvis

The functional innervation of the pelvis can be divided into supradiaphragmatic and infradiaphragmatic compartments. Supradiaphragmatic innervation of the pelvis is entirely visceral and involves the regulation and control of the bladder, uterus, and rectum. In addition, the autonomic nervous system controls the tone of the internal (ie, smooth muscle) sphincters of both the urethra and anus. Under sympathetic control, the muscular bladder and rectum relax and become low-pressure containers for excrement, as the smooth muscle sphincters contract. Once the parasympathetic system is activated, the bladder outlet, urethral sphincters, and anal sphincters relax, allowing for passage of urine and stool. The majority of sympathetic innervation of the pelvic organs originates from the hypogastric plexi that are found along the aorta and sacrum, while a minor amount is supplied by sacral sympathetic trunk. The parasympathetic innervation originates from the sacral spinal nerves. The autonomic innervation then passes through the pelvic plexi before distributing diffusely over the end organs. The autonomic innervation of the pelvis can be injured during labor and delivery, as well as with pelvic, vascular, or spinal surgical procedures. Important to note is the potential for overdistention injury of the bladder in patients who are unable to void postoperatively. Overdistention of even short durations can lead to permanent dysfunction of the parasympathetic innervation of the bladder, leaving the patient in chronic urinary retention [18].

The infradiaphragmatic motor innervation is almost entirely somatic and arises from the pudendal nerve. The pudendal nerve originates from the S2-4 nerve roots, exits the pelvis through the greater sciatic foramen, and re-enters the pelvis through the lesser sciatic foramen. Distally, it splits into multiple branches, which provide the cutaneous innervation of the external genitalia, the motor innervation of the urogenital diaphragm, and most importantly the innervation to the striated muscles of the urethra and anus. These muscles augment the smooth muscle function and maintain continence in the presence of severe stressors. A coordinated relaxation of the muscles must take place to allow for voluntary voiding and defecation.

## Summary

In conclusion, the female pelvis is a complex anatomic space with critical support and functional roles. Understanding how to achieve optimal exposure and establish the avascular spaces will allow the surgeon to approach complex pelvic problems confidently. Further knowledge of pelvic vasculature, lymphatics, and innervation will allow safe completion of surgical procedures and will be of utmost value when dealing with hemorrhagic emergencies. Finally, identifying key relationships between the gynecologic, urinary and gastrointestinal tracts will minimize inadvertent injuries.

## References

[1] Gallop DG. Opening and closing of the abdomen and wound healing. In: Gershenson DM, DeCherney AH, Curry SL, editors. Operative gynecology. Philadelphia: W.B. Saunders Company; 1993. p. 127–46.
[2] Meeks GR. Clinical anatomy of incisions. In: Mann WJ, Stovall TG, editors. Gynecologic surgery. San Francisco (CA): Churchill Livingstone; 1996. p. 121–68.
[3] Cherney LS. A modified transverse incision for low-abdominal operations. Surg Gynecol Obstet 1941;72:92–5.

[4] Nygaard IE, Squatrito RC. Abdominal incisions from creation to closure. Obstet Gynecol Surv 1996;51(7):429–36.
[5] Maylard AE. Direction of abdominal incisions. Br Med J 1907;5:895–901.
[6] Baggish MS. Abdominal incisions. In: Baggish MS, Karram MM, editors. Atlas of pelvic anatomy and gynecologic surgery. 2nd edition. Philadelphia: Elsevier; 2006. p. 77–91.
[7] Wheeless CR. Abdominal wall. In: Wheeless CR, editor. Atlas of pelvic surgery. 3rd edition. Philadelphia: Williams and Wilkins; 1997. p. 361–78.
[8] Luijendijk RW, Jeekel J, Storm RK, et al. The low transverse Pfannenstiel incision and the prevalence of incisional hernia and nerve entrapment. Ann Surg 1997;225:365–9.
[9] Whiteside JL, Barber MD, Walters MD, et al. Anatomy of ilioinguinal and iliohypogastric nerves in relation to trocar placement and low transverse incisions. Am J Obstet Gynecol 2003;189(6):1574–8.
[10] Curry SL. Embryology and anatomy of the female pelvis. In: Gershenson DM, DeCherney AH, Curry SL, editors. Operative gynecology. Philadelphia: W.B. Saunders Company; 1993. p. 19–27.
[11] Mishell DR, Stenchever MA, Droegemueller W, et al. Reproductive anatomy. In: Mishell DR, Stenchever MA, Droegemueller W, et al, editors. Comprehensive gynecology. 3rd edition. Philadelphia: Mosby-Year Book, Inc.; 1997. p. 41–72.
[12] Speroff L, Fritz MA. The ovary—embryology and development. In: Speroff L, Fritz MA, editors. Clinical gynecologic endocrinology and infertility. 7th edition. Philadelphia: Lippincott Williams & Wilkins; 2005. p. 97–111.
[13] Baggish MS. Identifying and avoiding ureteral injury. In: Baggish MS, Karram MM, editors. Atlas of pelvic anatomy and gynecologic surgery. 2nd edition. Philadelphia: Elsevier; 2006. p. 371–80.
[14] Lichtenegger W, Del Priore G. Anatomy. In: Smith JR, Del Priore G, Curtin J, et al, editors. An atlas of gynecologic oncology: investigation and surgery. London: Martin Dunitz; 2001. p. 9–17.
[15] Anderson JR, Genadry R. Anatomy and embryology. In: Berek JS, Adashi EY, Hillard PA, editors. Novak's gynecology. 12th edition. Philadelphia: Williams & Wilkins; 1996. p. 71–122.
[16] Grigorescu BA, Lazarou G, Olson TR, et al. Innervation of the levator ani muscles: description of the nerve branches to the pubococcygeus, iliococcygeus and puborectalis muscles. Int Urogynecol J Pelvic Floor Dysfunct 2008;19(1):107–16.
[17] Gallup DG, Freedman MA, Meguiar RV, et al. Necrotizing fasciitis in gynecologic and obstetric patients: a surgical emergency. Am J Obstet Gynecol 2002;187(2):305–10.
[18] Wein A. Lower urinary tract dysfunction in neurologic injury and disease. In: Wein A, Kavoussi L, Novic A, et al, editors. Campbell-Walsh urology. 9th edition. Philadelphia: Saunders Elsevier; 1997. p. 2011–45.

SURGICAL
CLINICS OF
NORTH AMERICA

Surg Clin N Am 88 (2008) 245–264

# Benign Gynecologic Conditions

## Kevin J. Boyle, MD*, Saioa Torrealday, MD

*Department of Obstetrics and Gynecology, Tripler Army Medical Center,*
*1 Jarrett White Road, Honolulu, HI 96859-5000, USA*

## Benign adnexal masses

Benign adnexal tumors are masses involving the ovary, fallopian tube, or surrounding uterine ligaments. Adnexal masses are a common and challenging problem faced by gynecologists. Although most adnexal masses are benign, their potential for malignancy drives the need for accurate diagnosis and treatment.

### Etiology

*Functional ovarian cysts*

Follicular cysts are the most common cystic structures seen on the normal ovary. Normal follicles typically are multiple and range in size from a few millimeters to several cm. Follicles become cystic once they reach a diameter greater than 3 cm. Follicular cysts are believed to grow in response to gonadotropins. It remains unknown whether follicular cysts form when dominant follicles fail to rupture and release their ova, or if they form when nondominant follicles fail to undergo the normal process of atresia. Follicular cysts usually are thin walled, contain clear fluid, and have maximum diameters of up to 15 cm [1].

Corpus luteum cysts develop from mature postovulatory Graafian follicles. Like follicular cysts, corpus luteum are not termed "cysts" until they reach a minimum size of 3 cm in diameter [1]. Most corpus luteum cysts remain asymptomatic and small with an average diameter of only 4 cm. Two to 3 days after ovulation, thin-walled capillaries normally invade the granulosa cell, and spontaneous bleeding fills the central cavity of the maturing

The views expressed in this article are those of the authors and do not reflect the official policy or position of the Department of the Army, Department of Defense, or the US Government.

\* Corresponding author.

*E-mail address:* kevin.j.boyle@us.army.mil (K.J. Boyle).

0039-6109/08/$ - see front matter. Published by Elsevier Inc.
doi:10.1016/j.suc.2007.12.001

*surgical.theclinics.com*

corpus luteum with blood. Usually this blood is absorbed from the central cavity to form a cystic space. When the hemorrhage is excessive, it overcomes the body's ability to absorb the blood, and the cystic space continues to grow. These cysts can become significantly large and cause discomfort as they enlarge. Eventually, if the intra-cystic pressure exceeds the capacity of the cyst's thin walls to contain the blood, these cysts rupture, potentially causing significant intraperitoneal hemorrhage. Because corpus luteum cysts secrete progesterone, menstrual bleeding may be normal or delayed, depending on how long the cysts' progesterone production stabilizes the endometrial lining. Halban's triad of spotting, unilateral pain, and a pelvic mass often is used to describe the presence of corpus luteum cysts [1].

Theca lutein cysts are the least common functional ovarian cysts. They almost always are bilateral and cause moderate to massive enlargement of the ovaries. These cysts arise from excessive or prolonged luteinization of the ovary by human chorionic gonadotropin (hCG). Multiple cysts can form on the ovary, each ranging in size from 1 to 10 cm. Iatrogenic stimulation of the ovaries with assisted reproductive regimens may initiate the formation of theca lutein cysts; conception tends to prolong and maintain their growth secondary to persistent hCG stimulation. In fact, any condition that causes sustained hCG production can lead to development of theca lutein cysts. Thus, it is common to discover these cysts during the later months of singleton gestations, in the earlier months of twin or higher multiple pregnancies, and occasionally concomitant with molar pregnancies, choriocarcinomas, and other hCG-secreting tumors [2].

## Endometriomas

Endometrial implants can form throughout the pelvis and quite frequently are found on the ovary (see section on endometriosis). Endometriosis of the ovary may become cystic and form an endometrioma. These cysts can be unilocular or multilocular and range in size from less than 1 cm to greater than 15 cm as they fill with blood and endometrial tissue. Endometriomas sometimes are referred to as "chocolate cysts" because of the color of the old blood that collects within [1].

## Inflammatory disease

Tubo-ovarian abscess can form in the presence of pelvic inflammatory disease (PID) (see later section). These masses typically are pus-filled cavities and often are loculated. The classic findings of cervical motion tenderness, abdominal/adnexal pain, elevated temperature, and leukocytosis suggest the presence of PID, but these symptoms vary considerably and usually are nonspecific [3]. If a mass is felt in a patient undergoing treatment for PID, or if symptoms remain unresponsive to antibiotic therapy, a tubo-ovarian abscess should be suspected, and further studies should be ordered. Because adolescents have the highest prevalence of PID, tubo-ovarian abscesses are seen most commonly within this age group.

*Benign neoplasms*

Mature teratomas (dermoid cysts) are cystic structures that histologically contain mature cells derived from all three germ layers. Benign teratomas are the most common ovarian neoplasm and account for more than 90% of germ cell tumors of the ovary [2]. Dermoids are detected most often during the reproductive years, but they can be found in all age groups. Benign teratomas are believed to arise from a single germ cell after the first meiotic division, and their chromosomal makeup is always 46XX [4]. Benign cystic teratomas can be single or multiple tumors that vary widely in size, ranging from a few millimeters to larger than 20 cm. In 1% to 2% of cases, mature teratomas undergo malignant transformation to form a cancer of squamous cell origin.

Fibromas are benign, solid neoplasms that arise from the undifferentiated fibrous stroma of the ovary. These tumors account for 20% of all solid ovarian tumors and comprise approximately 5% of benign ovarian neoplasms. Fibromas are slow-growing tumors with a malignant potential of less than 1%. These tumors can vary significantly in size and weight. Although most fibromas are unilateral, it is common to find more than one tumor within the affected ovary. The diameter of the fibroma may be clinically significant, because it correlates with the amount of ascites that often is a concurrent symptom. In Meigs' syndrome, which mimics malignancy, benign ovarian fibromas are associated with ascites and hydrothorax.

Benign serous cystadenomas account for approximately 25% of all benign ovarian tumors. They usually are large and unilocular with a cyst wall comprised of a single layer of cuboidal epithelium, frequently with cilia. They most likely arise from the invagination of the ovarian surface epithelium. These tumors are seen commonly in patients in their fourth or fifth decades of life and are bilateral in 15% of the cases.

Benign mucinous cystadenomas usually are much larger than serous tumors and more often are unilateral. Grossly these tumors are multiloculated and contain thick mucinous material. The cyst wall usually is smooth and lined by a single layer of columnar cells with mucin-containing cytoplasm and a centrally located nucleus. These tumors are most prevalent in the third to fifth decades of life.

Brenner tumors are rare neoplasms, contain benign transitional cells, and account for less than 2% of all ovarian tumors. They typically are found incidentally within mucinous cystadenomas and, less commonly, in serous cystadenomas and dermoid cysts. Brenner tumors are small, solid, and grayish-white in color. The transitional epithelium component is scattered with dense fibrous stroma. They usually are seen in the fifth to sixth decades of life [2].

*Clinical characteristics*

Although an adnexal mass is a common finding in the clinical setting, patients present with a wide variety of symptoms. Most adnexal masses are asymptomatic and are found incidentally on examination or through radiologic studies. The most common symptom tends to be pelvic pain, which may be secondary to the enlarging size of a mass or to peritoneal irritation by fluid or blood within the pelvis resulting from cyst rupture. Sometimes an enlarging abdomen or palpable mass may prompt evaluation. Other patients may present for care if a mass becomes large enough to produce pelvic pressure or dyspareunia or to compromise nearby organs, resulting in urinary frequency, urinary retention, or constipation.

*Diagnosis*

The definitive diagnosis of a pelvic mass can be made only with its removal and pathologic evaluation. The diagnosis often can be surmised, however, based on the patient's risk factors and patient's age at presentation and by the radiologic characteristics of the mass. A thorough history and physical examination should be performed on all patients. A bimanual examination often can determine the size and location of the mass. In addition, the pelvic examination can note the presence of adnexal or cervical motion tenderness. The characteristics of masses that should be documented carefully include tumor size, location, shape, mobility, bilaterally, associated tenderness, and any interval changes. Adequate pelvic examinations are difficult to perform on children; therefore abdominal examinations with supplementary studies often are used for thorough evaluation of masses in prepubertal patients.

Diagnostic studies are used to help determine the nature of the mass and denote any changes in size. Pelvic ultrasonography is the most useful initial study. It can detect a mass's location, size, and morphology accurately and identify the presence of ascites. CT and MRI are used to provide a more detailed description of the mass, to show the relationship of the mass to adjacent organs, or to assess for involvement of the paracervical or parametrial regions [5].

*Treatment*

Usually, functional ovarian cysts simply are observed for resolution, because most are self-limiting and disappear within 4 to 8 weeks [1]. If the cyst causes significant pain, persists beyond 8 weeks, or enlarges with observation, however, surgical management is warranted. Cystectomy, with preservation of the remaining ovary, is the preferred operative management of a functional cyst in women of reproductive age. Most functional cysts can be removed laparoscopically. Preoperative risks for malignancy that should be considered include the patient's age, the characteristics of the mass (complex masses with solid components, papillary projections, or external excrescences are of greatest concern), and the tumor volume. If the surgeon is concerned that a cyst might be malignant, laparotomy should be performed to facilitate intact removal and staging procedures as indicated. Additionally, laparotomy should be considered for functional cysts larger than 8 to 10 cm.

Most corpus luteum cysts are asymptomatic and can be observed. If the patient suffers severe pelvic pain associated with free peritoneal fluid, operative management may be necessary to remove the irritating blood/fluid from the abdominal and pelvic cavities. Rarely, patients may suffer significant blood loss from ruptured corpus luteum (hemorrhagic) cysts requiring emergent surgical control. Of note, the symptoms associated with corpus luteum cysts (abdominal pain, irregular spotting, and a pelvic mass) mimic those of an ectopic pregnancy. Thus, a sensitive serum hCG level to rule out the possibility of a pregnancy should be obtained.

Theca lutein cysts rarely require surgical intervention. Their thin walls make bleeding difficult to control if they are punctured. These cysts typically regress with the fall in hCG levels and are managed better with conservative observation [1].

Benign ovarian tumors are managed surgically with excision of the cyst and preservation of as much normal ovarian tissue as possible. Alternatively, in the peri- or postmenopausal patient, an oophorectomy may be performed. As with all adnexal masses, any concerns for malignancy may warrant an open procedure. All masses larger than 6 cm or with a solid component should undergo surgical excision. Similarly, masses found in postmenopausal women or any rapidly growing mass warrants removal.

To perform a cystectomy, an elliptic incision is made through the ovarian cortex overlying the mass, and the cyst wall is shelled out from the ovary. Once the cyst has been removed, the resulting dead space is re-approximated using an absorbable suture. The ovarian cortex then can be closed with either interrupted or running sutures. Some surgeons prefer to leave the ovarian cortex open, and this alternative is acceptable once homeostasis is assured [6].

## Leiomyomas

Uterine leiomyomas are well-circumscribed benign tumors of smooth muscle cell origin combined with some fibrous connective tissue elements. The most frequently encountered pelvic tumor, leiomyomas cause symptoms in approximately 20% of reproductive aged women [7]. The majority of myomas are found on the corpus of the uterus, but they also can be found attached to the oviducts, within the round ligaments, and on the cervix. Management of leiomyomas accounts for approximately one third of all gynecologic inpatient admissions, and definitive treatment of leiomyomas is the indication for roughly 30% of all hysterectomies performed in the United States [8,9]. Leiomyoma growth is estrogen dependent; therefore these tumors thrive during women's reproductive years. Women who have had lengthy and continuous estrogen exposure are at increased risk for developing myomas. This cohort includes women who experience early menarche or late menopause as well as nulliparous patients whose estrogen exposure has remained uninterrupted by pregnancy [10]. For unknown reasons, African American women have a threefold greater risk for developing leiomyomas than white, Asian, and Hispanic women [11].

*Etiology*

The etiology of leiomyomas is not understood completely. Myomas are thought to originate from the growth of a single muscle cell or myocyte, making each myocyte in the tumor monoclonal. Data suggest that myomas arise because of systematic and tumor-specific chromosomal abnormalities [12]. These aberrant chromosomes are thought to induce a cytogenetic mutation whose expression alters and increases the myoma response to steroid hormones. The increased steroid influence in turn enhances the growth potential of the myoma. The increased prevalence of leiomyomas within certain races, in affected twins, and among first-degree relatives supports the theory that some women have an inherited predisposition toward leiomyoma formation [13].

Uterine myomas typically are classified as submucosal (beneath the endometrium), intramural (within the myometrium), or subserosal (beneath the serosa) [14]. Initially, all myomas develop within the intramural segment. As they grow, they remain attached to the myometrium by a pedicle of variable thicknesses. The direction in which the myoma grows determines its ultimate location. Leiomyomas are hyperresponsive to estrogen because they contain a higher concentration of estrogen receptors than found within the normal myometrium. Collagen genes within myomas also overproduce under the influence of estrogen. This excessive collagen production accounts for the pale color and firm texture noted on gross inspection of leiomyomas.

The relationship between leiomyomas and leiomyosarcomas is uncertain. It is debatable whether myomas degenerate into sarcomas or whether sarcomas arise spontaneously within myomas, but the transformation of a leiomyoma to a malignant leiomyosarcoma has yet to be confirmed conclusively. Concomitant leiomyomas and leiomyosarcomas are well described, and the fact that these masses demonstrate different tumor markers suggests de novo development of the sarcoma rather than transformation of a benign tumor into its cancerous counterpart. At any rate, the risk of a myoma being or becoming malignant is low (between 0.04% and 0.7%), although this risk increases with the patient age [12]. Although definitive diagnosis of a leiomyosarcoma requires pathologic examination to confirm cellular atypia, increased mitotic activity, and the presence of coagulative necrosis, any rapidly growing myoma should raise concern for possible malignancy. Moreover, any growth of a myoma in a postmenopausal woman is worrisome [14].

*Clinical characteristics*

Most leiomyomas (fibroids) are asymptomatic. When symptoms do arise, they usually are related to the size, number, and location of the myomas. The most common symptoms are those of an enlarging pelvic mass: abnormal uterine bleeding and pelvic pressure or pain [15]. Subserosal and intramural myomas can become significantly large and often cause symptoms similar to those of a pregnant uterus. Myomas that compress the bladder can cause urinary symptoms of urgency or increased frequency. Similarly, myomas found on the posterior aspect of the uterus may disrupt defecation. Although all three types of myomas may cause abnormal uterine bleeding, severe bleeding most commonly is associated with submucosal fibroids. The resultant hemorrhage can lead to symptomatic iron deficiency anemia that may require blood transfusions. Abnormal bleeding typically presents as menorrhagia, but intermenstrual spotting and postcoital bleeding can be seen also.

Patients can present with pain caused by myomal degeneration (often termed "hyaline degeneration"). Rarely, pain arises because of torsion of a pedunculated fibroid. Special note should be made of the phenomena of red degeneration, also known as "necrobiosis." This type of degeneration is found usually, but not exclusively, during pregnancy and is associated with both pain and fever [16].

Occasionally myomas are found incidentally during evaluation for infertility or recurrent pregnancy loss. It is thought that myomas that distort the endometrial cavity can affect normal endometrial function and/or inhibit embryonic implantation, both are effects that can cause recurrent spontaneous abortion. Additionally, large tumors at or near the tubal ostia or pedunculated, subserosal tumors can compromise the patency of the fallopian tubes and induce tubal infertility. Ultimately, the association between myomas and infertility is both rare and weak [15]. Therefore, all other reasons for infertility should be ruled out before ascribing its cause to the presence of myomas.

*Diagnosis*

The definitive diagnosis of uterine myoma is based on surgical removal with pathologic evaluation of the tissue, but a thorough history and physical examination often may be sufficient to confirm the diagnosis. On bimanual pelvic examination, an enlarged, firm, irregular-shaped uterus may be palpated. It is important to differentiate a uterine myoma from an ovarian neoplasm. The mobility and size of the uterus is an important distinguishing factor. Myomas typically are mobile, and the uterus is enlarged, whereas ovarian neoplasms tend to be fixed with an adjacent uterus of normal size. Any question about the origin of a pelvic mass usually can be resolved with ultrasound. CT and MRI are expensive studies that rarely offer added benefit to pelvic ultrasound [17]. MRI, however, may be helpful to distinguish adenomyosis (invasion of endometrial tissue into the myometrium) from uterine myomas.

In cases of abnormal uterine bleeding, hysterosalpingography, saline sonography, or hysteroscopy may be the best techniques to identify a submucosal myoma. It also is important to consider other causes for abnormal uterine bleeding. Thus a sensitive pregnancy test should be obtained to rule out pregnancy, and, if the pregnancy test is negative, an endometrial biopsy should be performed to exclude endometrial hyperplasia or cancer. Likewise, a cervical Papanicolaou smear should be obtained to rule out cervical dysplasia as a cause of the patients' symptoms.

## Treatment

Asymptomatic pelvic masses thought to be myomas on examination or pelvic ultrasound can be managed expectantly. Serial physical examinations should be performed to assess for interval growth. A baseline pelvic ultrasound may be useful for future size comparisons. If symptoms develop, if the mass begins to grow rapidly, or if changes in bleeding patterns are noted, various treatment options should be offered.

Medical therapy with gonadotropin-releasing hormone (GnRH) agonists, such as leuprolide acetate (Lupron), has been used to treat myomas. Research has shown a decrease in myoma size by up to 50% with 3 to 6 months of GnRH agonist treatment [18]. GnRH agonists bind to the GnRH receptors in the hypothalamus to stimulate the release of stored gonadotropins and an initial increase in the luteinizing hormone (LH)/follicle-stimulating hormone levels. This spike is followed by chronic suppression of gonadal steroid secretion, resulting in a hypoestrogenic state. GnRH treatment is not always efficacious. First, the response to treatment is variable, with some patients experiencing a marked decrease in the size of the myoma(s) and others demonstrating little, if any, changes in the size of the tumors. Secondly, once treatment ends, the myoma tends to return to pretreatment size [19]. GnRH agonists have been used in women desiring hysterectomy to shrink the size of the tumors before operative resection. Often the uterus can be shrunk enough to allow vaginal hysterectomy in lieu of the abdominal approach, facilitate easier removal with a smaller mass, and decrease the potential blood loss during surgical resection. Similarly, GnRH agonists may be useful in treating perimenopausal women who do not desire surgery. Successful reduction in the size of the myoma can provide symptomatic relief throughout the perimenopausal transition. Once menopause is attained, it is unlikely that the myoma will grow back in the absence of treatment with exogenous hormone therapy [20].

The severity of the symptoms, the location of the myoma, and the reproductive desires of the patient all must be considered when surgical options are entertained [21]. A vaginal myomectomy may be performed in the presence of a pedunculated submucosal myoma. Once the base of the myoma is identified, the pedicle can be clamped and suture ligated, or, if the pedicle is small enough, the myoma simply can be twisted free. Other submucosal fibroids can be excised via hysteroscopic resection that can provide up to a 90% reduction in menorrhagia in affected women. Hysteroscopic resection is unlikely to be successful if more than half the myoma is intramural. If the vaginal or hysteroscopic approach is not feasible, abdominal myomectomy becomes the treatment of choice for patients who desire to maintain fertility or decline hysterectomy for other psychologic/cultural reasons. When myomectomies are performed for treatment of infertility or recurrent pregnancy loss, the American College of Obstetrics and Gynecology (ACOG) recommends that a complete infertility evaluation be documented that finds no other, more likely cause for the patients' symptoms. Disadvantages of myomectomies include the risk of recurrence that requires additional surgery, significant blood loss that may be associated with the procedure, and considerable postoperative adhesions that frequently form (particularly when myomas are located in the posterior aspect of the uterus).

Myomectomies typically are performed through Pfannenstiel or Maylard incisions as determined by the size of the myoma. The location of the myoma should be identified in relation to the uterine vessels, oviducts, and endocervical canal. A vasoconstrictive agent such as vasopressin often is injected along the myoma to help develop a plane of resection and to assist with hemostasis. The use of a tourniquet for hemostasis also has been described but us used less commonly. A single incision is made over the largest myoma, and the myoma is removed with sharp dissection and traction. If multiple myomas are present, they should be excised and delivered through the same uterine incision whenever possible. Using a series of delayed-absorbable sutures, the uterine defect is closed. The serosa is re-approximated with a "baseball" stitch using a smaller delayed-absorbable suture [22]. If the endometrial cavity is compromised during the myomectomy, women generally are discouraged from laboring with subsequent pregnancies, because they are thought to be at increased risk for uterine rupture [23]. Laparoscopic myomectomies are an option for select patients and offer the advantage of shorter recovery times than with open procedures. Many myomas are not amenable to laparoscopic resection, however, because larger uterine defects can be difficult to close laparoscopically.

Abdominal or vaginal hysterectomy is the definitive treatment for leiomyomas. There is no chance for recurrence, and often there is less blood loss than with myomectomy. Before hysterectomy, the surgeon must rule out both cervical and endometrial malignancies. Additional ACOG criteria for hysterectomy include (1) uterine size by abdominal palpation (typically greater than at 12-weeks' pregnancy), or (2) pelvic discomfort caused by the myoma, or (3) excessive uterine bleeding (menses lasting > 8 days or anemia caused by chronic blood loss) [23].

A newer procedure used for the treatment of myomas is minimally invasive uterine artery embolization. Embolic material (eg, gelatin sponge, silicone spheres, polyvinyl alcohol) is injected into the uterine artery supplying the myoma. The decreased blood supply results in myoma shrinkage and necrosis. Success rates are reported to be as high as 90% [24]. Uterine artery embolization should be offered to symptomatic patients who do not desire surgery. Contraindications to this procedure are desired fertility, allergy to contrast medium, an undiagnosed pelvic mass, or pelvic infection [25].

## Endometriosis

Endometriosis is a disease defined by the presence of endometrial glands and stroma located outside the uterine cavity. These ectopic implants can be found throughout the pelvis, on and within the ovaries, abutting the uterine ligaments, occupying the rectovaginal septum, invading the intestinal serosa, and along the parietal peritoneum. Endometrial implantation at distant sites such as the pleura, lung, within surgical scars, and along the diaphragm also have been reported. Although the exact prevalence of this disease remains unknown, it is believed to affect between 3% and 10% of women of reproductive age with an increased prevalence of up to 30% or more in infertile women [26].

### Etiology

Ulcerations on the surfaces of the bladder, intestine, and uterus indicative of endometriosis were first described more than 300 years ago. In 1860 von Rokitansky first definitively described lesions resembling endometrium outside the uterine cavity. With improvements in microcopy, Sampson [27] identified the growth of ectopic endometrial tissue as the cause of these lesions in 1920. Although endometriosis has been a well-defined disease process for hundreds of years, the exact mechanism by which it develops remains unknown. Multiple theories have been proposed to explain its pathogenesis, but none of them can account for the myriad presentations of this complex disease. Suggested theories ascribe endometriosis to aberrant implantation, ceolomic metaplasia, vascular and lymphatic dissemination, and pathogenic immune system responses.

The implantation theory, first postulated by Sampson [27], suggests that fragments of endometrial tissue flow retrograde through the fallopian tubes and then attach and proliferate at ectopic sites in the peritoneal cavity. This theory is supported by the anatomic distribution of endometriosis noted during laparoscopy. Endometriosis affects the pelvic organs in a stepwise manner based on their dependent position within the pelvis [28]. The ovaries and uterosacral ligaments are affected preferentially, followed by the posterior aspect of the uterus, the posterior cul-de-sac, and the posterior broad ligaments. Studies have shown that sloughed menstrual endometrial cells remain viable and have the capacity to implant at ectopic locations [29]. Cases of iatrogenically derived endometriosis resulting from mechanical transplantation of endometrium also support the implantation theory. There are numerous case reports of endometriosis in episiotomy scars following vaginal delivery and in laparotomy scars after cesarean section [30]. Similarly, endometriosis has occurred remote from pregnancy in umbilical incisions following laparoscopic tubal ligation and in needle tracks following amniocentesis

[31]. Retrograde menstruation, however, has been found to be a nearly universal phenomenon in women who have patent oviducts, and this theory cannot explain why only some women are predisposed to endometriosis but others remain disease free.

The ceolomic metaplasia theory is based on studies showing that germinal epithelia of the ovaries, endometrium, and peritoneum all originate from the same embryologic precursor [32]. This theory suggests that these totipotent cells are capable of transforming into endometrial cells when exposed to the necessary hormonal or immunologic stimuli. This theory is attractive in that it can explain the presence of endometriosis anywhere in the abdominal and thoracic cavities. It also has been used to explain the rare cases of endometriosis being found within the peritoneal cavities of male patients who have undergone orchiectomy and received exogenous estrogen therapy [33].

The vascular and lymphatic dissemination theory, also called "Halban's theory," suggests that endometrial cells can be transported to extrauterine sites via hematogenous or lymphatic spread [34]. There are extensive vascular and lymphatic communications between the uterus, ovaries, oviducts, pelvic and vaginal lymph nodes, kidney, and umbilicus [35]. This hematologic and lymphatic network would facilitate metastasis of endometrial cells via these routes. Vascular dissemination can explain the occurrence of endometriosis at sites distant to the pelvis including the retroperitoneal spaces, the pleura of the lung, the pericardium, within bone and muscles, and in peripheral nerves and brain parenchyma.

Last, there is thought that an immune component can be implicated in both the genesis and maintenance of ectopic endometrial tissue. With data suggesting that retrograde menstruation and implantation of endometrial fragments is the most likely means of developing endometriosis in the peritoneal cavity, alterations in the immune response to this tissue may explain why some women develop endometriosis and others do not. Women who have endometriosis have been found to have a greater predominance of macrophages within their peritoneal fluid than found in their disease-free counterparts [36]. The macrophages are thought to contribute to the pathogenesis of endometriosis by secreting growth factors and cytokines that either enhance the establishment of endometriosis and/or maintain viability of the ectopic tissue.

## Clinical characteristics

Clinical features of endometriosis vary, and presentation often depends on the site of implantation and severity of disease. Although most women who have endometriosis are asymptomatic, there is no good correlation between the extent of the disease and its resultant symptomatology. Women who have extensive disease can remain symptom free, and others who have only limited disease can be severely debilitated. The classic triad of dysmenorrhea, infertility, and dyspareunia often is used to describe endometriosis. Dysmenorrhea is the most commonly reported symptom, and it typically precedes the onset of menstruation. Between 30% and 50% of women who have endometriosis are infertile [37]. In these patients, the disease is thought to distort the pelvic anatomy, which, in turn, may impair ovulation, inhibit retrieval of oocytes by the tubal fimbria, and/or block sperm entry into the pelvic cavity. Additionally, the increased concentrations of both macrophages and prostaglandins found in the peritoneal fluid of affected women may impair oocyte, sperm, embryo, and fallopian tube function [37]. Associated dyspareunia often is seen in patients whose disease involves the uterosacral ligaments and/or has induced fixed uterine retroversion. Patients who have endometriosis also may present with a variety of other symptoms, including lower back pain, dyschezia, generalized pelvic pain, or dysuria.

## Diagnosis

A patient history demonstrating cyclical pain often suggests the presence of endometriosis. Bimanual pelvic examination may reveal pain with movement of the uterus, tenderness along the uterosacral ligaments, the presence of adnexal masses suggestive of endometriomas, a fixed and retroverted uterus, or nodularity in the rectovaginal septum. Although physical findings may support the diagnosis, a normal physical examination does not correlate with absence of disease.

Few laboratory tests or radiologic studies are useful when diagnosing endometriosis. For any female patient who presents with pain, a pregnancy test, complete blood cell count, and a urinalysis should be obtained to exclude abnormal gestations, pelvic infections, or cystitis. Serum antigen CA-125 levels may be elevated in severe cases of endometriosis; however this marker is not specific to this condition, nor is it sufficiently sensitive to identify lesser stages of the disease. Ultrasound may be helpful to determine the presence of ovarian endometriomas. These would appear as unilocular cystic structures within the ovary and demonstrate hazy borders and internal echoes [38].

The definitive diagnosis of endometriosis can be substantiated only by visualization of the pelvis via laparoscopy or laparotomy. Endometrial implants are notorious for their multiple appearances, and knowledge of these variations is necessary for correct diagnosis. The classic description is of a dark-pigmented lesion attributed to hemosiderin deposition. Other presentations of this disease include clear vesicles, flat plaques, white lesions, red lesions, powder burn lesions, chocolate ovarian cysts, and peritoneal windows. Peritoneal biopsy is desirable, because many other lesions can mimic endometriosis, and the positive predictive value of visual diagnosis is only around 45% [39].

During surgical evaluation the location and extent of disease should be documented and scored with the Revised American Society for

Reproductive Medicine Endometriosis scoring system. Use of this standardized form allows comparison of disease progression over time, more accurate description of the disease among different providers, and objective assessment of its response to treatment modalities [40].

## Treatment

Treatment for endometriosis is individualized to each patient and initiated when a patient complains of pain, experiences difficulty in conceiving, or presents with a pelvic mass. Factors to consider when deciding to initiate therapy include the patient's age, desired fertility, severity of symptoms, and other coexisting medical/surgical issues. Expectant management once was recommended for most women who had mild or moderate disease. Now, however, data show that patients who have dysmenorrhea and other pelvic pain benefit from surgical resection or destruction of visible implants with follow-on hormonal therapy. Additionally, surgical resection seems to lessen time to conception in the infertile population [38]. Potential benefits of cytoreductive therapy should be weighed against the risk of recurrence and iatrogenic adhesive disease as a result of surgery.

Medical management is the first-line therapy for women who have mild disease, and they are usually prescribed nonsteroidal anti-inflammatory agents (NSAIDs). Pelvic pain and dysmenorrhea may be manifestations of excess prostaglandin synthesis by the ectopic implants, and these symptoms can be diminished effectively with NSAID therapy. Because NSAIDs generally are well tolerated and are relatively safe, they should be tried as initial treatment for all patients who have mild pain symptoms [41].

Hormonal agents also are used to treat endometriosis. The goal of their use is induction of amenorrhea. Pregnant women who have a history of endometriosis are known to enjoy symptomatic relief with pregnancy-induced amenorrhea. Continuous use of oral contraceptive agents is prescribed in an attempt to produce a similar effect. Typical dosing is one tablet daily of a monophasic pill, which may need to be increased to two tablets a day to achieve amenorrhea. With prolonged therapy, glands and stroma undergo decidual reactions both within the uterus and in endometrial implants, and the patient's symptoms subside.

Progestin-only therapy also can induce amenorrhea, and medroxyprogesterone acetate is the most commonly prescribed agent. Oral medroxyprogesterone acetate, at 30 mg per day, or a 3-month treatment with intramuscular injection of 150 mg of depot medroxyprogesterone acetate (Depo-Provera) are two standard regimens used to treat pain symptoms. Progestins inhibit the pituitary release of LH; the fall in LH suppresses ovarian steroidogenesis; and the fall in ovarian hormone production promotes decidualization of the endometriotic stroma.

Danazol (Danocrine) is another option for hormonal treatment. Danazol is a synthetic derivative of 17 α-ethinyl testosterone and has both progestagenic and androgenic properties. Danazol inhibits GnRH secretion, which in turn prevents the midcycle LH surge. This chain of events ultimately results in the inhibition of ovarian steroidogenesis, which thwarts the growth of both normal and ectopic endometrium. Doses of 400 mg to 800 mg/d are recommended to achieve adequate suppression for symptomatic relief.

Because it also induces a hyperandrogenic state, danazol doses may need to be titrated to prevent adverse side effects. Weight gain, oily skin, acne, deepening of the voice, decreased breast size, and vasomotor symptoms can occur and may lead to discontinuation of therapy. Danazol is contraindicated in pregnancy because of its potential to virilize the external genitalia of a female fetus.

GnRH agonists such as leuprolide acetate (Lupron) are the primary medical treatment of endometriosis today. Because GnRH agonists initially increase the secretion of LH and follicle-stimulating hormone from the pituitary stores, patients should be cautioned that they may experience a transient worsening of their symptoms. With continued administration, there is a desensitization of the pituitary receptors leading to a reversible down-regulation of the pituitary-gonadal axis and decreased steroidogenesis. Side effects of GnRH agonists mimic those seen in hypoestrogenic states and include hot flashes, vaginal dryness, and decreased bone mineral density. Treatment usually is limited to 6 months' duration to avoid an excessive loss in bone mineral density [41]. Patients who have persistent symptoms or who need more than 6 months of treatment may require add-back therapy with progestins or combination low-dose estrogen and progestin. Additionally, all patients receiving GnRH therapy should be prescribed supplemental calcium and vitamin D.

Surgical management of endometriosis is indicated for patients who experience severe pain, have fertility issues, or have failed medical therapy. Laparoscopy is preferred to laparotomy. It provides superior visualization of the endometrial implants, allows inspection of the complete abdominal/pelvic cavity through small incisions, decreases the likelihood of postoperative adhesion formation, and usually affords the patient a shorter recovery time. Laparotomy is reserved for cases with extensive adhesions, endometriomas larger than 5 cm, and when the endometriosis infiltrates near the pelvic vasculature or the ureter or has penetrated into the bowel muscularis.

Conservative surgery is performed to preserve ovarian function and restore pelvic anatomy. Conservative procedures include excision, vaporization, and coagulation of endometrial implants, removal of ovarian endometriomas, and lysis of adhesions. Small superficial peritoneal implants less than 5 mm in diameter can be ablated with laser ($CO_2$) or bipolar cautery. Deeper lesions may need to be excised, usually with a margin around the lesion to remove concomitant microscopic disease. Superficial implants on the ovary also can be treated with laser ablation or fulguration using bipolar cautery [42].

Endometriomas smaller than 5 cm can be surgically resected via laparoscopy. A longitudinal incision is made in the cortex overlying the endometrioma with a monopolar microneedle or scalpel. The endometrioma is entered, and its contents are drained and suctioned, followed by copious irrigation. The ovarian cortex is stabilized with atraumatic forceps while the cyst wall of the endometrioma is grasped and excised from the surrounding normal ovarian tissue. Hydrodissection may facilitate removal of the cyst wall. If the endometrioma remains intact, sharp and blunt dissection can separate the cyst from the ovarian tissue. The cyst then is placed in a laparoscopic bag (endobag) and drained to facilitate its removal from the peritoneal cavity. Bipolar cautery is used to achieve homeostasis, and the ovarian bed can be left open to heal by secondary intention. Rarely, large defects are produced, or cautery cannot provide adequate homeostasis. In these instances, absorbable sutures are used to re-approximate the ovarian edges.

Large endometriomas necessitating laparotomy are removed in a similar fashion. A longitudinal incision is made over the endometriomas. Sharp and blunt dissection is performed to excise the endometrioma; ideally, it is removed intact. Should the endometrioma rupture intraoperatively, the pelvis should be irrigated copiously to avoid transient peritonitis. The ovarian defect is closed in two layers using purse-string sutures. The cortical edges then are re-approximated using an appropriately sized absorbable suture.

Definitive therapy for endometriosis consists of a total abdominal hysterectomy and bilateral salpingo-oophorectomy and is reserved for patients who have completed childbearing and have failed more conservative therapy. Unfortunately, up to one third of patients who initially are treated with conservative therapy end up requiring definitive surgery within the following 5 years. Most gynecologists remove the appendix at the time of this surgery. Despite comprehensive surgery, some patients suffer from persistent pain, and they may benefit from further adjunctive operative procedures including presacral neurectomy, resection of the uterosacral ligaments, and uterosacral nerve ablation [42]. Additional hormonal therapy may provide relief to patients who experience ovarian remnant syndrome or in whom it was impossible to resect residual endometrial tissue completely.

## Pelvic inflammatory disease

PID is an acute infection of the upper genital tract affecting any or all of the following: the endometrium (endometritis), the oviducts (salpingitis), the ovary (oophoritis), the uterine wall (myometritis), the broad ligaments (parametritis), or the pelvic peritoneum (peritonitis). In the United States, PID is the most frequent gynecologic condition warranting emergency department visits and hospitalizations among women of reproductive age. Although screening for sexually transmitted diseases has resulted in a decline in the incidence of PID during recent years, it still is estimated that annually 1.5 million women will suffer from this disease [43,44]. Thus, the epidemic of sexually transmitted disease and corresponding PID constitutes a major public health concern as well as a significant financial burden, particularly among adolescents and young adult females. Delay in diagnosis and treatment contributes to the inflammatory sequelae often seen in the upper reproductive tract. These inflammatory sequelae can cause patients to suffer significant long-term morbidity, such as tubal infertility, ectopic pregnancies, and chronic pelvic pain.

*Etiology*

PID is a polymicrobial ascending infection consisting of organisms that make up the bacterial flora of the vagina and cervix. The vaginal vaults of normal, healthy women are colonized by low numbers of a variety of potentially pathogenic organisms. The endocervical canal normally serves as a barrier to inhibit these potential pathogens from ascending into the upper genital tract. When there is a disruption in the mucosal surface of the endocervical canal, bacteria are able to ascend into the upper genital tract and colonize the endometrium, fallopian tubes, and surrounding organs. The two most common initiating pathogens are *Neisseria gonorrhea* and *Chlamydia trachomatis*. Other micro-organisms that comprise the vaginal flora (such as anaerobes, *Haemophilus influenzae*, gram-negative rods, and *Streptococcus agalactiae*) also have been associated with PID [45].

Approximately 85% of the cases are postcoital. The remaining 15% of infections are thought to be iatrogenic because they occur subsequent to procedures that disrupt the mucosal surfaces of the endocervical canal. Such procedures include endometrial biopsies, dilation and curettage, and placement of intrauterine devices.

Several risk factors predispose women to acute PID, and they are similar to the risk factors for contracting sexually transmitted diseases. Early age of first intercourse, large numbers of sexual partners, the use of nonbarrier contraception, age less than 25 years, prior sexually transmitted disease or PID infections, alcohol use, and being unmarried have been associated with both an increased incidence of sexually transmitted diseases and subsequent diagnosis of PID [46]. With the increasing popularity of intrauterine devices, the concurrent diagnosis of PID may be encountered. PID diagnosed within the first 3 weeks following IUD insertion may be attributable to the placement procedure itself, and most practitioners would recommend removal [47]. In other cases of concomitant PID with an IUD in place, the IUD does not necessarily need to be removed. Close follow-up is warranted, however, and a woman who fails to demonstrate rapid improvement in her symptoms after initiating therapy should have the IUD removed to ensure that it is not serving as a nidus for continued microbial colonization and infection.

*Clinical features*

Women who have PID can present with a wide range of nonspecific complaints. The most common clinical feature is lower abdominal pain.

This pain typically is bilateral and often is exacerbated by movement and/or intercourse. Abnormal uterine bleeding, particularly spotting or menorrhagia, is seen in up to one third of women who have PID. Purulent vaginal discharge, urethritis, vaginitis, and fevers and chills may be seen also. In a small segment of woman perihepatic inflammation, referred to as "Fitz-Hugh-Curtis syndrome," occurs causing right upper quadrant pain. Its presence is confirmed by laparoscopic visualization of filmy perihepatic adhesions. Fitz-Hugh-Curtis syndrome is believed to occur from the transperitoneal or vascular dissemination of either gonococcal or chlamydial organisms to the perihepatic region, inducing a local inflammatory response [48]. Its presence suggests fairly profound pathogenic inoculation. The onset of PID symptoms often occurs within the first 7 days of the menstrual cycle [49]. Menstruation disrupts the protective mucosal barrier of the endocervical canal, and the menstrual discharge also serves as an excellent culture media to allow colonization and overgrowth of infecting pathogens.

*Diagnosis*

The reference standard for diagnosing acute PID is direct visualization of the pelvic organs via laparoscopy [50]. Pelvic organs that appear indurated and edematous, or the presence of purulent material, pyosalpinx, or tubo-ovarian abscess, can diagnose PID definitively. Surgery often can be avoided, however, because a careful history and physical examination usually are sufficient to establish the diagnosis in the stable patient. Laparoscopy is indicated in patients who have an acute abdomen or who present with septic shock or when the diagnosis is uncertain based on symptoms alone.

The Centers for Disease Control and Prevention (CDC) recommends that physicians maintain a low threshold for diagnosing and treating PID because of its potential long-term morbidities [45]. Women who are at risk for PID and present with uterine, adnexal, or cervical motion tenderness without other attributable causes should be treated for presumptive PID. Findings on examination that support the diagnosis of PID include cervical or vaginal mucopurulent discharge, cervical motion tenderness, adnexal tenderness, and fever. Laboratory evaluation should include a pregnancy test, a complete blood cell count, an erythrocyte sedimentation rate, an HIV screening test, and DNA cultures for gonorrhea and chlamydia. An elevated erythrocyte sedimentation rate, leukocytosis, and the presence of gonorrhea or chlamydia support the diagnosis. Some clinicians also obtain an endometrial biopsy, which may detect endometritis. Empiric therapy should not be delayed while awaiting laboratory or pathology results. Imaging studies also are useful as an adjunct in diagnosing PID. Pelvic ultrasound can detect the presence of a tubo-ovarian abscess, tubo-ovarian complex, and thickened fluid within the oviduct (pyosalpinx) [45].

## Treatment

Because PID is a polymicrobial infection, empiric treatment regimens must provide broad-spectrum coverage. Treatment should be initiated as soon as the presumptive diagnosis has been made to prevent long-term sequelae. For patients who have mild to moderate PID, outpatient therapy with oral antibiotics can be considered, because clinical outcomes are similar between cohorts receiving oral and parenteral therapy. Recommended oral regimens include fluoroquinolones alone or a second- or third-generation parenteral cephalosporin with doxycycline. Metronidazole often is prescribed concurrently [45]. Patients who are treated with oral antibiotics should be followed closely. Patients who do not respond to oral therapy within 72 hours should be re-evaluated to confirm the diagnosis. If PID still is suspected, parenteral therapy should be considered.

The decision to hospitalize a patient who has PID for parenteral treatment is left to the discretion of the health care provider. CDC recommendations for hospitalizations include the inability to exclude a surgical emergency (eg, appendicitis); pregnancy; no response to oral antibiotics or inability to tolerate medications; presence of tubo-ovarian abscess; noncompliance; or severe illness, high fevers, nausea, or vomiting. Parenteral regimens suggested for hospitalized patients include intravenous cephalosporin combined with intravenous or oral doxycycline or intravenous clindamycin plus intravenous gentamicin. Parenteral therapy may be discontinued 24 hours after a patient improves clinically, but oral therapy with doxycycline should be continued until completion of a full 14-day regimen. When a tubo-ovarian abscess is present, clindamycin or metronidazole may be added to doxycycline to provide more anaerobic coverage [45]. A tubo-ovarian abscess need not be explored and drained surgically, but patients who have this condition often require extended antibiotic therapy. The abscess needs to be imaged periodically to assure its resolution. If the abscess fails to resolve, or if the patient's clinical picture does not improve with antibiotic therapy, surgical intervention should be considered. Surgery also is recommended when there is a high suspicion for other surgical emergencies, such as appendicitis. Overall, surgery therapy becomes necessary in approximately 25% of patients treated for tubo-ovarian abscess [51].

## References

[1] Droegemueller W. Benign gynecological lesions. In: Mishell DR Jr, editor. Comprehensive gynecology. 4th edition. St Louis (MO): Mosby; 2001. p. 479–525.
[2] Ioffe O, Simsir A, Silverberg S. Pathology. In: Berek JS, Hacker NF, editors. Practical gynecology oncology. 4th edition. Philadelphia: Lippincott; 2005. p. 188–236.
[3] Droegemueller W. Infections of the upper genital tract. In: Mishell DR Jr, editor. Comprehensive gynecology. 4th edition. St. Louis (MO): Mosby; 2001. p. 707–39.
[4] Tavossoli FA, Devillee P. WHO classification of tumours: pathology and genetics of tumours of the breast and female genital tract. Lyon (France): IARC Press; 2003. p. 170–81.

[5] Droegemueller W, Katz V. Diagnostic procedures. In: Mishell DR Jr, editor. Comprehensive gynecology. 4th edition. St Louis (MO): Mosby; 2001. p. 219–49.

[6] Sanflippo J, Rock J. Surgery for benign disease of the ovary. In: Rock JA, Jones HW III, editors. Te Linde's operative gynecology. 9th edition. Philadelphia: Lippincott; 2003. p. 639–60.

[7] Buttram V, Reiter R. Uterine leiomyomata: etiology, symptomatology, and management. Fertil Steril 1981;36:433–55.

[8] Lepine L, Hillis S, Marchbanks P, et al. Hysterectomy surveillance—United States, 1980–1993. MMWR CDC Surveill Summ 1997;46:1–15.

[9] Xhao SZ, Wong JM, Arguelles LM. Hospitalization costs associated with leiomyoma. Clin Ther 1999;21:563–75.

[10] Marshall LM, Spiegelman D, Goldman MB, et al. A prospective study of reproductive factors and oral contraceptive to risk of uterine leiomyomata. Fertil Steril 1998;70(3):432–9.

[11] Marshall LM, Spiegelman D, Barbieri RL. Variation in the incidence of uterine leiomyoma among premenopausal women by age and race. Obstet Gynecol 1997;90:967–73.

[12] Breech L, Rock J. Leiomyomata uteri and myomectomy. In: Rock JA, Jones HW III, editors. Te Linde's operative gynecology. 9th edition. Philadelphia: Lippincott; 2003. p. 753–98.

[13] Treloar SA, Martin NG, Dennerstein L, et al. Pathways to hysterectomy: insights from longitudinal twin research. Am J Obstet Gynecol 1992;167:82–8.

[14] Benda J. Pathology of smooth muscle tumors of the uterine corpus. Clin Obstet Gynecol 2001;44(2):350–63.

[15] Stovall D. Clinical symptomatology of uterine leiomyomas. Clin Obstet Gynecol 2001;44(2): 364–71.

[16] Berkely B, Bonney V. Uterine myomata complicating pregnancy, labour and the puerperium. In: A text-book of gynaeclogical surgery. London: Cassell and Co., LTD; 1913. p. 516–21.

[17] Droegemueller W. Endometriosis and adenomyosis. In: Mishell DR Jr, editor. Comprehensive gynecology. 4th edition. St. Louis (MO): Mosby; 2001. p. 531–63.

[18] Friedman AJ, Barbierie RL, Doubilet PM, et al. A randomized, double-blind trial of a gonadotropin releasing-hormone agonist (leuprolide) with or without medroxyprogesterone acetate in the treatment of leiomyomata uteri. Fertil Steril 1988;49(3):404–9.

[19] Adamson G. Treatment of uterine fibroids: current findings with gonadotropin-releasing hormone agonists. Am J Obstet Gynecol 1992;166(2):746–51.

[20] Chavez N, Stewart E. Medical treatment of uterine fibroids. Clin Obstet Gynecol 2001;40(2): 372–84.

[21] Davies A, Magos A. Indications and alternatives to hysterectomies. Baillieres Clin Obstet Gynaecol 1997;11(1):61–75.

[22] Guarnaccia M, Rein M. Traditional surgical approaches to uterine fibroids: abdominal myomectomy and hysterectomy. Clin Obstet Gynecol 2001;40(2):385–400.

[23] American College of Obstetrics and Gynecology practice bulletin: surgical alternatives to hysterectomy in the management of leiomyomas. Washington (DC): American College of Obstetrics and Gynecology; Number 16, May 2000.

[24] Ravina J, Ciraru-Vigneron N. Uterine artery embolization for fibroid disease: results of a 6-year study. Minim Invasive Ther Allied Technol 1999;8(6):441–7.

[25] Goodwin S, Wong C. Uterine artery embolization for uterine fibroids: a radiologist's perspective. Clin Obstet Gynecol 2001;40(2):412–24.

[26] American College of Obstetrics and Gynecology educational bulletin: endometriosis. Washington (DC): American College of Obstetrics and Gynecology; Number 184, September 1993.

[27] Sampson J. Peritoneal endometriosis due to the menstrual dissemination of endometrial tissue into the peritoneal cavity. Am J Obstet Gynecol 1927;14:422–69.

[28] Jenkins S, Olive DL, Haney AF. Endometriosis: pathogenic implications of the anatomic distribution. Obstet Gynecol 1986;67:335–8.

[29] Ridley J, Edwards I. Experimental endometriosis in the human. Am J Obstet Gynecol 1958; 76:783–90.
[30] Wittich A. Endometriosis in an episiotomy scar: review of the literature and report of case. J Am Osteopath Assoc 1982;82:22–3.
[31] Kaunitz A, Di Sant'Agnese P. Needle tract endometriosis: an unusual complication of amniocentesis. Obstet Gynecol 1979;54:753–5.
[32] Gruenwald P. Origin of endometriosis from the mesenchyme of the coelemic wall. Am J Obstet Gynccol 1942;44:470–4.
[33] Schrodt G, Alcorn MO, Ibenez J. Endometriosis of the male urinary system: a case report. J Urol 1980;124:722–3.
[34] Halban J. Metastatic hysteroadenosis. Wien Klin Wochenschr 1924;37:1205–6.
[35] Schenken R. Pathogenesis. In: Schenken RS, editor. Endometriosis: contemporary concepts in clinical management. Philadelphia: J.B. Lippincott; 1989.
[36] Hill JA, Farris HM, Schiff I, et al. Characterization of leukocyte subpopulations in the peritoneal fluid of women with endometriosis. Fertil Steril 1988;50:216–22.
[37] Burns W, Shencken R. Pathophysiology of endometriosis-associated infertility. Clin Obstet Gynecol 1999;42:586–610.
[38] Lucidi RS, Witz C. Endometrisois. In: Evans M, editor. Reproductive endocrine and infertility. The requisites in obstetrics and gynecology. Philadelphia: Mosby, Inc; 2007. p. 213–27.
[39] Walter A, Hentz J, Magtibay P, et al. Endometriosis: correlation between histology and visual findings at laparoscopy. Am J Obstet Gynecol 2001;184(7):1407–13.
[40] Hoeger M, Guzick D. An update on the clasification of endometriosis. Clin Obstet Gynecol 1999;42:611–9.
[41] Moghissi K. Medical treatment of endometriosis. Clin Obstet Gynecol 1999;42:620–32.
[42] Kim A, Adamson D. Surgical treatment options for endometriosis. Clin Obstet Gynecol 1999;42:633–44.
[43] Rein D, Kassler W, Irwin K, et al. Direct medical cost of pelvic inflammatory disease and its sequelae: decreasing, but still substantial. Obstet Gynecol 2000;95:397–402.
[44] Curtis K, Kieke B, Hillis S, et al. Visits to emergency departments for gynecological disorders in the United States, 1992–1994. Obstet Gynecol 1998;91:1007.
[45] Centers for Disease Control and Prevention. Sexually transmitted disease treatment guidelines, 2006. MMWR Morb Mortal Wkly Rep 2006;55:55–61.
[46] Suss A, Homel P, Hammerschlag M, et al. Risk factors for pelvic inflammatory disease in inner-city adolescents. Sex Transm Dis 2000;27:289–91.
[47] Grimes D. Intrauterine device and upper-genital-tract infection. Lancet 2000;356:1013.
[48] Wang S, Eschenbach D. Chlamydia trachomatis infection in Fitz-Hugh-Curtis syndrome. Am J Obstet Gynecol 1980;138:1034–8.
[49] Eschenbach D. Acute pelvic inflammatory disease: etiology, risk factors and pathogenesis. Clin Obstet Gynecol 1976;19:147.
[50] Sellors J, Mahony J, Goldsmith C, et al. The accuracy of clinical findings and laparoscopy in pelvic inflammatory disease. Am J Obstet Gynecol 1991;164:113–20.
[51] Weisenfeld H, Sweet R. Progress in management of tuboovarian abscesses. Clin Obstet Gynecol 1993;36:433–44.

SURGICAL
CLINICS OF
NORTH AMERICA

Surg Clin N Am 88 (2008) 265–283

# Gynecologic Emergencies

Grant D.E. McWilliams, DO[a],*, Micah J. Hill, DO[b],
Charles S. Dietrich III, MD[c]

[a]Department of OB/GYN, Tripler Army Medical Center, 1 Jarrett White Road,
Tripler AMC, HI 96859-5000, USA
[b]Department of OB/GYN, Blanchfield Army Community Hospital, 650 Joel Drive,
Fort Campbell, KY 42223, USA
[c]Department of OB/GYN, Gynecologic Oncology Service, Tripler Army Medical Center,
1 Jarrett White Road, Tripler AMC, HI 96859-5000, USA

The purpose of this article is to assist general surgeons in clarifying their thoughts and decision making when confronted with an acute abdomen in a female patient. In this setting, the etiology may include gastrointestinal, urologic, gynecologic, or obstetric considerations. During evaluation of a patient in the clinic or emergency room setting, if there is concern for a gynecologic issue, specifically a neoplastic process, a gynecology or a gynecology/oncology consult should be placed. The article focuses on the gynecologic causes, although many of the acute findings can be duplicated on physical examination in a patient who has appendicitis, mesenteric lymphadenitis, cystitis, or renal calculi. The structure for each section details common gynecologic emergencies and covers differential diagnosis, signs and symptoms, laboratory results, radiographic tests, and treatment options. Topics covered are ectopic pregnancies, adnexal torsion, tubo-ovarian abscess, hemorrhagic ovarian cysts, gynecologic hemorrhage (specifically abnormal uterine bleeding), and vulvar and vaginal trauma.

## Ectopic pregnancies

### Differential diagnosis

When evaluating a patient who has a potential ectopic pregnancy, it is paramount to remember that it is possible for an intrauterine pregnancy

The views expressed in this manuscript are those of the authors and do not reflect the official policy or position of the Department of the Army, Department of Defense, or the US Government.

* Corresponding author.
  *E-mail address:* grant.mcwilliams@us.army.mil (G.D.E. McWilliams).

0039-6109/08/$ - see front matter. Published by Elsevier Inc.
doi:10.1016/j.suc.2007.12.007

*surgical.theclinics.com*

to coexist with an appendicitis, ruptured hemorrhagic ovarian tumors, adnexal torsion, or endometriosis. Until a viable intrauterine pregnancy is excluded, caution should be practiced during the evaluation.

## Etiology

The most common cause of ectopic pregnancy is salpingitis, usually resulting from pelvic infections. If a fallopian tube has acute or chronic inflammation decreasing the luminal diameter, the fertilized oocyte, or embryo, may have difficulty navigating the tubal length into the intrauterine environ. Comparatively smaller spermatozoa can often travel distally resulting in fertilization. If the ensuing delay in passage exceeds 7 days of gestational age, then implantation occurs in the fallopian tube rather than in the uterus. Almost 50% of patients who underwent a salpingectomy for an ectopic pregnancy had a clinical history or histopathologic findings consistent with acute salpingitis [1]. Other causes include altered ciliary motility within the oviduct from hormonal imbalances or tobacco abuse, altered tubal architecture from pelvic masses, tubal adhesions from prior surgeries, and abnormal embryonic development. Table 1 shows the relative risk for ectopic pregnancies with selected patient histories [2].

## Signs and symptoms

Weckstein [3] evaluated the most common symptoms patients who have ectopic pregnancies present with and found abdominal pain, amenorrhea, and irregular vaginal bleeding to be most prevalent. On physical examination, the most common findings include ipsilateral adnexal tenderness, abdominal tenderness, and an adnexal mass. These findings have been confirmed by Lawlor and Rubin [4–11] and can be reviewed in Tables 2 and 3. Not all patients who have an ectopic pregnancy, even those who have a hemoperitoneum, have rebound tenderness or peritoneal signs. Also of note, vigorous pressure during bimanual examination can cause a previously unruptured ectopic pregnancy to rupture; therefore, gentle examination is required.

Table 1
Relative risk for ectopic pregnancies

| History | Relative risk (95% CI) |
| --- | --- |
| Ectopic pregnancy | 7.7 (1.9–31.5) |
| Pelvic infection | 7.5 (3.5–16.0) |
| Two or more induced abortions | 2.6 (0.9–7.4) |
| Pelvic surgery | 2.6 (1.4–4.6) |
| One induced abortion | 1.3 (0.6–2.7) |

Table 2
Symptoms of ectopic pregnancy

| Symptoms | Patients who have symptoms (%) |
|---|---|
| Abdominal pain | 56–100 |
| Amenorrhea | 62–84 |
| Vaginal bleeding | 55–84 |
| Dizziness, fainting | 17–31 |
| Pregnancy symptoms | 10–25 |
| Urge to defecate | 5–15 |
| Passage of tissue | 5–10 |

## Diagnosis

Diagnosis of an ectopic pregnancy is based on physical examination, laboratory assessment, and transvaginal ultrasound findings. If acute bleeding is occurring, there may not be an initial drop in the patient's hemoglobin; therefore clinical suspicion in a hemodynamically unstable patient may warrant surgical diagnosis. If the patient is clinically stable, then it is appropriate to follow her with serial laboratory tests and physical examinations until diagnosis is confirmed. Recommended laboratory evaluations include a complete blood count (CBC), quantitative β-human chorionic gonadotropin (β-hCG), and blood type to assess the need for RhoGAM. Progesterone levels have been used historically, but with the availability of sensitive β-hCG assays, this test is no longer routinely used. Quantitative β-hCG levels should be drawn on initial examination, and repeated in 48 hours if the patient is stable or if the diagnosis remains unclear. Studies have shown that 85% of normal pregnancies have a β-hCG increase of 66% or more within 48 hours [12], as opposed to only 13% of ectopic pregnancies that demonstrate increases exceeding 66%. In measuring serial quantitative β-hCGs, an increase of 1000 mIU/mL in 2 days has been used to differentiate a normal pregnancy from an ectopic pregnancy with a predictive value of 90%, sensitivity of 86%, and specificity of 93% [13,14].

Transvaginal ultrasound has proved invaluable in assessing early pregnancy complaints, including vaginal bleeding and pelvic pain. Combined

Table 3
Signs of ectopic pregnancy

| Sign | Patients who have signs (%) |
|---|---|
| Adnexal tenderness | 75–90 |
| Abdominal tenderness | 80–95 |
| Adnexal mass | 50 |
| Uterine enlargement | 20–30 |
| Orthostatic changes | 10–15 |
| Fever | 5–10 |

with β-hCG levels, ultrasound has allowed earlier diagnosis and treatment of abnormal gestations. The cutoff quantitative β-hCG value at which an intrauterine pregnancy should be visualized on transvaginal ultrasound ranges between 1500 and 2000 mIU/mL. Caution should be taken because an intrauterine twin pregnancy can have higher β-hCG values than a singleton pregnancy and is not visualized at singleton threshold levels. Furthermore, pseudosacs commonly seen with ectopic pregnancies can often be confused with early intrauterine gestational sacs. If the patient is stable, serial quantitative β-hCG levels and ultrasound evaluations are helpful as interval changes are often more important than a single assessment. Other ultrasound findings that may suggest an ectopic pregnancy include an adnexal mass, especially if it is separate from the ovary, and pelvic fluid. In the unstable patient, a focused abdominal sonogram for trauma examination can reliably identify intra-abdominal hemorrhage.

Although ultrasound has minimized the need for culdocentesis, this simple procedure can help triage patients requiring surgical intervention. During vaginal examination, a spinal needle is inserted through the posterior vaginal fornix parallel to the uterine axis into the posterior cul-de-sac. If non-clotting blood is aspirated, the likelihood of an ectopic pregnancy is high.

Although it may be more difficult to differentiate an ectopic pregnancy from an inevitable abortion, once the diagnosis of an abnormal gestation is confirmed through abnormal β-hCG levels, a dilation and curettage can be performed and the tissue sent to pathology for examination of chorionic villi. A frozen section is 93% sensitive in identifying chorionic villi [15]. If no villi are present, a stronger suspicion should be made for an ectopic pregnancy. A repeat β-hCG 24 hours after a dilation and curettage should show a decrease in levels by approximately 50%.

In asymptomatic patients who have appropriately rising β-hCG levels, serial pelvic ultrasounds can be obtained weekly. These patients should be followed until an intrauterine pregnancy showing cardiac activity is identified. On transvaginal ultrasound, there are certain milestones that can be measured to ascertain normal embryologic development (Table 4) [15–17]. If measurements of the gestational sac are irregular, this may indicate an abnormal gestation and the patient may be offered a dilation and curettage to evaluate for products of conception.

Table 4
Size of gestational sac and expected visualization on pelvic ultrasound

| Gestational sac (mm) | Expected ultrasound findings | Gestational age |
| --- | --- | --- |
| 2–3 | Gestational sac | 4 wk 1 d to 4 wk 3 d |
| 5–12 | Fetal pole | 5–6 wk |
| 13–18 | Fetal cardiac activity | 6 wk 0 d to 6 wk 4 d |

## Treatment

Algorithms are useful in the emergency room setting, although not all possible methods of treatment can be limited to an algorithm and consultation with an obstetrician/gynecologist is recommended. A sample can be seen in Fig. 1; however, in review of this algorithm it is imperative to keep in mind that with pregnancy, specifically with a multiple gestation, there is no guaranteed cutoff for a quantitative value.

Historically, almost all identified ectopic pregnancies were treated surgically. In the past decade, the advent of a methotrexate regimen has offered a medical alternative for patients. Expectant management is also an option, but is not routinely recommended given the risks associated with rupture and intra-abdominal hemorrhage remote from medical resources.

There is a debate between laparotomy versus laparoscopy as to the best method of entrance into the abdominal cavity. Laparoscopic approaches have been shown to have fewer postoperative pelvic adhesions, less estimated blood loss, a decreased length in hospital stay, and improved recovery time. Laparoscopy has a minimally increased risk for persistent ectopic pregnancy, however, and is not appropriate for hemodynamically unstable patients who have brisk intra-abdominal bleeding. Surgical options for tubal ectopic pregnancies include salpingostomy versus salpingectomy. Many providers perform a salpingostomy in hopes of preserving the fallopian tube. Vasopressin can be injected along the superior portion of the

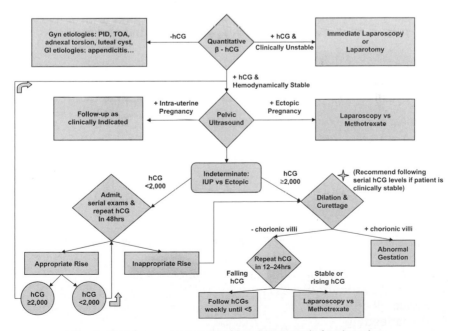

Fig. 1. Ectopic management algorithm. Symptomatic female patient.

fallopian tube, and a linear incision is performed with monopolar cautery along the site of the ectopic. The pregnancy can be removed with blunt graspers or the suction irrigator can be used to perform hydrodissection. A salpingectomy should be performed if the fallopian tube has had previous damage, such as a previous ectopic pregnancy, to obtain hemostasis, if the patient has undesired future fertility, or if the patient has already decided to pursue in vitro fertilization for future pregnancies. At any time during the evaluation or while in the operating room it is advisable to convert from a laparoscopy to an exploratory laparotomy if the patient becomes hemodynamically unstable, there is difficulty entering the abdomen, or there is concern for visualization. Rarely, an ectopic pregnancy can be located in sites other than the fallopian tubes, including the ovary, uterine cornua, cervix, or another abdominal location. As such, the surgeon should be prepared to alter the surgical approach as indicated.

Methotrexate has had great success in treating ectopic pregnancies while preserving the tubular architecture. It is dosed by body surface area at 50 mg/m$^2$. The success rate for single-dose methotrexate can be as high as 91.5%. It acts by inactivating dihydrofolate reductase leading to decreased tetrahydrofolate levels. Patients should be counseled to stop taking prenatal vitamins while on methotrexate as they contain high doses of folic acid and can limit the success rate. The indications and contraindications for methotrexate use are listed in Box 1. The single-dose protocol is listed in Table 5. The best predictor of success for methotrexate therapy ($\sim$90%) is if the initial β-hCG is less than 5000 mIU/mL. Recent data shown in Table 6 demonstrate that future fertility outcomes are relatively equivalent in patients undergoing methotrexate therapy or laparoscopic salpingostomy [18].

---

**Box 1. Indications and contraindications for methotrexate use**

*Indications*
Unruptured pregnancy
Ectopic mass <3.5 cm
No fetal cardiac activity
β-hCG<15,000 mIU/mL

*Contraindications*
Abnormal renal function (CrCl<60)
Hepatic dysfunction (liver function tests >2.5 times the upper limit
    of normal)
Absolute neutrophil count <1500, platelets <100
Active pulmonary diseases
Peptic ulcer disease
Breastfeeding

Table 5
Single-dose protocol for methotrexate

| Day | Laboratory tests | Actions |
|---|---|---|
| 1 | β-hCG, ALT, Cr, CBC, type and screen | MTX 50 mg/m$^2$ IM<br>RhoGAM 300 μg IM if Rh negative |
| 4 | β-hCG | |
| 7 | β-hCG, ALT, Cr, CBC | If change in β-hCG has not decreased by ≥15% from day 4–7, second course of MTX may be provided |
| Weekly | β-hCG | Follow up β-hCG until <5 |

*Abbreviations:* ALT, alanine amino transferase; CBC, complete blood count; Cr, creatinine; MTX, methotrexate.

## Adnexal torsion

### Differential diagnosis

Patients who have adnexal torsion often present with intermittent acute abdominal pain. The differential diagnosis to keep in mind while examining the patient includes ruptured corpus luteum, adnexal abscess, acute appendicitis, ectopic pregnancy, and bowel obstruction.

### Etiology

Adnexal torsion is almost always associated with an enlarged ovarian mass. The risk is greatest when the tumor measures approximately 8 to 12 cm [19]. There is an increased incidence in adnexal torsion in patients undergoing in vitro fertilization as the ovarian follicles become hyperstimulated [20]. Pregnancy may also predispose a patient to adnexal torsion. As the uterus enlarges out of the pelvis (around 10–12 weeks) and into the abdominal cavity, it may push the ovaries anteriorly causing torsion. Ovarian tumors account for 50% to 60% of torsion cases, and of these, mature cystic teratomas (dermoid tumors) are most frequently involved.

### Signs and symptoms

Patients presenting with adnexal torsion complain of an acute, intermittent, unilateral pelvic pain. This pain may be exacerbated by positional shifts. Approximately 70% of patients have associated gastrointestinal complaints to include nausea and vomiting, which can lead some providers to include in their differential appendicitis, bowel obstruction, or mesenteric

Table 6
Comparison of systemic methotrexate and laparoscopic salpingostomy

| Outcome measurements | Relative risk |
|---|---|
| Primary treatment success | 1.20 (0.93–1.40) |
| Tubal preservation | 0.98 (0.87–1.10) |
| Spontaneous intrauterine pregnancy | 0.89 (0.42–1.90) |

ischemia [21]. The episodes may have intermittently persisted for the past few days to weeks. On physical examination, a tender, unilateral adnexal mass is appreciated in roughly 70% of patients [22]. This tender mass becomes enlarged because in a partial torsion, there is enough arterial pressure for blood to flow into the adnexa. The venous blood is unable to return, however, because of the pressure dampening of the torsion. If the torsion persists or progresses, then the arterial blood flow is unable to oxygenate the ovary and the tissue begins to undergo necrosis. Many women only develop a fever once necrosis ensues.

## Diagnosis

Diagnosis is often made by ruling out other causes and by having a strong clinical suspicion. A pregnancy test can help exclude an ectopic pregnancy; a GC/chlamydia culture may help rule out pelvic inflammatory disease (PID). Unless necrosis has started, however, it is unlikely that a drop in hemoglobin or an elevated white count will be seen. A pelvic ultrasound with color Doppler flow can be highly predictive of an adnexal torsion [23]. A normal Doppler flow should not exclude the possibility of torsion in a patient who has an acute abdomen, however. An abdominal and pelvic CT can be performed in a patient to evaluate other causes, but is unable to evaluate blood flow in the adnexa [24]. The diagnosis and treatment of adnexal torsion are made on surgical evaluation.

## Treatment

The treatment of adnexal torsion is surgical reduction. More recently, studies have evaluated a more conservative surgical approach to patients who have adnexal torsion. Instead of performing a salpingo-oophorectomy, a laparoscopic evaluation with a gentle untwisting of the ovary and an oophoropexy can be performed. Oophoropexy involves surgically tacking the ovarian stroma to the pelvic sidewall with sutures [25]. This procedure has a success rate of approximately ~88%. In the setting of severe vascular compromise, unilateral salpingo-oophorectomy should be performed. Zweizig and colleagues [26] demonstrated that in patients of reproductive age (<40 years) who had adnexal torsions, conservative surgical management allowed patients to retain their fallopian tubes and ovaries without an increased risk for morbidity. These findings have been confirmed by further studies [27,28]. Care should be taken in removal of the adnexal mass to include reduction of the torsion before excision. The ureter runs inferiorly and laterally to the infundibulopelvic ligament and can be tented upward from the torsion process.

In a pregnant patient, there have been successful cases of laparoscopic adnexal torsion reduction. The incidence of adnexal torsion in pregnancy is 1 in 5000 pregnancies [29]. Many authors recommend entering in an open manner as opposed to Verres needle or in a direct approach; however, there has been documentation of complications in all three approaches [30].

In pregnant patients, precautions should be taken as the uterus may be in the abdominal cavity and surgical pneumoperitoneum poses the risk for decreased uterine blood flow secondary to increased intra-abdominal pressure [31]. Fetal cardiac activity should be documented before and after the procedure and the patient should be positioned in the dorsal supine position with left lateral tilt during the operation. The pregnant patient should be counseled on risks, including premature, preterm rupture of membranes, and preterm delivery [32].

## Tubo-ovarian abscess

### Differential diagnosis

PID can result in significant morbidity, not only in the initial presentation but also, more importantly, concerning the long-term sequelae. PID is diagnosed clinically based on having three physical findings (major criteria) plus one additional finding (minor criteria) from a laboratory or radiographic result (Box 2) [33]. Patients who have infections of the upper genital tract may present in a similar fashion as those who have an ectopic pregnancy, hemorrhagic corpus luteal cyst, appendicitis, or endometriosis/endometrioma.

PID may be treated on an outpatient basis; however, there are some indications for hospitalization of patients who have an acute PID picture (Box 3) [34]. When evaluating a patient who has an adnexal mass and an acute abdomen in a setting of PID, a tubo-ovarian abscess should be considered.

---

**Box 2. Criteria for diagnosis of pelvic inflammatory disease**

*All three are required*
Direct abdominal tenderness
Cervical motion tenderness
Adnexal tenderness

*Additionally, one or more findings should be present*
Temperature >38°C
Leukocytosis >10,500
Erythrocyte sedimentation rate >15 mm/h
Gram stain of endocervix—positive for Gram-negative intracellular diplococci
Positive culture of *Chlamydia trachomatis* or *Neisseria gonorrhea*
Mucopurulent material from cervix, or noted from peritoneal cavity by culdocentesis or laparoscopy
Pelvic abscess or complex on bimanual examination or on pelvic ultrasound

---

---

**Box 3. Indications for hospitalization of patients who have pelvic inflammatory disease**

Presence of tubo-ovarian complex or abscess
Pregnancy
All adolescents (compliance with therapy unpredictable)
Immunodeficiency
Uncertain diagnosis and surgical emergencies
Gastrointestinal symptoms (nausea and vomiting)
History of operative or diagnostic procedures
Inadequate response to outpatient therapy
Peritonitis in upper quadrants
Presence of an intrauterine device

---

*Etiology*

A subtle difference between the classic definition of an abscess and a tubo-ovarian abscess is that instead of a collection of pus developed in a newly created space, the tubo-ovarian abscess is a collection of pus contained by adherence of adjacent organs. The organisms responsible are polymicrobial organisms, although the two most common bacteria are *Neisseria gonorrhoeae* and *Chlamydia trachomatis*. Many times these bacteria coexist and when found should be treated with adequate antibiotic coverage.

*Signs and symptoms*

The most common presenting signs and symptoms are shown in Table 7 [35]. Approximately 90% of patients present with the chief complaint of abdominal pain and approximately ~75% of those patients have an elevated white count.

Table 7
Signs and symptoms of patients undergoing medical or surgical treatment

| Symptom/finding | Medically treated (N = 175) | Surgically treated (N = 57) |
|---|---|---|
| Acute pain | 158 (90%) | 48 (84%) |
| Chronic pain | 29 (17%) | 14 (25%) |
| Fever/chills | 86 (49%) | 31 (53%) |
| Vaginal discharge | 53 (30%) | 11 (19%) |
| Abnormal uterine bleeding | 37 (21%) | 11 (19%) |
| Nausea | 44 (25%) | 17 (30%) |
| Vomiting | 23 (13%) | 13 (23%) |
| Temperature $>100°F$ | 102 (58%) | 37 (65%) |
| White blood cell count $> 10,000/\mu L$ | 114 (72%) | 44 (77%) |

## Diagnosis

Diagnosis of a tubo-ovarian abscess is made by incorporating the criteria used for PID and radiographic findings on pelvic ultrasound, CT scan, or MRI. Often a complex adnexal mass with thickened walls and central fluid is noted. Pelvic ultrasounds may provide detailed findings of the uterus, adnexa, and ovaries. CT scan findings can show a tubo-ovarian complex with regular margins and internal findings similar to that seen in hemorrhagic ovarian cysts or endometriomas.

## Treatment

Traditionally, patients who have a tubo-ovarian complex are admitted to the hospital and started on intravenous (IV) antibiotics for a "cooling-off" period of 48 to 72 hours [36]. After cervical cultures are obtained, broad-spectrum antibiotics should be started. A commonly used regimen includes clindamycin, gentamicin, and ampicillin [37]. Because an abscess has low oxygen, anaerobic bacteria are frequently found and have been cultured in greater than 60% of patients. Clindamycin works well in this environment and in combination with an aminoglycoside is considered the standard treatment of choice for a tubo-ovarian abscess. Ampicillin is added to cover for enterococcus. If the patient does not clinically improve on broad-spectrum antibiotics, drainage should be considered [38]. Following 48 hours of antibiotics, interventional radiology may be consulted for drain placement. The drain should be left in place for at least 48 hours regardless of drainage, because early removal can result in reaccumulation of purulent material. Catheter placement may be preferentially placed transvaginally, or if the abscess is unable to be reached from the pouch of Douglas, transabdominal percutaneous placement has also shown good results [39]. The abscess fluid should be sent for culture and sensitivities. Simultaneous antibiotics and immediate catheter placement have also been described with good results [40].

Initial operative intervention may be considered in patients who have life-threatening infections, ruptured tubo-ovarian abscesses, or for removal of persistent, symptomatic masses in women who have no further desire for future fertility. During surgical evaluation, findings consistent with Fitz-Hugh-Curtis syndrome can be found in 5% to 10% of patients. Adhesions from the anterior portion of the liver to the anterior abdominal wall, noted as "violin strings," are evidence of the ascending perihepatic inflammation that can occur. In most cases, laparotomy is necessary secondary to dense inflammatory pelvic adhesions.

Today, the mortality in the United States for a ruptured tubo-ovarian abscess is between 5% and 10% even with modern medical and operative therapy. Because of the sequelae that can follow PID, specifically a patient who develops a tubo-ovarian abscess, it is essential to include treatment and education of all partners, thus reducing the risk for reinfection.

### Hemorrhagic ovarian cysts

*Differential diagnosis*

Patients who have hemorrhagic ovarian cysts often present with an acute abdomen. Diagnoses to consider in the differential include acute appendicitis, ectopic pregnancy, ruptured endometrioma, ovarian torsion, or a ruptured hemorrhagic cyst.

*Etiology*

Approximately 2 to 4 days after ovulation, the ovary becomes increasingly vascular. With neovascularization, blood from the vascular theca zone often fills the cavity of the cyst. Often, the cyst reabsorbs the blood; however, if the amount of bleeding is large or a cyst ruptures the bleeding may continue, producing a hemoperitoneum. Increased caution should be taken in patients who are anticoagulated.

*Signs and symptoms*

Pertinent history should include when the patient's last menstrual period took place. Pain can occur with ovulation of a follicular cyst, otherwise known as mittelschmerz syndrome. Enlarging ovarian follicles often produce a colicky or dull unilateral tenderness in the lower abdomen or pelvic region. Rarely, patients may present with hypovolemia and hemodynamic instability. A bimanual examination should be performed to evaluate the size of the cyst and tenderness. On physical examination, a corpus luteal cyst can mimic an ectopic pregnancy. Originally described by Halban, a triad of symptoms includes a delay in menses, followed by spotting, unilateral pelvic pain, and a small, tender, adnexal mass. Hallatt and colleagues [41] retrospectively reviewed charts in 173 patients who presented to the emergency room (ER) and were subsequently found to have ruptured corpus luteal cysts. Their symptoms on presentation are shown in Table 8.

*Diagnosis*

Diagnosis of a hemorrhagic or ruptured cyst is often made by narrowing the differential. Transvaginal ultrasound often demonstrates an adnexal

Table 8
Symptoms with ruptured corpus luteal cysts

| Symptom | No. (%) |
|---|---|
| Abdominal pain | 173 (100) |
| Abdominal pain onset with intercourse | 29 (17) |
| Pain starting within past 24 h | 94 (54) |
| Pain starting in the past 1–7 d | 40 (23) |
| Gastrointestinal symptoms: nausea, vomiting, or diarrhea | 60 (35) |

mass; however, the ovary may be normal in size if rupture has decompressed any cysts. In these cases, a large amount of pelvic fluid is usually noted. A quantitative pregnancy test can rule out an ectopic pregnancy. A CBC should be taken to assess the current blood count. An elevated white count is rarely seen in a ruptured luteal cyst. Once pregnancy is ruled out, an abdominal/pelvic CT with contrast can further assist in evaluating other potential causes, including acute appendicitis.

*Treatment*

Initial management of a suspected follicular or hemorrhagic cyst is supportive management and continued observation with a repeat pelvic ultrasound in approximately 4 to 6 weeks to document resolution. Oral contraceptive medication can be started in patients to halt further ovulation. Indications for immediate operative intervention include a large amount of peritoneal fluid found on a transvaginal ultrasound, hemodynamic instability, and severe pain. Delayed operative management is indicated for patients in whom pain is not improving with conservative management or for persistent tumors to rule out a neoplastic process. A cystectomy is recommended as opposed to a unilateral salpingo-oophorectomy in reproductive-aged women. Laparoscopic evaluation is usually feasible; however, if cancer is suspected, laparotomy may be necessary to ensure intact removal and for staging purposes. Intraoperative spillage of a malignant tumor does not necessarily worsen prognosis, but it does necessitate adjuvant chemotherapy. If the cyst is benign, a ruptured cyst may still cause postoperative abdominal pain secondary to chemical peritonitis.

**Gynecologic hemorrhage, specifically abnormal uterine bleeding**

*Differential diagnosis*

Gynecologic hemorrhage usually presents in two main cohorts: those who have abnormal uterine bleeding (AUB) with an organic cause and those who have a cause based on ovulation, or more specifically, the anovulatory patterns of a patient's menstrual cycle. The most important cause to rule out is a malignant process, specifically in a patient who has postmenopausal bleeding or risk factors for endometrial cancer. An endometrial biopsy should be performed on these patients and if an adequate sampling is not obtained, the patient should be taken to the operating room (OR) for a dilation and curettage.

*Etiology*

AUB can occur as menorrhagia (bleeding greater than 7 days or 80 mL occurring at regular intervals) or metrorrhagia (uterine bleeding occurring at irregular intervals). AUB is treated based on the root cause. Fig. 2 can be used to assist in breaking down the diagnosis into its compartment causes. As each cause can be different from the others, many providers order multiple laboratory tests and a transvaginal ultrasound and perform an endometrial biopsy before providing the patient medications, because many of the medications are hormonal and can affect the tissue samples.

*Signs and symptoms*

Many patients have a history of AUB and develop symptomatic anemic from the blood loss. The normal menstrual cycle has an interval between onset of menses of 28 days (±7 days). If the interval occurs before 21 days or after 35 days it is considered abnormal. The average length of menses is 4 days and menses lasting longer than 7 days are considered abnormally long. There is no definition of how little blood loss a woman may have during her menstrual cycle, but some authors have found that women who have menstrual blood loss greater than 80 mL during their cycle have significantly lower hemoglobin, hematocrit, and iron levels [42]. Almost half of women who lose more than 80 mL of blood consider their cycles to be small or moderate in quantity. Each woman's definition of her menstrual cycle is heavily variable and the definition of AUB may largely be subjective in nature. Because of the difficulty patients have quantifying their bleeding habits, queries should include how often the patient changes her pads or how often she goes through a box of pads, the type of pad worn, clots expressed with her bleeding, if her cycle is affecting her lifestyle, or if she has to use a back-up method (eg, a tampon in addition to a pad).

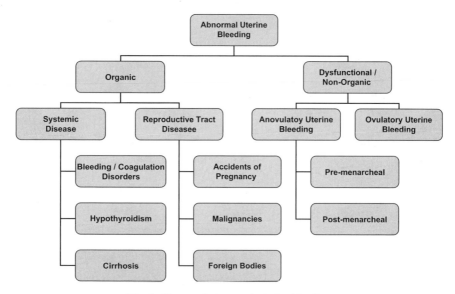

Fig. 2. Causes of abnormal uterine bleeding.

*Diagnosis*

In finding the cause of a patient's bleeding, laboratory evaluation can include a CBC, coagulation panel, liver function tests, thyroid-stimulating hormone, and a pregnancy test. Malignancy or infection should be ruled out. On pelvic examination the following should be performed: pap smear, gonorrhea/chlamydia culture, and an endometrial biopsy. If the biopsy returns insufficient or a suspicion for endometrial cancer is present, a dilation and curettage should be performed. This procedure may help with the patient's symptomatic bleeding in addition to its diagnostic benefits. Radiographic tests include a pelvic ultrasound, with or without a saline sonogram, to evaluate the endometrial lining for polyps and the myometrium for leiomyomas. If a foreign body is present, such as an IUD, it should be removed and sent for culture.

*Treatment*

Treatment of AUB is directed toward the root cause. AUB is classically broken into organic and nonorganic causes. Patients who have organic causes of bleeding can be subdivided into those who have a systemic abnormality or an abnormality in the reproductive tract. Adolescent patients who have AUB are at an increased risk for having a coagulation defect and laboratories should be obtained to include a CBC, von Willebrand factor, and evaluation for a prothrombin deficiency. Claessens and Cowell [43] noted that 20% of adolescent females hospitalized for AUB were linked to coagulation defects. In a patient who has hypothyroidism, initiation of L-thyroxine has been shown to resolve AUB [44]. Patients who have a history of alcoholism or liver cirrhosis have a decreased ability to metabolize estrogens. These patients should be evaluated in coordination with gastroenterology.

A common cause of AUB is pregnancy, which groups together patients who have a threatened, incomplete, or missed abortion and those who have an ectopic pregnancy. Many of these patients can be followed with serial β-hCG levels and transvaginal ultrasound. It is important to remember that if the patient is clinically stable, the trend of the β-hCG levels should be followed, because many patients may continue to have an intrauterine pregnancy although nothing is visualized on the initial transvaginal ultrasound. If the β-hCG values are decreasing or have plateaued after a 48-hour period, it is reasonable to consent the patient for a dilation and curettage. If there is concern that the patient may also have a gestational trophoblastic neoplastic process, the patient should also be counseled on the risk for hysterectomy during a dilation and curettage secondary to uncontrolled bleeding.

Any patient at risk for endometrial cancer should have endometrial sampling to rule out malignancy. This risk group includes patients older than 35 years of age and those who have unopposed estrogen use, obesity, or chronic anovulation. After an intrauterine pregnancy is ruled out, an endometrial biopsy can be performed in the clinic or in the ER with an endometrial Pipelle. If the patient is unable to tolerate the procedure, she may be taken back to the OR for a dilation and curettage. The curettage has shown some short-term benefit for patient's symptoms, but the symptoms will likely reoccur. A transvaginal ultrasound can also be performed to evaluate the thickness of the endometrial lining. If the pathology report returns as a malignant process, consultation to the gynecologic oncology service is recommended. If other benign findings are noted (such as intrauterine polyps or leiomyomas), then the patient may benefit from a diagnostic and operative hysteroscopy.

In a patient who is clinically unstable, medical supportive care includes blood product transfusion and high-dose estrogen for stabilization of the endometrial lining. Once stabilization of the endometrial lining occurs, the patient should be counseled that her next menstrual cycle will likely be heavier than usual. Table 9 lists IV and oral regimens used to control persistent uterine bleeding that necessitates hospitalization. The patient usually responds to the hormonal therapy within 6 to 12 hours. The patient should be informed about the side effects of high-dose estrogen, including nausea and increased thrombotic events. Patients should be placed on an antiemetic regimen and given leg stockings and intermittent self-compression devices for deep vein thrombosis prophylaxis. If an anatomic cause is found, the patient may be taken back to the OR for definitive surgical therapy after stabilization of the bleeding has occurred from hormonal therapy. If the patient continues to desire future fertility, she may be placed on long-term progesterone therapy, such as Depo-Provera, in lieu of definitive surgical management.

## Vulvar and vaginal trauma

### Etiology

Hematomas of the vulva and vagina are usually secondary to blunt trauma. They often correspond to a saddle injury, such as a fall on a bicycle; high-pressure injuries, such as skiing or water slides; or automobile

Table 9
Medication regimen for stabilization of abnormal uterine bleeding

| Medication | Dosage and route | Regimen |
| --- | --- | --- |
| Premarin | 25 mg IV | Every 4 h or until bleeding stops |
| Premarin | 2.5 mg, 1 tablet by mouth | Three times a day × 7 d, then daily OCP × 3 wk |
| OCP | 1 tablet by mouth | Four times a day × 7 d, then daily × 3 wk |
| OCP | 1 tablet by mouth | Three times a day × 3 d, then twice a day × 3 d, then once daily |

*Abbreviation:* OCP, oral contraceptive pills.

accidents. Hematomas not involved with blunt trauma can also be seen with a rupture of a varicosity in the late antepartum period, during labor, or early postpartum period when there is venous pelvic congestion. Sexual abuse should be strongly considered when the trauma includes hymenal or labial tearing in a pediatric or adolescent patient.

*Signs and symptoms*

Patients presenting with vulvar hematomas typically have an obvious painful mass in the labial region. Vaginal hematomas may not be readily apparent on external examination; however, patients usually complain of vaginal pressure and may have difficulty voiding or defecating.

*Diagnosis*

If a patient is admitted with recent trauma, pelvic fractures should be ruled out initially. In the setting of blunt or penetrating injury, especially with associated pelvic fractures, trauma to the bladder, bowel, and peritoneal cavity must also be considered. If gross or microscopic hematuria is found, a CT scan with a voiding cystourethrogram should be obtained before placement of a Foley catheter.

Before examination, intravenous, topical, or regional anesthesia may be required. Careful notation of the hematoma size and location should be made. Rectovaginal examination is important to assess extension into the retroperitoneal spaces. In the pediatric patient, the parent's assistance is recommended to help position the child for the examination. Visualization is best obtained with the child either in a frog-leg position or lying down in a knee-to-chest position. The vaginal vault should be well irrigated with warm saline and any foreign bodies removed.

A CBC may be drawn in the setting of hemodynamic instability or rapidly expanding hematoma. For the vast majority of patients, little benefit is found in obtaining laboratory or radiographic data unless the injury is traumatic and there is concern for ureteral or sigmoid injury.

*Treatment*

Management of vulvar and vaginal hematomas is usually conservative unless the hematoma exceeds 10 cm in diameter or if it is rapidly expanding. Most hematomas are venous in origin; however, a rapidly expanding hematoma could indicate an arterial injury and attempts should be made to identify this vessel for ligation. In the case of a slowly expanding hematoma, the culprit is more likely venous. Venous hematomas are typically self-limiting in nature and more difficult to control surgically than arterial hematomas.

Of note, vaginal hematomas have the ability to expand into the retroperitoneal pelvic spaces allowing for significant blood loss. Most patients respond to ice packs and compression. In cases wherein the bleeding site cannot be identified, interventional radiology can perform embolization. If necessary a cystoscopy can be performed to evaluate function of the ureters. A Foley catheter should be placed because urinary retention can occur with significant hematoma expansion. In the setting of a chronic, expanding hematoma, debridement and placement of a drain is recommended. The patient should be aware that complete resolution may take several weeks. Once healed, there is usually minimal scarring or sequelae.

## References

[1] Westrom L, Bengtsson LP, Mardh PA. Incidence, trends, and risks of ectopic pregnancy in a population of women. Br med J (Clin Res Ed) 1981;282(6257):15–8.

[2] Levin AA, Schoenbaum SC, Stubblefield PG, et al. Ectopic pregnancy and prior induced abortion. Am J Public Health 1982;72(3):253–6.

[3] Weckstein LN. Current perspectives on ectopic pregnancy. Obstet Gynecol Surv 1985;40(5): 259–72.

[4] Lawlor HK, Rubin BJ. Early diagnosis of ectopic pregnancy. West J Med 1993;159(2):210–1.

[5] Alsuleiman SA, Grimes EM. Ectopic pregnancy: a review of 147 cases. J Reprod Med 1982; 27(2):101–6.

[6] Brenner PF, Roy S, Mishell DR. Ectopic pregnancy. A study of 300 consecutive surgically treated cases. JAMA 1980;243(7):673–6.

[7] Gonzalez FA, Waxman M. Ectopic pregnancy. A retrospective study of 501 consecutive patients. Diagn Gynecol Obstet 1981;3(3):181–6.

[8] Gonzalez FA, Waxman M. Ectopic pregnancy. A prospective study on differential diagnosis. Diagn Gynecol Obstet 1981;3(2):101–9.

[9] Kitchin JD, Wein RM, Nunley WC, et al. Ectopic pregnancy: current clinical trends. Am J Obstet Gynecol 1979;134(8):870–6.

[10] McBride JR, Wait RB. Ectopic pregnancy: a review of 212 cases. Tex Med 1980;76(5):37–9.

[11] Sandevi R. Diagnosis of ectopic pregnancy. Diagn Gynecol Obstet 1981;3(1):15–8.

[12] Kadar N, Caldwell BV, Romero R. A method of screening for ectopic pregnancy and its indications. Obstet Gynecol 1981;58(2):162–6.

[13] Gronlund B, Marushak A. Serial human chorionic gonadotropin determination in the diagnosis of ectopic pregnancy. Aust N Z J Obstet Gynaecol 1983;22(3):312–4.

[14] Spandorfer SD, Sawin SW, Benjamin I, et al. Postoperative day 1 serum human chorionic gonadotropin level as a predictor of persistent ectopic pregnancy after conservative surgical management. Fertil Steril 1998;70(1):172–4.

[15] Coulam CB, Britten S, Soenksen DM. Early (34-56 days from last menstrual period) ultrasonographic measurements in normal pregnancies. Hum Reprod 1996;11(8):1771–4.

[16] Rossavik IK, Torjusen GO, Gibbons WE. Conceptual age and ultrasound measurements of gestational sac and crown-rump length in in-vitro fertilization pregnancies. Fertil Steril 1988; 49(6):1012–7.

[17] Hadlock FP, Shah YP, Kanon DJ, et al. Fetal crown-rump length: reevaluation of relation to menstrual age (5-18 weeks) with high-resolution real-time US. Radiology 1992;182(2):501–5.

[18] Dias Pereira G, Hajenius PJ, Mol BW, et al. Fertility outcome after systemic methotrexate and laparoscopic salpingostomy for tubal pregnancy. Lancet 1999;353(9154):724–5.

[19] Stenchever MA, Droegemueller W, Herbst, et al. Comprehensive gynecology. 4th edition. Philadelphia: Mosby; 2001. p. 519.

[20] Robson S, Kerin JF. Acute adnexal torsion before oocyte retrieval in an in vitro fertilization cycle. Fertil Steril 2000;73(3):650–1.

[21] Houry D, Abbott JT. Ovarian torsion: a fifteen-year review. Ann Emerg Med 2001;38(2): 156 9.

[22] Bayer AI, Wiskind AK. Adnexal torsion: can the adnexa be saved? Am J Obstet Gynecol 1994;171(6):1506–10.

[23] Albayam F, Hamper UM. Ovarian and adnexal torsion: spectrum of sonographic findings with pathologic correlation. J Ultrasound Med 2001;20(10):1083–9.

[24] Hiller N, Appel Baum L, Simanovsky N, et al. CT features of adnexal torsion. AJR Am J Roentgenol 2007;189(1):124–9.

[25] Nagel TC, Sebastian J, Malo JW. Oophoropexy to prevent sequential or recurrent torsion. J Am Assoc Gynecol Laparosc 1997;4(4):495–8.

[26] Zweizig S, Perron J, Grubb D, et al. Conservative management of adnexal torsion. Am J Obstet Gynecol 1993;168(6 Pt 1):1791–5.

[27] Cohen SB, Wattiez A, Seidman DS, et al. Laparoscopy versus laparotomy for detorsion and sparing of twisted ischemic adnexa. JSLS 2003;7(4):295–9.

[28] Oelsner G, Bider D, Goldenberg M, et al. Long-term follow-up of the twisted ischemic adnexal managed by detorsion. Fertil Steril 1993;60(6):976–9.

[29] Al-Fozan H, Tulandi T. Safety and risks of laparoscopy in pregnancy. Curr Opin Obstet Gynecol 2002;14(4):375–9.

[30] Stepp K, Falcone T. Laparoscopy in the second trimester of pregnancy [review]. Obstet Gynecol Clin North Am 2004;31(3):485–96, vii.

[31] Fatum M, Rojansky N. Laparoscopic surgery during pregnancy. Obstet Gynecol Surv 2001; 56(1):50–9.

[32] Agarwal N, Parul, Kriplani A, et al. Management and outcome of pregnancies complicated with adnexal masses. Arch Gynecol Obstet 2003;267(3):148–52.

[33] Hager WD, Eschenbach DA, Spence MR, et al. Criteria for diagnosis and grading of salpingitis. Obstet Gynecol 1983;61(1):113–4.

[34] Modified from centers for disease control and prevention: 1998 guidelines for treatment of sexually transmitted diseases. MMWR Morb Mortal Wkly Rep 1997;47:81.

[35] Landers DV, Sweet RL. Tubo-ovarian abscess: contemporary approach to management. Rev Infect Dis 1983;5(5):876–84.

[36] Landers DV, Sweet RL. Current trends in the diagnosis and treatment of tubo-ovarian abscess. Am J Obstet Gynecol 1985;151(8):1098–110.

[37] McNeeley SG, Hendrix SL, Mazzoni MM, et al. Medically sound, cost-effective treatment for pelvic inflammatory disease and tuboovarian abscess. Am J Obstet Gynecol 1998; 178(6):1272–8.

[38] Corsi PJ, Johnson SC, Gonik B, et al. Transvaginal ultrasound-guided aspiration of pelvic abscesses. Infect Dis Obstet Gynecol 1999;7(5):216–21.

[39] Shulman A, Maymon R, Shapiro A, et al. Percutaneous catheter drainage of tubo-ovarian abscesses. Obstet Gynecol 1992;80(3 Pt 2):555–7.

[40] Aboulghar MA, Mansour RT, Serour GI. Ultrasonographically guided transvaginal aspiration of tuboovarian abscesses and pyosalpinges: an optional treatment for acute pelvic inflammatory disease. Am J Obstet Gynecol 1995;172(5):1501–3.

[41] Hallatt JG, Steele CH Jr, Snyder M. Ruptured corpus luteum with hemoperitoneum: a study of 173 surgical cases. Am J Obstet Gynecol 1984;149(1):5–9.

[42] Hallberg L, Hogdahl AM, Nilsson L, et al. Menstrual blood loss—a population study. Variation at different ages and attempts to define normality. Acta Obstet Gynecol Scand 1966; 45(3):320–51.

[43] Claessens EA, Cowell CA. Acute adolescent menorrhagia. Am J Obstet Gynecol 1981; 139(3):277–80.

[44] Wilansky DL, Greisman B. Early hypothyroidism in patients with menorrhagia. Am J Obstet Gynecol 1989;160(3):673–7.

SURGICAL
CLINICS OF
NORTH AMERICA

Surg Clin N Am 88 (2008) 285–299

# Ovarian Cancer

Nishan Chobanian, MD[a],*,
Charles S. Dietrich III, MD[b]

[a]*Gynecologic Oncology, Saint John's Mercy Medical Center, 607 S. New Ballas Road,
Saint Louis, MO 63101, USA*
[b]*Gynecologic Oncology, Department of Obstetrics and Gynecology, Tripler Army Medical
Center, 1 Jarrett White Road, Honolulu, HI 96859-5000, USA*

## Epidemiology

The overall incidence of ovarian cancer in the United States has remained constant for the last 30 years. The age-specific incidence of ovarian cancer rises with age, peaking in the eighth decade [1,2]. The incidence is relatively rare before it peaks at 57 per 100,000 in the 70- to 74-year age group [3]. The overall lifetime risk of developing ovarian cancer is estimated to be 1 in 70 (1.43%). Rates are highest among white women in Europe and the United States; lower rates are observed in women from Central and South America [4]. The incidence of ovarian cancer generally is lower among black women in the United States than among white women.

The molecular events leading to the development of epithelial ovarian cancer are not known currently. Epidemiologically developed risk factors that have been identified include family history, nulliparity, early menarche and late menopause, increasing age, and residence in North America [5].

Most ovarian cancers are the result of sporadic mutations. Approximately 10% of cases are attributed to a familial disposition. Women who carry deleterious mutations of the *BRCA1* or *BRCA2* gene are the largest subset at risk for ovarian cancer. For women who have *BRCA1* (17q21 chromosome) mutations, the risk of ovarian cancer begins to rise in their late 30s and is estimated to result in a lifetime risk of 25% to 40% [6]. Women who carry *BRCA2* (13q12 chromosome) gene mutations also are

The views expressed in this article are those of the authors and do not reflect the official policy or position of the Department of the Army, Department of Defense, or the US Government.
  * Corresponding author.
  *E-mail address:* chobnh@stlo.mercy.net (N. Chobanian).

at substantial risk of developing ovarian cancer (15%–25%), although the risk does not seem to rise until the late 40s [6,7]. Both *BRCA1* and *BRCA2* are tumor-suppressor genes inherited in an autosomal dominant mode. Finally, ovarian cancer also is one of the cancers considered part of the hereditary nonpolyposis colorectal cancer syndrome. For women who have this syndrome, the lifetime risk of developing ovarian cancer is estimated at 10% to 12% [8]. The genes most commonly involved are the DNA mismatch repair genes *hMSH2* or *MLH1*. The resulting loss of the ability to repair DNA mismatches is a phenomenon called "microsatellite instability." Other cancers associated with this syndrome include endometrial cancer (40%–60% risk), gastrointestinal cancers, and urinary tract malignancies.

## Screening

Screening is defined as the identification of unrecognized disease by the application of test or examinations to apparently well persons to sort out those who probably have a particular disease from those who do not. The 5-year survival rate for early-stage ovarian cancer is estimated to be almost 90%. This 5-year survival rate drops precipitously to 30% for advanced-stage disease. Unfortunately, 75% of patients present with advanced stages (stage III or IV). The currently used screening modalities in ovarian cancer include ultrasonic imaging, serum CA-125 values, and rectovaginal pelvic examinations.

Because of the low prevalence of ovarian cancer (50 cases per 100,000 women) and a documented sensitivity of approximately 50%, the positive predictive value for transvaginal ultrasound is reported at less than 10%. Nonetheless, some authors have reported success with ultrasound-based screening. In a study by van Nagell and colleagues [9] screening 25,327 women from 1987 to 2005, annual transvaginal ultrasound screening was associated with a decrease in disease stage at detection and with as a decrease in case-specific ovarian cancer mortality. Using a morphology index (based on the combination of tumor volume and complexity) defining high-risk tumors, 364 patients (1.4%) underwent surgical evaluation identifying 51 malignancies. Forty-four primary ovarian cancers were noted, and 36 (81.8%) of these were detected at stage I/II disease. Only nine women developed ovarian cancer within a year of a negative screen (false-negative screens), making the negative predictive value greater than 99%. The 5-year survival rate of patients who had ovarian cancer in the screened population was 77.2%. The cost of this success was that an average of seven patients underwent surgical intervention for benign pathology for each malignancy detected.

CA-125–based screening also has been disappointing. The CA-125 antigen is derived from the coelomic epithelium. Overexpression occurs in several conditions, including nonmucinous epithelial ovarian cancer, uterine leiomyomas, pregnancy, infection, postoperative inflammation, and endometriosis, limiting the screening capabilities of this test. Helzlsour and colleagues [10] performed a case-controlled study in 1993 in which more than 20,000 blood specimens were obtained. The sensitivity of CA-125 in identifying ovarian cancer was a dismal 57.4% at 2 years. Skates and colleagues [11], in an attempt to improve the sensitivity of CA-125 screening, developed an algorithm using serial CA-125 measurements. Because CA-125 levels correlate with tumor volume, and tumor growth is exponential in early disease, his algorithm had a positive predictive value of 16%.

Preliminary data were presented by Petricoin and colleagues [12] on the use of protein spectrum analysis (proteomics). They reported a sensitivity of 100% and a specificity of 95% for identifying patients who had ovarian cancer. Further analysis, to this point, has been unable to support these data.

It is clear that newer screening modalities are necessary to enhance the early detection of ovarian cancer. Future modalities include a number of potential tumor markers including lysophosphatidic acid (LPA) and CA-125II, as well as proteomics.

## Prevention

Because the screening modalities available clearly are suboptimal, the prevention of this disease currently plays a vital role in decreasing the site-specific mortality rate. The "incessant ovulation" hypothesis of ovarian carcinogenesis was presented by Fathalla in 1972 [13]. He postulated that cellular injury occurs with each ovulation, and disordered repair can lead to neoplastic transformation.

This theory is supported by the numerous findings suggesting the protective effect of parity and multiple births. A pooled analysis of three European studies found that, compared with nulliparous women, parous women have a relative risk of 0.7 for developing ovarian cancer [14]. Additionally, case-controlled studies have repeatedly demonstrated that oral contraceptive users have a 30% to 60% decreased risk of developing ovarian cancer. This risk reduction is maximized after 5 years of use.

For the subset of women who have a genetic predisposition (*BRCA1*, *BRCA2*, MLH1, and *MSH2* carriers), risk-reducing bilateral salpingo-oophorectomy (RRSO) has demonstrated a 71% to 96% reduction in the risk of subsequent ovarian, primary peritoneal, and fallopian tube cancers [13,14]. Importantly, occult ovarian and fallopian tube cancers have been detected in 2% to 10% of surgical specimens during RRSO. Thus, it is imperative that washings be obtained and that the pathologic specimens be sectioned serially and examined by a gynecologic pathologist. Additionally, in premenopausal women, RRSO is associated with a 50% to 68% reduction in the development of subsequent breast cancer [7].

Some controversy exists as to the addition of a hysterectomy to the RRSO procedure. The disadvantage is the risk associated with a more invasive procedure, because the current trend is to perform the RRSO laparoscopically. The addition of a hysterectomy does provide a few advantages, however. First, the removal of the intramural portion of the fallopian tube eliminates the risk of a malignancy developing in this segment. There has been no evidence to date, however, of fallopian tube carcinoma arising in the intramural portion of the tube after an RRSO procedure. Further advantage relates to hormone administration. For women who have *BRCA* mutations, the lifetime risk of developing breast cancer peaks at about 60%. For these women, the relative risk of developing endometrial cancer while taking tamoxifen is 2.53. Hysterectomy eliminates this excess risk. Finally, hormone replacement therapy is facilitated, and risks are diminished without the necessary progestin component in patients without a uterus.

Patients who are identified as having a genetic predisposition for ovarian cancer and who refuse surgical intervention need to be informed of the risks involved. Nonsurgical methods of risk reduction include the use of oral contraceptive pills and routine screening including CA-125 and transvaginal ultrasonography.

## Natural history

Ovarian cancer spreads via three primary routes. First, and most commonly, there is direct extension. The tumor typically invades the ovarian capsule, and cells exfoliate and directly invade contiguous organs including the bladder, rectum, uterus, or peritoneum. Next, tumor cells can spread via lymphatic dissemination to the pelvic and/or para-aortic lymph nodes. Lymph node metastases may be present in up to 20% of early-stage ovarian cancers and are very common in advanced-stage disease. Finally, ovarian cancer cells may spread throughout the entire upper abdomen. This process occurs when exfoliated tumor cells are disseminated via the clockwise movement of ascetic fluid, the peristalsis of the small intestines, or diaphragmatic respiratory motion.

Seventy-five percent of patients diagnosed as having ovarian cancer present with advanced (stage III or IV) disease. The overwhelmingly accepted theory for this advanced presentation is the lack of screening tools for this disease and the nonspecific symptoms present during the early stages. The retrospective study performed by Sackett [15] revealed that, on average, patients who had ovarian cancer delayed seeking medical attention for 9 months. Furthermore, there was an additional delay of 9 months until these patients received a pelvic examination or ultrasound. A recent study by Smith and Anderson [16] demonstrated that more than 75% of patients who had ovarian cancer present early in their disease process with a constellation of symptoms, not limited to but including abdominal pain and swelling, gastrointestinal symptoms, or pelvic pain or mass. In 2007, the Gynecologic Cancer Foundation, the Society of Gynecologic Oncologists, and the American Cancer Society released a consensus statement highlighting symptoms that, if present on a daily basis for several weeks, should prompt medical attention and gynecologic evaluation. These symptoms include bloating, urinary urgency, pelvic or abdominal pain, and difficulty eating [17].

## Borderline ovarian tumors

Tumors with low malignant potential (borderline tumors) comprise 5% to 20% of all ovarian cancers. Pathologically, these tumors differ from invasive tumors based on a lack of stromal invasion. They occur predominately in younger women and typically present at earlier stages than their invasive counterparts. The tumors are diagnosed as stage I in 82% of patients and have a 5-year survival rate of 99% [2]. Even when diagnosed at advanced stages, survival approaches 80% to 95%.

These tumors typically are identified during an operative intervention for an adnexal mass. Frozen-section analysis is accurate approximately 80% of the time. Based on the frozen-section results, conservative/fertility-sparing staging (unilateral salpingo-oophorectomy) may be performed as a treatment for borderline tumors. Appendectomy should be included when the lesion is mucinous in origin. Staging is necessary in case the preliminary pathology underestimates the final diagnosis. Metastatic disease usually is confined to the abdomen. Most implants also have borderline features, but some can demonstrate an invasive component. Borderline tumors with invasive implants identified during staging have a threefold increased risk of recurrence (45%) but have no impact on survival.

The therapy for borderline tumors is optimal cytoreduction. The use of adjuvant therapy in these lesions is controversial. Typically, they are slow-growing lesions with late recurrences up to 10 years after initial diagnosis. The current accepted standard is the use of adjuvant chemotherapy (carboplatin/paclitaxel) in cases in which there is residual macroscopic postoperative disease or if invasive implants are identified. Consideration should be given to completion of the procedure (hysterectomy and unilateral salpingo-oophorectomy) after childbearing.

## Early-stage disease

Only 25% of patients are diagnosed with localized early-stage disease (International Federation of Gynecology and Obstetrics stages I or II) (Box 1). Comprehensive surgical staging is necessary for all patients suspected of having early-stage disease grossly. This procedure includes thorough evaluation of the entire pelvic and abdominal peritoneal contents.

---

**Box 1. International Federation of Gynecology and Obstetrics staging of ovarian carcinoma**

*Stage I: tumor confined to the ovaries*
IA Growth limited to one ovary, no growth on the surface, capsule intact
IB Growth limited to both ovaries
IC Surface involvement, capsule rupture, malignant ascites, positive washings

*Stage II: pelvic extension*
IIA Extension to the uterus or fallopian tubes
IIB Extension to other pelvic tissues (including rectosigmoid colon)
IIC Surface involvement, capsule rupture, malignant ascites, positive washings

*Stage III: implants beyond the pelvis (including the small bowel and omentum), positive lymph nodes, serosal liver implants*
IIIA Microscopic seeding of abdominal peritoneal surfaces
IIIB Implants ≤ 2 cm or smaller
IIIC Implants larger than 2 cm, positive retroperitoneal or inguinal nodes
*Stage IV: Distant metastases including malignant pleural effusions and parenchymal liver metastases*

---

Additionally, the following procedures are necessary for a complete staging: abdominal-pelvic washings, total abdominal hysterectomy, bilateral salpingo-oophorectomy, omentectomy, multiple peritoneal biopsies (pelvic sidewalls, paracolic gutters, colonic and bladder serosa, diaphragm, and any adhesions) and pelvic/para-aortic lymph node sampling. Young and colleagues [18] reported that disease is upstaged in almost 22% of patients when the proper staging procedure is performed. Furthermore, Chen and Lee [19] provided evidence that lymphadenectomy in patients who had stage I ovarian cancer improved 5-year disease-specific survival rates by almost 10%.

There is some suggestion that conservative staging can be performed in young women who have early-stage disease who wish to preserve their fertility. In these patients the unaffected ovary and uterus are preserved. The obstetric and oncologic outcomes have been shown to be reasonably good in patients who have conservatively treated early-stage epithelial ovarian cancer. Maltaris and colleagues [20] reported on 282 patients treated in this fashion. There were 113 pregnancies with 87 term deliveries, and there were 33 relapses with 16 disease-specific deaths (4%). The necessary conditions for the conservative staging procedure, as defined by Plante [21], include a unilateral, well-differentiated, well-encapsulated tumor without ascites. Because of the relatively high incidence of bilaterality with serous ovarian tumors (30%), it is important to examine the contralateral ovary thoroughly and to perform biopsies of any suspicious lesions.

The recommendation for adjuvant therapy for early-stage disease is derived from two major studies, the European Organization for Research and Treatment of Cancer (EORTC) trial and a trial by the British Medical Research Council [22]. Analysis of these studies demonstrated a significant survival benefit for the chemotherapy arm (82% versus 74%). To identify the optimal treatment regimen better, the Gynecologic Oncology Group (GOG) performed trial 157. In this trial, 321 eligible patients (stages IA, IB, grade 3, IC and II) were assigned randomly to three or six cycles of the standard chemotherapeutic regimen (carboplatin and paclitaxel). There was a decrease in recurrence in the six-cycle arm (27% versus 19%), although this decrease was not found to be statistically significant. The six-cycle regimen also was associated with a significantly increased risk of anemia, granulocytopenia, and neurotoxicity [23].

### Advanced epithelial ovarian cancer

The most common presentation (75%) for epithelial ovarian cancer is in the advanced stages (stage III/IV; see Box 1). In this setting, optimal cytoreductive surgery and platinum-based chemotherapy have been established as the most important components when treating advanced epithelial ovarian cancer. The initial report purporting the benefits of cytoreduction was Griffiths' [24] in 1975. A survival benefit was reported for patients who had stage II/III epithelial ovarian cancer whose largest residual remnant disease was smaller than 1.5 cm. Numerous retrospective analyses have supported this original contention [25,26]. Even today, however, there is no universally accepted standard for optimal cytoreduction, although most gynecologic oncologists advocate less than 1.0 cm of residual disease. More recent evidence derived from the completed GOG clinical trials 52, 158, and 172 has defined complete removal of gross residual disease as the treatment option conferring the survival benefit [27]. Eisenkop and colleagues [28], in a study of patients who had stage III and IV disease, demonstrated that 5-year survival was significantly improved with microscopic reduction (52%) compared with macroscopic reduction to less than 1.0 cm (29%). The theoretic and proven benefits of optimal debulking include removal of resistant clones, removal of large devascularized tumor beds (allowing more effective chemotherapeutic delivery), and removal of bulky disease (allowing improved appetite) [29]. Furthermore, as tumor volume is reduced, a greater proportion of remaining cancer cells is transitioned to the growth phase of the cell cycle, making them more susceptible to cytotoxic therapy.

The need for concomitant intestinal surgery to obtain optimal debulking in advanced epithelial ovarian cancer is high because of the proximity of the ovary to the recto-sigmoid and the pattern of intraperitoneal dissemination. The gynecologic oncology literature reports the risk of anastomotic leak after recto-sigmoid resection to be 0.8% to 3.2% in [30]. In the colorectal literature, a distance from the anal verge of less than 7 cm is an important risk factor for a leak. In ovarian cancer debulking operations, however, the majority of recto-sigmoid resections are above this level. Other identified risk factors for anastomotic leak are the presence of fecal contamination, pelvic radiation, tension on the anastomosis, uremia, and malnutrition (albumin < 3.0 g/dL) [31]. Richardson's study [30] analyzed several variables, including carcinomatosis, length of operating time, tobacco use, and malnutrition, for an association with anastomotic leak. Consequently, the operating surgeon should consider a diverting colostomy in malnourished patients who have ovarian cancer requiring a recto-sigmoid resection for completion of optimal cytoreduction.

Despite the proven benefits of optimal cytoreduction, many patients do not have maximal cytoreductive effects with their initial operation. Many factors contribute to this lack of benefit, including surgeon experience, comorbid medical conditions, and extensive disease. For these patients, interval debulking surgery or neoadjuvant chemotherapy has been advocated. The EORTC conducted a randomized trial on 319 patients who had suboptimal initial debulking. Following three courses of chemotherapy, patients who did not have progressive disease were assigned randomly to an interval debulking procedure followed by adjuvant chemotherapy versus continued chemotherapy. The group that underwent interval debulking showed a 33% reduction in death at 2 years [32]. Although no randomized trials have compared neoadjuvant therapy with the standard approach, many retrospective reviews have shown promising survival rates. Mazzeo and colleagues [33] reviewed 45 patients who had unresectable disease and who were treated with platinum-based neoadjuvant chemotherapy followed by interval debulking and adjuvant chemotherapy. Complete macroscopic debulking was achieved in 53.3% of these patients. The EORTC currently is conducting a randomized trial of neoadjuvant chemotherapy and delayed primary surgery, which should help define this role better.

The current standard adjuvant chemotherapy regimen for ovarian cancer includes six cycles of carboplatin (area under the curve, 6–7.5) and paclitaxel ($175$ mg/m$^2$). Eighty percent of patients achieve complete clinical remission with this regimen. Unfortunately, the majority ultimately will die of recurrent disease. A number of recent studies initiated by the GOG have investigated the role of intraperitoneal chemotherapy as the front-line adjuvant therapy for patients who attain optimal cytoreduction at initial debulking surgery (Southwest Oncology Group 8501, GOG 104, GOG 114, and GOG 172). The results from these randomized phase III trials have culminated in a recent National Cancer Institute clinical statement advocating the use of intraperitoneal chemotherapy in this clinical situation. The most convincing evidence is derived from the recent GOG 172 study. In this investigation, intravenous cisplatin (75 $mg/m^2$ over 24 hours) and paclitaxel (135 $mg/m^2$ over 24 hours) was compared with intraperitoneal cisplatin (100 $mg/m^2$) plus paclitaxel (135 $mg/m^2$ intravenously over 24 hours on day 1 and 60 $mg/m^2$ intraperitoneally on day 8) for six cycles, delivered every 21 days. The study enrolled 429 eligible patients and identified a 25% reduction in the risk of death for the intraperitoneal group. Additionally, the median overall survival for the intraperitoneal group was significantly better than for the intravenous group (65.6 versus 49.7 months). This intraperitoneal regimen has yet to be recognized as the standard of care. The regimen is extremely toxic, and only 86 women (42%) completed all six cycles of the intraperitoneal regimen. The most common reasons cited for discontinuation included cisplatin-induced toxicities, poorly tolerated abdominal distention and pain, and intraperitoneal catheter–related issues [34].

Future studies for treating advanced ovarian cancer probably will focus on targeted biologic therapies. Of particular note, bevacizumab has shown potential promise. Bevacizumab is a recombinant antibody to vascular endothelial growth factor. It has been shown to improve overall survival in colorectal and lung cancer and to lengthen progression-free survival in breast and renal cancers. In phase II trials in heavily pretreated ovarian cancer patients, the response rate to bevacizumab ranges from 16% to 35% [35]. Bevacizumab currently is being incorporated with carboplatin and paclitaxel for front-line adjuvant treatment in the ongoing GOG protocol 218. One of the main concerns with bevacizumab is the potential for life-threatening gastrointestinal perforations. In a culmination of the available literature, this risk is 5.4% in the ovarian cancer population [35]. Patients who have bowel involvement, prior radiation exposure, and recent surgery seem to have the highest risk.

## Recurrent ovarian cancer

Unfortunately, almost 65% of patients who have advanced-stage ovarian cancer relapse within 2 years of initial therapy [36]. The therapeutic options for the recurrent setting are based on treatment responses and interval from treatment. Ovarian cancer that recurs within 6 months is classified as platinum-resistant disease; recurrence after 6 months is considered platinum sensitive. Numerous studies have demonstrated an improved response to chemotherapeutic agents in the platinum-sensitive patients. The current recommended standard in these patients is a platinum/taxane combination. For individuals who have platinum-resistant disease, there are numerous options for chemotherapy, including topotecan, docetaxel, liposomal doxorubicin, gemcitabine, and etoposide. Responses range from 15% to 20% in this patient subset. The choice of particular agent is based on the patient's health status, current disease status, and toxicities.

In addition to chemotherapeutic intervention in the recurrent setting, there is some support in the literature for secondary cytoreduction; however, there is no current consensus concerning its role. A large number of studies have evaluated the role of cytoreductive surgery, and nearly all report a significant survival advantage for patients undergoing optimal cytoreduction in the recurrent setting [37]. Controversies include which patients should undergo this procedure and which subset will benefit from this potentially morbid procedure. Chi and colleagues [38] reported on 157 patients at Memorial Sloan-Kettering Cancer Center who underwent secondary cytoreduction and concluded that disease-free interval and the number of recurrence sites should be taken into account before proceeding. If the disease-free interval was between 6 and 12 months, the median survival time was 30 months following surgery. On the other hand, if the disease-free interval was longer than 30 months, the median survival time was 51 months. Patients who had a single site of recurrence faired better than those who had multiple sites (60 months versus 42 months), and patients who had residual disease 0.5 cm or smaller had better survival than patients who residual cancer greater than 0.5 cm (56 months versus 27 months) [38].

The management of patients who have recurrent epithelial ovarian cancer also involves an understanding of the management of bowel obstructions. Many patients who have recurrent ovarian cancer develop intestinal obstructions as a result of the direct intra-abdominal spread of disease. Although most bowel obstructions result from disease progression, postoperative adhesions and radiation fibrosis also are potential causes. The majority of obstructions are isolated to the small intestine (54%), but 31.7% are in the large bowel, and 14.3% in both the colon and small intestine [39]. The decision regarding medical versus surgical management can be difficult. No randomized trials have compared these two treatment modalities directly. Initial treatment includes nonsurgical management unless an acute abdomen is noted clinically. The typical regimen of bowel rest (using a nasogastric tube), taking nothing by mouth, and intravenous fluid hydration is successful in only 1% to 15% of these cases [40]. The diagnosis of a bowel obstruction in the recurrent setting usually is associated with incurable disease. The majority of patients survive an average of only 65.5 days after the diagnosis of obstruction in this setting [41]. Thus, it is important to consider preoperatively the patient's remaining treatment options, overall medical condition, and current tumor burden. There are no current universal, reliably consistent indicators of good prognosis after surgical intervention. A number of retrospective analyses have advocated using prospective indicators such as age, tumor status, nutritional status, ascites, prior radiotherapy, the extent of prior chemotherapy, and the presence of distant metastases [42]. The reality is that the operating surgeon must incorporate an understanding of the procedure with an understanding of the disease process in deciding whether to proceed with surgical management.

In the palliative setting, patients who have bowel obstruction can benefit immensely from gastrostomy placement. This procedure eliminates the need for nasogastric decompression and potentiates home management of symptoms. Many patients are able to maintain some oral intake despite obstruction, improving comfort for the terminally ill. Although gastrostomy tubes can be placed by open laparotomy, in many cases a percutaneous technique also is feasible with only local anesthesia and sedation. In reported series, only 7% to 11% of percutaneous attempts were unsuccessful [43].

## Nonepithelial ovarian cancer

Most ovarian cancers are epithelial in origin. Nonepithelial ovarian lesions include germ cell tumors and stromal cell tumors. Germ cell tumors comprise approximately 15% to 20% of ovarian neoplasms; stromal tumors account for 5% to 10%.

Germ cell tumors represent 20% of all ovarian tumors and 2% to 3% of ovarian malignancies. They are subclassified as dysgerminoma, endodermal sinus tumor, embryonal cell carcinoma, and teratoma (mature and immature). These neoplasms have a peak incidence in the third decade and decline dramatically in incidence thereafter. Most have unique tumor markers that can help predict the histology preoperatively and assist in postoperative management and surveillance (Table 1).

Dysgerminoma is the most common germ cell tumor in adolescent females (40% of all germ cell tumors). The peak age of incidence is 19 years. Most patients present with pain and an abdominopelvic mass. There is a propensity for early stage at presentation: 67% present as stage IA. Although the incidence of bilaterality is 10% to 15%, most patients can be treated with fertility-sparing surgery. Because of the propensity for lymphatic dissemination, a conservative staging procedure (as discussed previously for epithelial ovarian cancer) should be performed. Adjuvant treatment (bleomycin, etoposide, and cisplatin, BEP) has been derived from the

Table 1
Tumor markers for germ cell and stromal ovarian malignancies

| Tumor type | Tumor marker |
| --- | --- |
| Germ cell tumors | |
|   Dysgerminoma | LDH, occasionally β-hCG |
|   Endodermal sinus tumor | AFP |
|   Embryonal carcinoma | β-hCG, occasionally AFP |
|   Immature teratoma | Occasionally AFP |
| Stromal tumors | |
|   Granulosa cell tumor | Inhibin |
|   Sertoli-Leydig tumor | Testosterone |

*Abbreviations:* AFP, alfa-fetoprotein; β-hCG, beta human chorionic gonadotropin; LDH, lactate dehydrogenase.

testicular cancer literature and is reserved for all patients except for those who have stage IA disease. The overall survival is excellent at 85%.

Endodermal sinus and embryonal cell tumors are much less common than dygerminomas and very rarely are bilateral (< 1%). These tumors also may be treated with a conservative staging approach. Adjuvant treatment (BEP) should be administered to all patients, regardless of stage. The overall survival rates, 70% for endodermal sinus tumors and 40% for embryonal cell tumors, are somewhat lower than that of patients who have dysgerminoma. These tumors tend to be aggressive, and intra-abdominal metastases are common. Debulking is believed to be of benefit.

Immature teratomas are rare, comprising only 1% of ovarian tumors. These tumors rarely are bilateral (< 2%) and have a propensity for peritoneal dissemination and lymphatic spread. The histologic grading, which is determined by the degree of immature neural elements, is the most important factor in survival. Treatment is similar to that for other germ cell tumors, with conservative staging and adjuvant BEP chemotherapy for all but stage IA, grade 1 immature teratomas. The overall survival rate is 63%.

The most common malignant stromal tumors are granulosa cell tumors (adult and juvenile) and Sertoli-Leydig cell tumors. The granulosa cell tumors are more commonly adult type (95%). The presentation is variable, including pain, mass on pelvic examination, or postmenopausal vaginal bleeding. Granulosa cell tumors produce excess estrogen leading to concurrent endometrial hyperplasia in 35% of patients and endometrial cancer in 10%. Treatment includes complete hysterectomy and staging as well as tumor debulking. For premenopausal patients, conservative staging is acceptable, but thorough evaluation of the endometrium with dilation and curettage should be performed to exclude simultaneous uterine pathology. Ninety percent of granulosa cell tumors present at an early stage and have an excellent disease-free survival rate (90%). For patients presenting with stage II disease or greater, four cycles of adjuvant BEP is the current recommended therapy.

Sertoli-Leydig tumors comprise less than 0.2% of ovarian tumors. The average age at diagnosis is 25 years. Extraovarian spread at diagnosis is rare (2%–3%). These tumors are characterized by the presence of a testicular structure that produces androgens. Consequently, presenting symptoms include menstrual disorders, virilization, and abdominal pain. Virilization occurs in 35% of patients who have these tumors. The most important predictor of outcome is the stage at presentation, with 97% of patients presenting at stage I. As is the case with the granulosa cell tumors, conservative staging with endometrial sampling is indicated for young women who desire to preserve their fertility. For patients who have completed childbearing, complete surgical staging is indicated. Currently, there is no evidence indicating the efficacy of debulking surgery in Sertoli-Leydig cell tumors. Postoperatively, adjuvant chemotherapy (BEP) is indicated for all patients who have disease advanced beyond stage I.

# Summary

Epithelial ovarian cancer is the foremost gynecologic malignancy in terms of patient deaths. Formerly known as the "silent killer," ovarian cancer has a spectrum of nonspecific symptoms that, when recognized, may allow earlier detection and increased survival. Currently, the majority of patients present at an advanced disease stage, and survival is poor. The current standard treatment regimen employs optimal cytoreductive surgery and adjuvant chemotherapy. Early-stage disease is treated successfully with this regimen, and the 5-year survival rate is excellent. For patients presenting with advanced-stage disease (75%), initial clinical response/remission is excellent, but clinical recurrence is almost a certainty. Once ovarian cancer recurs, there is no longer a chance for cure, and all subsequent treatments are palliative. There is and has been a great emphasis on developing effective screening protocols, but to date there is no recommended successful screening tool for this disease. Recurrent disease frequently presents within a year or two of definitive initial treatment. Current treatment options include chemotherapy with or without secondary cytoreductive surgery. The responses generally are poor, and most patients ultimately die of the disease.

The nonepithelial ovarian cancers tend to occur in a younger population of patients. They typically present with earlier stages of disease and have an excellent survival potential when detected early. Most patients desiring future fertility can be treated successfully with a conservative staging procedure with or without adjuvant chemotherapy.

# References

[1] American Cancer Society. Cancer facts and figures, 2007. Estimated new cancer cases and deaths by sex for all sites. Available at: http://www.cancer.org/downloads/stt/CFF2007EstCsDths07.pdf. Accessed November 10, 2007.

[2] Ozols RF, Rubin SC, Thomas GM. Epithelial ovarian cancer. In: Hoskins WJ, Perez CA, Young RC, editors. Principles and practice of gynecologic oncology. Philadelphia: Lippincott Williams & Wilkins; 2000. p. 981–1057.

[3] Yancik R, Ries LG, Yates JN. Ovarian cancer in the elderly: analysis of surveillance. Am J Obstet Gynecol 1986;154:639.

[4] Ferlay J. Cancer incidence, mortality and prevalence. IARC Cancer Base No 5. Lyon: IARC Press; 2000.

[5] Daly M, Obrans GI. Epidemiology and risk assessment for ovarian cancer. Semin Oncol 1998;25:255.

[6] Schmeler KM, Sun CC, Bodurka DC, et al. Prophylactic bilateral salpingo-oophorectomy compared with surveillance in women with BRCA mutations. Obstet Gynecol 2006;108(3):515–20.

[7] SGO Committee Opinion. Clinical practice committee statement on prophylatic salpingo-oophorectomy. Gynecol Oncol 2005;98:179–81.

[8] Chen L, Yang KY, Little SE, et al. Gynecologic cancer prevention in Lynch syndrome/hereditary nonpolyposis colorectal cancer families. Obstet Gynecol 2007;110(1):18–24.

[9] van Nagell JR, DePriest PD, Ueland FR, et al. Ovarian cancer screening with annual transvaginal sonography: findings of 25,000 women screened. Cancer 2007;109(9):1887–96.

[10] Helzlsouer KJ, Bush TL, Alberg AJ, et al. Prospective study of serum CA 125 as marker for ovarian cancer. J Am Med Assoc 1993;269:1123–6.

[11] Skates SJ, Feng-Ji X, Yin-Hua Y, et al. Toward an optimal algorithm for ovarian cancer screening with longitudinal tumour markers. Cancer 1995;76:S2004–10.

[12] Petricoin EF, Ardekani AM, Hit BA, et al. Use of proteomic patterns in serum to identify ovarian cancer. Lancet 2002;359:572–7.

[13] Fathalla MF. Factors in causation and incidence of ovarian cancer. Gynecologic Surveys 1972;27:151–68.

[14] Rebbeck TR, Lynch HT, Neuhasen SL, et al. Prophylactic oophorectomy in carriers of BRCA1 or 2 mutations. N Engl J Med 2002;346:1616–22.

[15] Sackett D. Clinical epidemiology of what, who and whither. J Clin Epidemiol 1985;55(12):1161–6.

[16] Smith EM, Anderson B. The effects of symptoms and delay in seeking diagnosis on stage of disease at diagnosis among females with cancers of the ovary. Cancer 1985;56(11):2727–32.

[17] Ovarian cancer symptoms consensus statement. Chicago (IL): Gynecologic Cancer Foundation; 2007.

[18] Young R, Decker D, Wharton JT. Staging laparotomy in early ovarian cancer. J Am Med Assoc 1983;250:3072–6.

[19] Chen S, Lee L. Incidence of para-aortic and pelvic lymph node metastasis in epithelial carcinoma of the ovary. Gynecol Oncol 1983;16:95–100.

[20] Maltaris T, Boehm D, Dittrich R, et al. Reproduction beyond cancer: a message of hope for young women. Gynecol Oncol 2006;103:1109–21.

[21] Plante M. Fertility preservation in the management of gynecologic cancers. Curr Opin Oncol 2000;12:497–500.

[22] Bolis G, Colombo N, Percorelli S, et al. Adjuvant treatment for early epithelial ovarian cancer: results of two randomized clinical trials comparing cisplatin to no further treatment or chromic phosphate. GICOG. Ann Oncol 1995;6:887–93.

[23] Bell J, Brady M, Lage J, et al. A randomized phase III trial of 3 versus 6 cycles of carboplatin and paclitaxel in early stage epithelial ovarian cancer: a gynecologic oncology group study. Gynecol Oncol 2006;102:432–9.

[24] Griffiths CT. Surgical resection of tumor bulk in the primary treatment of ovarian cancer. Natl Cancer Inst Monogr 1978;42:131–6.

[25] Wharton JT, Herson J. Surgery for common epithelial tumors. Cancer 1981;48:582–9.

[26] Seifer DB, Kennedy AW, Webster KD, et al. Outcome of primary cytoreductive surgery for advanced epithelial ovarian cancer. Cleve Clin J Med 1988;55:555–600.

[27] Eisenkop SM, Spiritos NM, Wei-Chien ML. Optimal cytoreduction for advanced epithelial ovarian cancer. Gynecol Oncol 2006;103:329–35.

[28] Eisenkop SM, Friedman RL, Wang HJ. Complete cytoreductive surgery is feasible and maximizes survival in patients with advanced epithelial ovarian cancer: a prospective study. Gynecol Oncol 1998;69:103–8.

[29] Bhoola S, Hoskins WJ. Diagnosis and management of epithelial ovarian cancer. Obstet Gynecol 2006;107:1399–410.

[30] Richardson DL, Mariani A, Cliby WA. Risk factors for anastomotic leak after recto-sigmoid resection for ovarian cancer. Gynecol Oncol 2006;103(2):667–72.

[31] Mourton SM, Temple LK, Abu-Rustum NR, et al. Morbidity of rectosigmoid resection and primary anastomosis in patients undergoing primary cytoreductive surgery for advanced epithelial ovarian cancer. Gynecol Oncol 2005;99(3):608–14.

[32] van der Berg M, van Lent M, Buse M, et al. The effect of debulking surgery after induction chemotherapy on the prognosis in advanced epithelial ovarian cancer. N Engl J Med 1995;332:629–34.

[33] Mazzeo F, Berliere M, Kerger J, et al. Neoadjuvant chemotherapy followed by surgery and adjuvant chemotherapy in patients with primary unresectable, advanced-stage ovarian cancer. Gynecol Oncol 2003;90:163–9.

[34] Alberts DS, Delforge A. Maximizing the delivery of intraperitoneal therapy while minimizing drug toxicity and maintaining quality of life. Semin Oncol 2006;33(6 suppl 12):S8–17.

[35] Han ES, Monk BJ. What is the risk of bowel perforation associated with bevacizumab therapy in ovarian cancer? Gynecol Oncol 2007;105:3–6.

[36] Delgado G, Oram DH, Petril ES. Stage III epithelial ovarian cancer: the role of maximal surgical reduction. Gynecol Oncol 1984;18:293–8.

[37] Karlan BY, Bristow RE, Mutch DG, et al. Updates in current clinical practice—recurrent ovarian cancer 2007;1(3). Available at: www.partnersmeded.com. Accessed November 1, 2007.

[38] Chi DS, McCaughty K, Diaz JP, et al. Guidelines and selection criteria for secondary cytoreductive surgery in patients with recurrent, platinum-sensitive epithelial ovarian carcinoma. Cancer 2006;106(9):1933–9.

[39] Chu CS, Rubin SC. Second look laparotomy for epithelial ovarian cancer. Int J Gyn Cancer 2001;14:727–41.

[40] Glass RL, LeDuc RJ. Small intestinal obstruction for carcinomatosis. Surgery 1980;87:611–5.

[41] Gaducci A, Cosio S, Fanucchi AA, et al. Malnutrition and cachexia in ovarian cancer patients: pathophysiology and management. Anticancer Res 2001;21:2941–8.

[42] Krebs HB, Goplerud DR. Surgical management of bowel obstruction in advanced ovarian cancer. Obstet Gynecol 1983;61:327–30.

[43] Chu CS, Rubin SC. Management of intestinal obstruction in the terminal patient and management of ascites. In: Gershenson DM, McGuire WP, Gore M, et al, editors. Gynecologic cancer: controversies in management. Philadelphia: Elsevier; 2004. p. 727–41.

ELSEVIER
SAUNDERS

Surg Clin N Am 88 (2008) 301–317

SURGICAL
CLINICS OF
NORTH AMERICA

# Gynecologic Malignancies

## Bradford P. Whitcomb, MD

*Department of Obstetrics and Gynecology, Tripler Army Medical Center,*
*1 Jarrett White Road, Honolulu, HI 96859-5000, USA*

## Gynecologic malignancies

The specialty of gynecologic oncology was established in the late 1960s to early 1970s to improve the well being of women with cancer [1]. The pioneers in this field set out to establish an evidence-based approach to the care of women with gynecologic cancer, combining the modalities of surgery, chemotherapy, and radiation. Quality of life has become the cornerstone of care for these patients, in addition to advancing survival through surgical technology, collaborative research trials, and molecular approaches to early diagnosis and management. This article addresses the epidemiology, screening, preventive strategies, diagnosis, staging, surgical care, adjuvant therapy, prognosis, and recurrence management of three common gynecologic malignancies encountered in the operating arena: endometrial, cervical, and vulvar cancer.

## Vulvar cancer

### Epidemiology

Vulvar cancer was first described in 1769 by Morgagni [2]. Early descriptions of surgical technique reported radical vulvar resection with femoral and iliac nodes en bloc [3]. Taussig [4] published his series of cases, collected between 1911 and 1940, which were comprised of different surgical approaches from less invasive to more radical. He determined that the most radical approach had the best survival; however, the mortality rate in this subset was 7%. Taussig also described success in doing the procedure with separate groin incisions rather than en bloc. Through various historical

---

The views expressed in this manuscript are those of the author and do not reflect the official policy or position of the Department of the Army, Department of Defense, or the United States Government.

*E-mail address:* bradford.whitcomb@us.army.mil

0039-6109/08/$ - see front matter. Published by Elsevier Inc.
doi:10.1016/j.suc.2008.01.004

studies, it was determined that there was a marked improvement in survival, based on node negative disease, when inguinal and pelvic node dissection were undertaken [5]. This paved the way for more modern approaches to studying vulvar cancer and the current treatment recommendations described in this section.

Vulvar carcinoma, the vast majority having a squamous histology, represents 4% of female genital tract cancers and 0.6% of all cancers in women. The American Cancer Society (ACS) estimates 3,490 new cases and 880 deaths attributed to this disease in 2007 [6]. Average age at diagnosis is 70; however, there is a bimodal peak, with younger women having human papilloma virus (HPV)-related development of vulvar intraepithelial neoplasia (VIN) and cancer.

*Screening*

Annual pelvic examination and directed examination for vulvar complaints are currently the only methods for early detection of vulvar dysplasia and carcinoma.

*Prevention*

Limiting the number of partners, smoking cessation, annual gynecologic examination, and HPV vaccination are all components of disease prevention and early diagnosis. Risk factors prompting screening and preventive measures include VIN, age, immunosuppression, and lichen sclerosis et atrophicus.

*Diagnosis*

Women with new vulvar lesions should have punch biopsy or excision for diagnosis. Patients with chronic vulvar dermatologic conditions or chronic pruritus should also have representative biopsy.

*Staging*

Table 1 outlines the International Federation of Gynecologists and Obstetricians (FIGO) staging classification for vulvar cancer.

*Treatment*

Preinvasive disease (VIN II–III) is treated with laser ablation or surgical excision (wide local excision). Cure rates are very high for this disease, with an approximate 100% survival rate. However, because there is no direct treatment for HPV, recurrent dysplasia is possible unless immunologic clearance of the virus occurs.

Stage IA (microinvasive) vulvar cancer is treated surgically with wide local excision. No lymphadenectomy is required. Stage IB vulvar cancer

Table 1
FIGO staging for carcinoma of the vulva (surgical staging)

| FIGO stage | Criteria |
| --- | --- |
| 0 | Carcinoma in situ (vulvar intraepithelial neoplasia III, preinvasive) |
| IA | Confined to vulva/perineum, ≤ 2 cm greatest dimension, stromal invasion ≤ 1 mm |
| IB | Confined to vulva/perineum, ≤ 2 cm greatest dimension, stromal invasion > 1 mm |
| II | Confined to vulva/perineum > 2 cm greatest dimension |
| III | Tumor involves lower urethra, vagina, anus, and/or unilateral groin nodes |
| IVA | Tumor involves bladder or rectal mucosa, upper urethral mucosa, fixed to bone, and/or bilateral groin nodes |
| IVB | Any distant metastatic disease, including pelvic nodes |

*Data from* Benedet JL, Bender H, Jones H 3rd, et al. FIGO staging classifications and clinical practice guidelines in the management of gynecologic cancers. FIGO Committee on Gynecologic Oncology. Int J Gynaecol Obstet 2000 Aug;70(2):209–62.

(with clinically negative nodes, no lymphvascular space involvement or LVSI, and less than 5-mm depth of invasion) is treated with radical local excision and unilateral inguinofemoral lymphadenectomy [7,8]. Radical vulvectomy with bilateral inguinofemoral node dissection can also be performed when criteria are not met for more conservative approaches. Reduction in morbidity with similar outcomes has been shown for radical vulvectomy with separate groin incisions rather than the classic radical en bloc excision [9]. It has also been determined retrospectively that groin dissection is not superior to groin radiation for clinically negative lymph nodes [10]. This is important to those who refuse surgical groin dissection. The margin of excision for early stage disease is important for determining the need for postoperative radiation or re-excision. One study has demonstrated no recurrences for those with margins of 8 mm or more [11].

Stage II disease is approached with radical vulvectomy and bilateral inguinofemoral lymphadenectomy. Again, separate groin incisions are the preferred approach to reduce morbidity. Adjuvant groin-vulvar-pelvic radiation should be contemplated for LVSI, close margins (less than 8 mm), deep invasion (greater than 5 mm), and positive groin nodes [9,12–14].

Stage III vulvar cancer is treated with radical surgical resection and bilateral inguinofemoral lymphadenectomy, then adjuvant radiation or chemoradiation. If this cannot be accomplished, primary chemoradiation to the vulva-groin-pelvis can be performed with survival in approximately 47% to 84% of cases [15–18]. Similarly, if the tumor is resectable, stage IV disease can be treated with radical excision and bilateral groin dissection, sometimes requiring exenteration. Alternatively, preoperative radiation to decrease morbidity of an exenterative procedure, followed by surgery, is a reasonable approach to this extensive locoregional disease [19]. Postoperative pelvic radiation should be performed in patients with more than one positive inguinofemoral node, regardless of stage [20]. Metastatic disease (stage IVB) is considered incurable, but can be treated with study protocol or platinum-containing chemotherapy regimens with or without palliative surgery and radiation.

### Prognosis

The major distinguishing pathologic predictor of survival is inguinofemoral lymph node status. If negative, the 5-year survival is 90%; if positive, the survival is 50% to 60%. When the primary tumor is less than 2 cm with negative nodes, the survival is 98% [21]. Risk factors for nodal spread include LVSI, stage, thickness, depth of invasion, patient age, nodal status, and grade [14,21–24]. Table 2 lists the 5-year survival rate for respective FIGO stages.

### Recurrence

Local recurrence of vulvar cancer should be treated with radical local excision, chemoradiation, or a combination of the two approaches. If the non-metastatic disease is greater than 2 years from original therapy, survival is greater than 50% with treatment [25,26]. Patients with metastatic disease at diagnosis (stage IVB) or recurrence should be offered palliative chemotherapy, preferably as part of a clinical trial as no specific regimen has demonstrated superiority to date.

## Cervical cancer

### Epidemiology

Cervical cancer is one of the leading causes of cancer death worldwide. In the United States the incidence and mortality are significantly less because of screening and availability of treatment. The ACS estimates 11,150 new cases and 3,670 deaths from cervical cancer in 2007 [6]. Worldwide, however, cervical cancer remains the leading cause of death from gynecologic malignancy. The median age at diagnosis is approximately 48 in the United

Table 2
Vulvar cancer survival by FIGO stage

| FIGO stage | 5-year survival |
| --- | --- |
| I | 90% |
| II | 77% |
| III | 51% |
| IV | 18% |

*Data from* Hacker NF. Vulvar cancer. In: Berek JS, Hacker NF, editors. Practical gynecologic oncology, 3rd edition. Philadelphia: Lippincott Williams and Wilkins; 2000. p. 553–96.

States [27]. The vast majority of cervical cancer (99.7%) is associated with the human papilloma virus [28]. High-risk viral subtypes increase the risk of developing high grade cervical dysplasia and cancer. Increased number of sexual partners, early age at first coitus, low socioeconomic status, immunocompromise, smoking, diethylstilbestrol exposure, history of chlamydia, long-term oral contraceptive use, possible family histology, and multiparity are all reported risk factors [29]. The majority of cervical cancers are squamous in histology, with adenocarcinoma being the second most common histologic type.

*Screening*

Because invasive cervical cancer has a preinvasive condition (cervical intraepithelial neoplasia), screening is an effective tool in risk reduction. Regular Pap smear screening, as done in the United States, has dramatically reduced incidence and mortality from this disease. Identification of high-risk types of HPV has improved the sensitivity and specificity of the Pap smear test in certain circumstances (ASCUS/AGUS). Following an abnormal screening test, women are evaluated with colposcopy and directed biopsies to determine the extent of the disease. The majority of women who have abnormal Pap smears will not ever develop cervical cancer because of this rigorous process. The American Society of Colposcopy and Cervical Pathology has published practice guidelines based on National Institutes of Health (Bethesda) consensus conferences that can be referenced at www.asccp.org. Underdeveloped countries have limited or no access to screening exams or follow up, therefore cervical cancer rates are markedly higher and mortality significant in the population of these countries from this disease.

*Prevention*

The first HPV vaccination has recently been approved by the United States Food and Drug Administration (Gardasil, Merck). This is a quadravalent vaccine (HPV 6, 11, 16, 18), which is highly immunogenic and reduces rates of cervical intraepithelial neoplasia significantly, with an efficacy near 100% in women previously not exposed to these viral subtypes. This vaccine is recommended for girls and women aged 9 to 26, and is comprised of a three-vaccine series given at 0, 2, and 6 months. Because prevention ideally should begin before sexual activity ensues, the recommendation from the Centers for Disease Control and Prevention and other medical authorities is to begin the series by 11 years old, or as early as 9 years [30].

*Diagnosis*

Patients with microscopic cervical cancer are usually asymptomatic. Locally advanced disease presents with postcoital, intermenstrual, or postmenopausal bleeding. More rarely, these patients present with pain or

306

malodorous discharge. Pelvic examination, Pap smear, and biopsy of any abnormal lesions are required for diagnosis. The Pap smear alone is inaccurate at detecting invasive disease, with a false-negative rate of up to 50% [31]. Physical examination should include surveillance for metastatic disease (general physical examination), and detailed speculum and bimanual or rectovaginal examination. Rectal or rectovaginal examination is used to determine parametrial extension in cervical cancer. If invasive disease is suspected by Pap smear results, but there is not a gross lesion, colposcopy, directed biopsies, and sometimes conization are required for confirmation.

*Staging*

Cervical cancer is clinically staged (Table 3), where limited radiologic and examination findings can be included. This is because of the prevalence of this disease in underserved countries where technology is not available to perform all tests. In the United States, it is recommended, however, that CT imaging be

Table 3
FIGO staging for carcinoma of the cervix (clinical staging)

| FIGO stage | Criteria |
| --- | --- |
| 0 | Carcinoma in situ (cervical intraepithelial neoplasia III, preinvasive) |
| I | Confined to cervix |
| IA | Microscopic lesions (any macroscopic lesion is considered IB, even if superficially invasive) |
| IA1 | Invasion $\leq$ 3 mm depth, $\leq$ 7 mm width |
| IA2 | Invasion $>$ 3 mm, $\leq$ 5 mm depth, $\leq$ 7 mm width |
| IB | Any macroscopic lesion confined to cervix, any lesion $>$ Stage IA |
| IB1 | $\leq$ 4 cm lesion |
| IB2 | $>$ 4 cm lesion |
| II | Beyond cervix but not to pelvic sidewall OR upper two thirds vaginal involvement |
| IIA | No parametrial involvement |
| IIB | Parametrial involvement |
| III | Extension to pelvic sidewall, lower one third vaginal involvement, OR hydronephrosis/nonfunctioning kidney without other etiology |
| IIIA | Involvement of lower one third of vagina, no sidewall extension |
| IIIB | Sidewall extension OR hydronephrosis/nonfunctioning kidney |
| IV | Extension beyond true pelvis OR involvement of bladder or rectal mucosa |
| IVA | Adjacent organ involvement |
| IVB | Distant metastasis |

*Data from* Benedet JL, Bender H, Jones H 3rd, et al. FIGO staging classifications and clinical practice guidelines in the management of gynecologic cancers. FIGO Committee on Gynecologic Oncology. Int J Gynaecol Obstet 2000 Aug;70(2):209–62.

obtained for treatment planning and prognostication. More recently, the use of positron emission tomography (PET) or PET/CT has been advocated in cervical cancer staging and for treatment planning [32]. MRI can also be useful in certain circumstances where parametrial involvement is difficult to determine clinically and in pregnant women diagnosed with cervical cancer [33]. Surgical staging with exploration and pelvic or para-aortic lymphadenectomy is more accurate than clinical staging, with upstaging in approximately 24% of patients and downstaging in 14% [34]. Surgical staging in cervical cancer is controversial among gynecologic oncologists. The literature is contradictory with regard to survival benefit of lymphadenectomy, especially with microscopic nodal disease. Additionally, there may be significant delays in chemoradiation therapy after a patient is taken for surgery, and the inherent risk of surgical morbidity [35,36].

## Initial treatment: surgery, radiation, and chemotherapy

The treatment for cervical cancer is based upon the extent of local disease. Early stage disease is usually treated with radical hysterectomy and pelvic lymphadenectomy, but can be treated with primary radiation therapy with similar outcomes (stages IB to IIA) [37]. However, radiation complications (including loss of ovarian function, bowel stricture, and fistula formation) are oftentimes unacceptable. Patients with significant comorbidity may be selected for primary radiation. One exception to radical hysterectomy is in patients with stage IA1 squamous cell cancer (microinvasive) and no LVSI. This selected population is appropriately treated for cure with simple, extrafascial hysterectomy without lymphadenectomy. Alternatively, patients desiring future fertility can be treated with conization of the cervix alone with close follow up [38]. A more recent approach to fertility-sparing surgery is the radical trachalectomy, which removes the cervix, parametrial tissue, and upper vagina, while preserving the uterus for future childbearing. A permanent cervical cerclage and assisted reproductive technologies are required in this setting. Prognosis appears to be acceptable in this group regarding survival, recurrence, and pregnancy outcomes [39]; however, the procedure is performed at few institutions by specially trained surgeons.

When the cancer has progressed beyond the cervix, but without distant metastasis (stages II through IVA), primary chemoradiation therapy is used. The radiation therapy is delivered by a combination of teletherapy and brachytherapy to achieve an adequate dose to the cervix, parametria, and pelvic lymph nodes. Chemotherapy (cisplatin) is given weekly for 6 weeks concomitantly with radiation therapy as a radiosensitizing agent. Significantly improved survival in those receiving this combination versus radiation alone was demonstrated in multiple randomized trials in the 1990s [40–45].

Hysterectomy is performed after radiation therapy in patients with residual disease. Combining surgery and chemoradiation, however, increases morbidity. Patients with locally advanced cervical cancer, who have grossly positive lymph nodes, appear to benefit from surgical debulking of the nodes before chemoradiation therapy [35,46].

Distant metastatic cervical cancer (stage IVB) has a poor prognosis, and is palliated with chemotherapy that provides a limited survival benefit. The combination cisplatin and topotecan versus cisplatin alone revealed a survival of 9.4 months versus 6.5 months [47]. This was the first trial that demonstrated significantly improved outcomes using combination chemotherapy. Currently, a trial is underway by the Gynecologic Oncology Group (GOG 204) comparing various combinations of chemotherapy in this unfortunate group of patients.

*Adjuvant therapy*

Postoperative chemoradiation is recommended for patients who have had radical hysterectomy with the following risk factors on final pathology: parametrial involvement, close or positive vaginal margins, and positive lymph nodes. Patients with certain tumor characteristics should also receive postoperative radiation. A randomized GOG trial, revealed that patients with stage IB cervical cancer and certain combinations of risk factors (LVSI, tumor size, depth of stromal invasion), have a significant reduction in recurrence risk, and a trend toward improved survival, if they receive postoperative pelvic radiation [48].

*Prognosis*

See Table 4 for 5-year survival rates.

*Recurrence*

Recurrent cervical cancer has a dismal prognosis if not limited to the pelvis. If the recurrent disease is limited to the central pelvis without other

Table 4
Cervical cancer survival by FIGO stage

| FIGO stage | 5-year survival |
| --- | --- |
| IA1 | 94.6% |
| IA2 | 92.6% |
| IB1 | 80.7% |
| IB2 | 79.8% |
| IIA | 76.0% |
| IIB | 73.3% |
| IIIA | 50.5% |
| IIIB | 46.4% |
| IVA | 29.6% |
| IVB | 22.0% |

*Data from* Benedet J, Odicino F, Maisonneuve P, et al. Carcinoma of the cervix uteri: annual report on the results of treatment in gynecologic cancer. J Epidemiol Biostat 2001;6:7–43.

metastasis, and if no pelvic sidewall involvement is identified, there is the possibility of long-term survival. If the patient in this category has not had radiation therapy, this modality is recommended for locally confined recurrent disease. In previously radiated patients, pelvic exenteration (anterior, posterior, or total) offers survival rates of 20% to 60%. Prognostic factors include time from initial radiation therapy to exenterative surgery, pelvic sidewall involvement, mass size, node status, margins, and adjacent organ spread [49–54]. With nonresectable disease, overall survival is less than 1 year. Minimal benefit can be achieved with palliative combination chemotherapy, as seen in a recent trial with cisplatin plus topotecan. Unfortunately, this benefit only resulted in a median survival of 9.4 months [47].

## Endometrial cancer

### Epidemiology

Cancer of the uterine corpus is the most common gynecologic malignancy in the United States. The ACS estimates that in 2007 there will be 39,080 new cases of uterine corpus cancer and 7,400 deaths [6]. The majority of these cases are endometrial adenocarcinomas. Pre- and postmenopausal women are at risk for developing this cancer. Of endometrial cancers in the United States, 70% are diagnosed between the ages of 45 and 74. The lifetime risk of developing endometrial cancer is approximately 1 in 40 [56]. This disease is more common in urbanized nations. In 1988, the staging for this cancer changed from clinical to surgical, enabling clinicians a more defined approach to therapy and prognostication.

The main risk factor for endometrial adenocarcinoma is increased exposure to estrogen. Therefore, late menopause, low parity, obesity, unopposed estrogen therapy, anovulation, and polycystic ovarian syndrome all increase the risk. Young, premenopausal patients who have any of these risk factors associated with abnormal menses, should be evaluated with similar vigilance as the woman with postmenopausal bleeding. Rarely, estrogen-excreting tumors occur that require further evaluation. Tamoxifen, caused by estrogenic effect at the receptor, increases the risk of endometrial cancer as well (relative risk 2.2–7.5) [55–57]. Finally, hereditary nonpolyposis colon cancer (HNPCC) increases risk of endometrial cancer diagnosis. Smoking and oral contraceptive use decrease the risk of endometrial cancer.

### Screening

No serum, radiologic, or pathologic evaluation has been shown to be effective as a screening tool. Even in tamoxifen users, routine screening with ultrasound or endometrial biopsy is not recommended for the asymptomatic patient [58,59]. However, patients with risk factors such as HNPCC, chronic anovulation, and unopposed estrogen exposure, should be evaluated regularly with endometrial sampling. The ideal interval has not been established for testing.

## Prevention

Preventive strategies should focus on diminishing the environmental risk factors, notably diet, exercise, and avoidance of unopposed estrogen therapy. Additionally, oral contraceptive use is associated with a significant risk reduction. Smoking also reduces the risk of endometrial cancer by diminishing circulating estrogens, but is clearly not a part of any preventive strategy. Detailed family history is important in early detection strategies for patients at risk for HNPCC.

## Diagnosis

Early detection of malignancy or premalignant lesions is critical in planning appropriate treatment and improving outcomes. Early stage endometrial cancer (limited to the uterus) is curable in greater than 90% of cases. Additionally, the majority of cases are diagnosed as stage I because of the readily detectable symptom of uterine bleeding. Endometrial biopsy is usually performed as an office procedure; however, operative intervention with cervical dilation and curettage is sometimes necessary for cervical stenosis or persistent abnormal bleeding. The most accurate office biopsy device for detection of cancer is the Pipelle [60]. Ultrasound for measuring endometrial stripe thickness has also been recommended; however, in menopausal women there is a 4% risk of missing endometrial cancer and a high rate of false-positive results [61].

Once the diagnosis has been made, surgical staging and treatment is recommended. There are some populations that may not accept or be candidates for surgery, namely women desiring fertility and patients with significant comorbidity. If future childbearing is desired, a thorough counseling session involving gynecologic oncology and reproductive endocrinology and infertility is encouraged. Patients with grade I endometrioid histology may respond to high-dose progestational therapy; however, there is a risk of recurrent lesion or even, rarely, of progression to disease beyond the uterus.

## Staging

FIGO established endometrial cancer staging in 1971. This was a clinical staging system based on examination findings, limited imaging and tests such as proctoscopy and cystoscopy. This staging is currently only used for patients who are not able to have surgery. The surgical staging system was established in 1988 by FIGO (Table 5). The histologic grade of tumor is mandatory in staging endometrial cancer, as grade significantly affects prognosis and treatment. More than 70% of patients will be stage I after surgery, 12.5% stage II, 13.3 stage III, and 4% stage IV [62].

Table 5
FIGO staging for carcinoma of the corpus uteri (surgical staging)

| FIGO stage | Criteria |
| --- | --- |
| 0 | Carcinoma in situ (preinvasive) |
| I | Tumor confined to the uterine corpus |
| IA | No myometrial invasion (endometrium only) |
| IB | Invasion to $\leq$ 50% myometrium |
| IC | Invasion > 50% myometrium |
| II | Cervical involvement |
| IIA | Endocervical gland involvement |
| IIB | Cervical stromal invasion |
| III | Locoregional spread of tumor |
| IIIA | Uterine serosa, adnexa, or pertitoneal washings/ascites positive for tumor |
| IIIB | Vaginal involvement |
| IIIC | Pelvic and/or paraaortic lymph nodes |
| IVA | Bladder or bowel mucosal invasion |
| IVB | Distant metastasis |

*Data from* Benedet JL, Bender H, Jones H 3rd, et al. FIGO staging classifications and clinical practice guidelines in the management of gynecologic cancers. FIGO Committee on Gynecologic Oncology. Int J Gynaecol Obstet 2000 Aug;70(2):209–62.

## Surgery

CT scan of the abdomen and pelvis are infrequently required for detection of metastatic disease. Physical examination and laboratory findings will dictate the need for further investigation. Laboratory work should include complete blood count, metabolic panel with creatinine, and hepatic function. Chest x-ray should also be performed. CA-125 level can be used for patients suspected of having advanced disease to evaluate response to therapy and to detect recurrence.

Surgery includes laparotomy with pelvic washings, thorough exploration, total hysterectomy with removal of cervix, bilateral oophorectomy, and pelvic and paraaortic lymph node dissection. Some controversy exists over whether to stage patients with grade 1 disease and grossly superficial or no invasion; however, many tumors will be upgraded on final pathology, therefore lymphadenectomy is usually performed regardless of gross invasion [63,64]. Grade 1 lesions with greater than 50% myometrial invasion or gross cervical extension should definitely have thorough surgical staging. With grade 3 endometrioid or other high-risk histology (clear cell, papillary serous, carcinosarcoma) an omental biopsy, and sometimes serial peritoneal biopsies, are performed to exclude microscopic disease. If the cervix is grossly involved, radical hysterectomy with or without adjuvant radiation is recommended to improve survival [65]. If stage IV disease is detected, surgical cytoreduction might have a benefit based on retrospective data [66,67]. Laparoscopic lymphadenectomy with laparoscopically-assisted vaginal hysterectomy is also an accepted approach to surgical staging. Survival (with 33–45 month follow up) is similar when comparing laparotomy and laparoscopy [68]. There is a significant reduction in hospital stay with lapa-roscopy, and diminished recovery from surgery. Surgery alone or surgery with adjuvant radiation offer improved outcome over radiation alone [69,70].

*Adjuvant therapy*

If patients have had adequate surgical staging, stages IA and IB, grades 1 and 2 endometrial cancer are considered low risk and can be followed safely without adjuvant radiation [71–75]. Patients with poor prognostic factors who have not had thorough surgical staging (ie, no lymphadenectomy) should receive adjuvant pelvic radiation or reoperation for staging. Subjects with intermediate risk disease (stages IB, IC, IIA, IIB) were randomized to receive external beam radiotherapy (EBRT) versus no further treatment in GOG study 99 (392 subjects). In this study, there were significantly fewer re-currences in the EBRT group, most profoundly seen in the "high intermedi-ate risk" group (defined as subjects less than or equal to 50 years with grade 2–3 histology, lymph-vascular space invasion, and outer one third myome-trial invasion; greater than 50 years with 2 risk factors; and greater than 70 years with any risk factor); however, there was no statistically significant improved overall survival [76]. Stage II patients receive radiation therapy. Stage III and IV patients usually receive adjuvant chemotherapy with or without radiation. GOG study 122 revealed improved progression-free and overall survival in subjects receiving chemotherapy with cisplatin and doxorubicin versus whole abdominal radiation; however, they also had sig-nificantly increased acute toxicity [77]. Current research strategies include both volume directed radiation (EBRT plus or minus extended field radia-tion) and combination chemotherapy with doxorubicin and cisplatin versus doxorubicin, cisplatin and paclitaxel (GOG 184). In addition, an ongoing trial (GOG 209) is investigating combination chemotherapy with carbopla-tin plus paclitaxel versus doxorubicin, cisplatin, and paclitaxel. Different chemotherapy combinations are used for malignant mixed müllerian tumor, sarcoma, and papillary serous carcinoma than for the more common endo-metrioid adenocarcinoma.

*Prognosis*

Numerous prognostic indicators are known for endometrial adenocarci-noma. These include age, histology (serous, endometrioid, clear cell, papil-lary serous, malignant mixed müllerian tumor), grade, myometrial invasion, LVSI, tumor size, abdominal washings cytology, hormone receptor status, and DNA ploidy. African Americans have a significant increased risk of death from endometrial cancer, which may be a result of disparity in treat-ment; however, this difference persisted in advanced or recurrent disease when similar treatment was provided [78]. The 5-year survival by stage for endometrial adenocarcinoma is outlined in Table 6.

Table 6
Endometrial cancer survival by FIGO stage

| FIGO stage | 5-year survival |
| --- | --- |
| I | 86% |
| II | 66% |
| III | 44% |
| IV | 16% |

*Data from* Pettersson F, editor. Annual report on the results of treatment in gynecologic cancer, vol. 22, Stockholm, 1994, International Federation of Gynecology and Obstetrics.

## *Recurrence*

Patients with gynecologic malignancy should be followed routinely after diagnosis and initial treatment. The recommended course of surveillance is every 3 months for the first 2 years, then every 6 months for the following 3 years. Thereafter, annual examination is appropriate. The majority of recurrences occur at the vaginal cuff. When this is detected as isolated disease, there is a significant salvage rate. The patients who had prior radiation are more likely to fail this local radiation therapy and more likely to present with a distant recurrence [79]. Combination chemotherapy (doxorubicin, cisplatin, paclitaxel, and possibly carboplatin and paclitaxel) is used in distant or widespread recurrent disease. The overall response rate for the former regimen is approximately 57%, with a median survival of 15 months [80]. Pelvic exenteration for isolated central pelvic recurrence is feasible, and offers long term remission in 20% of patients [81].

## References

[1] Averette HE, Wrennick A, Angioli R. History of gynecologic oncology subspecialty. Surg Clin North Am 2001;81(4):747–51.
[2] Marsden D, Hacker N. Contemporary management of primary carcinoma of the vulva. Surg Clin North Am 2001;81(4):799–813.
[3] Speert H. Obstetric and gynecologic milestones illustrated. New York: Parthenon Publishing Group; 1996. p. 157.
[4] Taussig FJ. Cancer of the vulva: an analysis of 155 cases. Am J Obstet Gynecol 1940;40: 764–79.
[5] Way S. The surgery of vulvar carcinoma: an appraisal. Clin Obstet Gynecol 1978;5:623–8.
[6] Jemal A, Siegel R, Ward E, et al. Cancer statistics, 2007. CA Cancer J Clin 2007;57:43–66.
[7] Malfetano JH, Piver MS, Tsukada Y, et al. Univariate and multivariate analyses of 5-year survival, recurrence, and inguinal node metastases in stage I and II vulvar carcinoma. J Surg Oncol 1985;30(2):124–31.
[8] Stehman FB, Bundy BN, Dvoretsky PM, et al. Early stage I carcinoma of the vulva treated with ipsilateral superficial inguinal lymphadenectomy and modified radical hemivulvectomy: a prospective study of the Gynecologic Oncology Group. Obstet Gynecol 1992;79(4):490–7.
[9] Hoffman MS, Roberts WS, Lapolla JP, et al. Recent modifications in the treatment of invasive squamous cell carcinoma of the vulva. Obstet Gynecol Surv 1989;44(4):227–33.
[10] Petereit DG, Mehta MP, Buchler DA, et al. Inguinofemoral radiation of N0,N1 vulvar cancer may be equivalent to lymphadenectomy if proper radiation technique is used. Int J Radiat Oncol Biol Phys 1993;27(4):963–7.

[11] Heaps JM, Fu YS, Montz FJ, et al. Surgical-pathologic variables predictive of local recurrence in squamous cell carcinoma of the vulva. Gynecol Oncol 1990;38(3):309–14.

[12] Faul CM, Mirmow D, Huang Q, et al. Adjuvant radiation for vulvar carcinoma: improved local control. Int J Radiat Oncol Biol Phys 1997;38(2):381–9.

[13] Perez CA, Grigsby PW, Chao KC, et al. Irradiation in carcinoma of the vulva: factors affecting outcome. Int J Radiat Oncol Biol Phys 1998;42(2):335–44.

[14] Sedlis A, Homesley H, Bundy BN, et al. Positive groin lymph nodes in superficial squamous cell vulvar cancer. A Gynecologic Oncology Group study. Am J Obstet Gynecol 1987;156(5): 1159–64.

[15] Russell AH, Mesic JB, Scudder SA, et al. Synchronous radiation and cytotoxic chemotherapy for locally advanced or recurrent squamous cancer of the vulva. Gynecol Oncol 1992; 47(1):14–20.

[16] Berek JS, Heaps JM, Fu YS, et al. Concurrent cisplatin and 5-fluorouracil chemotherapy and radiation therapy for advanced-stage squamous carcinoma of the vulva. Gynecol Oncol 1991;42(3):197–201.

[17] Koh WJ, Wallace HJ, Greer BE, et al. Combined radiotherapy and chemotherapy in the management of local-regionally advanced vulvar cancer. Int J Radiat Oncol Biol Phys 1993;26(5):809–16.

[18] Thomas G, Dembo A, DePetrillo A, et al. Concurrent radiation and chemotherapy in vulvar carcinoma. Gynecol Oncol 1989;34(3):263–7.

[19] Boronow RC, Hickman BT, Reagan MT, et al. Combined therapy as an alternative to exenteration for locally advanced vulvovaginal cancer. II. Results, complications, and dosimetric and surgical considerations. Am J Clin Oncol 1987;10(2):171–81.

[20] Homesley HD, Bundy BN, Sedlis A, et al. Radiation therapy versus pelvic node resection for carcinoma of the vulva with positive groin nodes. Obstet Gynecol 1986;68(6):733–40.

[21] Homesley HD, Bundy BN, Sedlis A, et al. Assessment of current International Federation of Gynecology and Obstetrics staging of vulvar carcinoma relative to prognostic factors for survival. (A Gynecologic Oncology Group study). Am J Obstet Gynecol 1991;164(4):997–1003 [discussion 1003–4].

[22] Boyce J, Fruchter RG, Kasambilides E, et al. Prognostic factors in carcinoma of the vulva. Gynecol Oncol 1985;20(3):364–77.

[23] Binder SW, Huang I, Fu YS, et al. Risk factors for the development of lymph node metastasis in vulvar squamous cell carcinoma. Gynecol Oncol 1990;37(1):9–16.

[24] Homesley HD, Bundy BN, Sedlis A, et al. Prognostic factors for groin node metastasis in squamous cell carcinoma of the vulva (A Gynecologic Oncology Group study). Gynecol Oncol 1993;49(3):279–83.

[25] Podratz KC, Symmonds RE, Taylor WF, et al. Carcinoma of the vulva: analysis of treatment and survival. Obstet Gynecol 1983;61(1):63–74.

[26] Shimm DS, Fuller AF, Orlow EL, et al. Prognostic variables in the treatment of squamous cell carcinoma of the vulva. Gynecol Oncol 1986;24(3):343–58.

[27] Ries LAG, Melbert D, Krapcho M, et al, editors. SEER Cancer Statistics Review, 1975-2004, Bethesda, MD: National Cancer Institute. Available at: http://seer.cancer.gov/csr/1975_2004/. Accessed January 8, 2008.

[28] Walboomers JM, Jacobs MV, Manos MM, et al. Human papillomavirus is a necessary cause of invasive cervical cancer worldwide. J Pathol 1999;189:12–9.

[29] Tortolero-Luna G, Franco EL. Epidemiology of Cervical, Vulvar, and Vaginal Cancers. In: Gershenson DM, McGuire WP, Gore M, et al, editors. Gynecologic cancer: controversies in management. Philadelphia: Elsevier, Ltd.; 2004. p. 9–10.

[30] Markowitz LE, Dunne EF, Saraiya M, et al. Quadrivalent Human Papillomavirus Vaccine: Recommendations of the Advisory Committee on Immunization Practices (ACIP). MMWR Recomm Rep 2007;56(RR-2):1–24.

[31] Sasieni PD, Cuzick J, Lynch-Farmery E, et al. Estimating the efficacy of screening by auditing smear histories of women with and without cervical cancer. Br J Cancer 1996;73:1001–5.

[32] Grigsby PW, Siegel BA, Dehdashti F. Lymph node staging by positron emission tomography in patients with carcinoma of the cervix. J Clin Oncol 2001;19:3745–9.

[33] Wagenaar HC, Trimbus JB, Postema S, et al. Tumor diameter and volume assessed by magnetic resonance imaging in the prediction of outcome for invasive cervical cancer. Gynecol Oncol 2001;82:474–82.

[34] Lagasse LD, Creasman WT, Shingleton HM, et al. Results and complications of operative staging in cervical cancer: experience of the Gynecologic Oncology Group. Gynecol Oncol 1980;9:90–8.

[35] Cosin JA, Fowler JM, Chen M, et al. Pretreatment surgical staging of patients with cervical cancer. The case for lymph node sampling. Cancer 1998;82:2241–8.

[36] Koh W, Rose PG. Locally Advanced Cervical Cancer. In: Gershenson DM, McGuire WP, Gore M, et al, editors. Gynecologic cancer: controversies in management. Philadelphia: Elsevier, Ltd.; 2004. p. 177–9.

[37] Landoni F, Maneo A, Colombo A, et al. Randomised study of radical surgery versus radiotherapy for stage Ib-IIa cervical cancer. Lancet 1997;350:535–40.

[38] Roman LD, Felix JC, Muderspach LI, et al. Risk of residual invasive disease in women with microinvasive squamous cancer in a conization specimen. Obstetrics & Gynecology 1997;90: 759–64.

[39] Burnett AF, Roman LD, O'Meara AT, et al. Radical vaginal trachelectomy and pelvic lymphadenectomy for preservation of fertility in early cervical carcinoma. Gynecol Oncol 2003; 88:419–23.

[40] Whitney CW, Sause W, Bundy BN, et al. Randomized comparison of fluorouracil plus cisplatin versus hydroxyurea as an adjunct to radiation therapy in stage IIB–IVA carcinoma of the cervix with negative para-aortic lymph nodes: a Gynecologic Oncology Group and Southwest Oncology Group study. J Clin Oncol 1999;17(5):1339–48.

[41] Morris M, Eifel PJ, Lu J, et al. Pelvic radiation with concurrent chemotherapy compared with pelvic and para-aortic radiation for high-risk cervical cancer. N Engl J Med 1999; 340(15):1137–43.

[42] Rose PG, Bundy BN, Watkins EB, et al. Concurrent cisplatin-based radiotherapy and chemotherapy for locally advanced cervical cancer. N Engl J Med 1999;340(15):1144–53.

[43] Keys HM, Bundy BN, Stehman FB, et al. Cisplatin, radiation, and adjuvant hysterectomy compared with radiation and adjuvant hysterectomy for bulky stage IB cervical carcinoma. N Engl J Med 1999;340(15):1154–61.

[44] Thomas GM. Improved treatment for cervical cancer—concurrent chemotherapy and radiotherapy. N Engl J Med 1999;340(15):1198–200.

[45] Pearcey R, Brundage M, Drouin P, et al. Phase III trial comparing radical radiotherapy with and without cisplatin chemotherapy in patients with advanced squamous cell cancer of the cervix. J Clin Oncol 2002;20(4):966–72.

[46] Kim PY, Monk BJ, Chabra S, et al. Cervical cancer with paraaortic metastases: significance of residual paraaortic disease after surgical staging. Gynecol Oncol 1998;69:243–7.

[47] Long HJ, Bundy BN, Grendys EC, et al. Randomized phase III trial of cisplatin with or without topotecan in carcinoma of the uterine cervix: a Gynecologic Oncology Group study. J Clin Oncol 2005;23:4626–33.

[48] Sedlis A, Bundy BN, Rotman MZ, et al. A randomized trial of pelvic radiation therapy versus no further therapy in selected patients with stage IB carcinoma of the cervix after radical hysterectomy and pelvic lymphadenectomy: a Gynecologic Oncology Group study. Gynecol Oncol 1999;73:177–83.

[49] Brunschwig A. What are the indications and results of pelvic exenteration? JAMA 1965;194: 274–9.

[50] Shingleton HM, Soong SJ, Gelder M, et al. Clinical and histopathologic factors predicting recurrence and survival after pelvic exenteration for cancer of the cervix. Obstet Gynecol 1989;73:1027–34.

[51] Stanhope CR, Webb MJ, Podratz KC, et al. Pelvic exenteration for recurrent cervical cancer. Clin Obstet Gynecol 1990;33:897–909.

[52] Berek JS, Howe C, Lagasse LD, et al. Pelvic exenteration for recurrent gynecologic malignancy: Survival and morbidity analysis of the 45-year experience at UCLA. Gynecol Oncol 2005;99:153–9.

[53] Barber HR, Jones W. Lymphadenectomy in pelvic exenteration for recurrent cervix cancer. JAMA 1971;215:1945–9.

[54] Stanhope CR, Symmonds RE. Palliative exenteration—what, when, and why? Am J Obstet Gynecol 1985;152:12–6.

[55] Fisher B, Costantino JP, Redmond CK, et al. Endometrial cancer in tamoxifen-treated breast cancer patients: findings from the National Surgical Adjuvant Breast and Bowel Project (NSABP) B-14. J Natl Cancer Inst 1994;86:527–37.

[56] Fornander T, Hellstrom A, Moberger B. Descriptive clinicopathologic study of 17 patients with endometrial cancer during or after adjuvant tamoxifen in early breast cancer. J Natl Cancer Inst 1993;85:1850–5.

[57] Cohen I, Bernheim J, Azaria R, et al. Malignant endometrial polyps in postmenopausal breast cancer tamoxifen-treated patients. Gynecol Oncol 1999;75(1):136–41.

[58] Barakat RR, Gilewski TA, Almadrones L, et al. Effect of adjuvant tamoxifen on the endometrium in women with breast cancer: a prospective study using office endometrial biopsy. J Clin Oncol 2000;18(20):3459–63.

[59] Gerber B, Krause A, Muller H, et al. Effects of adjuvant tamoxifen on the endometrium in postmenopausal women with breast cancer: a prospective long-term study using transvaginal ultrasound. J Clin Oncol 2000;18(20):3464–70.

[60] Dijkhuizen FP, Mol BW, Brolmann HA, et al. The accuracy of endometrial sampling in the diagnosis of patients with endometrial carcinoma and hyperplasia: a meta-analysis. Cancer 2000;89:1765–72.

[61] Tabor A, Watt HC, Wald NJ. Endometrial thickness as a test for endometrial cancer in women with postmenopausal vaginal bleeding. Obstet Gynecol 2002;99:663–70.

[62] Creasman WT, Odicino F, Maisonneuve P, et al. Carcinoma of the corpus uteri. J Epidemiol Biostat 2001;6:47–86.

[63] Obermair A, Geramou M, Gucer F, et al. Endometrial cancer: accuracy of the finding of a well differentiated tumor at dilation and curettage compared to the findings at subsequent hysterectomy. Int J Gynecol Cancer 1999;9:383–6.

[64] Petersen RW, Quinlivan JA, Casper GR, et al. Endometrial adenocarcinoma—presenting pathology is a poor guide to surgical management. Aust N Z J Obstet Gynaecol 2000;40(2):191–4.

[65] Cornelison TL, Trimble EL, Kosary CL. SEER data, corpus uteri cancer: treatment trends versus survival for FIGO stage II, 1988-1994. Gynecol Oncol 1999;74(3):350–5.

[66] Bristow RE, Zerbe MJ, Rosenshein NB, et al. Stage IVB endometrial carcinoma: the role of cytoreductive surgery and determinants of survival. Gynecol Oncol 2000;78(2):85–91.

[67] Chi DS, Welshinger M, Venkatraman ES, et al. The role of surgical cytoreduction in Stage IV endometrial carcinoma. Gynecol Oncol 1997;67(1):56–60.

[68] Holub Z, Jaor A, Bartos P, et al. Laparoscopic surgery for endometrial cancer: long-term results of a multicentric study. Eur J Gynaecol Oncol 2002;23:305–10.

[69] Surwit EA, Joelsson I, Einhorn N. Adjunctive radiation therapy in the management of stage I cancer of the endometrium. Obstet Gynecol 1981;58(5):590–5.

[70] Grigsby PW, Perez CA, Camel HM, et al. Stage II carcinoma of the endometrium: results of therapy and prognostic factors. Int J Radiat Oncol Biol Phys 1985;11(11):1915–23.

[71] Carey MS, O'Connell GJ, Johanson CR, et al. Good outcome associated with a standardized treatment protocol using selective postoperative radiation in patients with clinical stage I adenocarcinoma of the endometrium. Gynecol Oncol 1995;57(2):138–44.

[72] Elliot P, Green D, Coats A, et al. The efficacy of postoperative vaginal irradiation in preventing vaginal recurrence in endometrial cancer. Int J Gynecol Cancer 1994;4(2):84–93.

[73] Poulsen HK, Jacobsen M, Bertelsen K, et al. Adjuvant radiation therapy is not necessary in the management of endometrial carcinoma stage I, low-risk cases. Int J Gynecol Cancer 1996;6(1):38–43.

[74] Fanning J, Evans MC, Peters AJ, et al. Adjuvant radiotherapy for stage I, grade 2 endometrial adenocarcinoma and adenoacanthoma with limited myometrial invasion. Obstet Gynecol 1987;70(6):920–2.

[75] Fanning J. Treatment for early endometrial cancer. Cost-effectiveness analysis. J Reprod Med 1999;44(8):719–23.

[76] Keys HM, Roberts JA, Brunetto VL, et al. A phase III trial of surgery with or without adjunctive external pelvic radiation therapy in intermediate risk endometrial adenocarcinoma: a Gynecologic Oncology Group study. Gynecol Oncol 2004;92(3):744–51.

[77] Randall ME, Filiaci VL, Muss H, et al. Randomized phase III trial of whole-abdominal irradiation versus doxorubicin and cisplatin chemotherapy in advanced endometrial carcinoma: a Gynecologic Oncology Group Study. J Clin Oncol 2006;249(1):36–44.

[78] Maxwell GL, Tian C, Risinger J, et al. Racial disparity in survival among patients with advanced/recurrent endometrial adenocarcinoma: a Gynecologic Oncology Group study. Cancer 2006;107(9):2197–205.

[79] Creutzberg CL, van Putten WL, Koper PC, et al. Survival after relapse in patients with endometrial cancer: results from a randomized trial. Gynecol Oncol 2003;89(2):201–9.

[80] Fleming GF, Brunetto VL, Cella D, et al. Phase III trial of doxorubicin plus cisplatin with or without paclitaxel plus filgrastim in advanced endometrial carcinoma: a Gynecologic Oncology Group Study. J Clin Oncol 2004;22(11):2159.

[81] Barakat RR, Goldman NA, Patel DA, et al. Pelvic exenteration for recurrent endometrial cancer. Gynecol Oncol 1999;75(1):99–102.

SURGICAL
CLINICS OF
NORTH AMERICA

Surg Clin N Am 88 (2008) 319 341

# Gynecologic Laparoscopy

Christopher P. DeSimone, MD[a],*,
Frederick R. Ueland, MD[a]

[a]Division of Gynecologic Oncology, Department of Obstetrics and Gynecology,
University of Kentucky Markey Cancer Center, 800 Rose Street,
333 Whitney-Hendrickson Building, Lexington, KY 40536-0298, USA

Laparoscopy for the gynecologist began in earnest in the 1980s. In the previous decade, laparoscopy was used mainly for diagnostic procedures in the female pelvis. Physician acceptance and a rapid evolution of instrumentation have enabled laparoscopy to flourish in recent years. The shorter recovery time and aesthetic advantages also have fueled patient advocacy. The first widely accepted gynecologic laparoscopy procedure was the tubal ligation. The small incisions and rapid recovery were appealing to the patient, and surgeons preferred the magnified optics. By the mid 1970s, many women were choosing sterilization, and the number of laparoscopic tubal ligations was on the rise [1]. Gynecologic surgeons began to explore other applications, including diagnostic procedures for pelvic pain, ectopic pregnancies, and appendicitis. In the early 1980s, additional operative procedures were introduced including adnexal surgery, uterine myomectomy, and hysterectomy. In the following decade, advanced operations for pelvic organ prolapse, urinary incontinence, and gynecologic cancers were performed. From simple beginnings, laparoscopy now is integrated completely into the field of gynecologic surgery.

This article is a survey of gynecologic laparoscopy for the general surgeon. It presents a review of pelvic anatomy, general tenets for gynecologic laparoscopy, instrumentation, specific gynecologic procedures, robotic applications, and potential complications.

## Pelvic anatomy

A systematic, anatomic approach is recommended for laparoscopic surgery in the female pelvis. The examination should begin with a survey of

---

\* Corresponding author.
*E-mail address:* cpdesi00@uky.edu (C.P. DeSimone).

doi:10.1016/j.suc.2007.12.008

the midline structures (uterus, bladder, and rectum) and progress to the right and left adnexa (Figs. 1 and 2). A normal uterus has a smooth, homogenous appearance and ranges in size from 4 to 8 cm in the longitudinal dimension. At the lateral fundus of the uterus are the utero-ovarian ligaments and fallopian tubes. The utero-ovarian ligament contains a rich anastomotic network of veins and arterioles from both the uterine and ovarian arteries (Fig. 3). Posteriorly, the uterine fundus tapers to the cervix and upper vagina. A thoughtful inspection of the posterior uterus is important early in the evaluation to identify any rectosigmoid attachment, particularly in patients who have endometriosis, previous pelvic surgery, pelvic inflammatory disease, or a history of sigmoid diverticular disease. The rectovaginal space can be entered by incising the peritoneum between the uterosacral ligaments adjacent to the posterior cervix and vagina. This incision helps mobilize the rectum and allows visualization of the rectovaginal fascia, the endopelvic fascia between the rectum and vagina. Anteriorly, the bladder extends midway up the uterine fundus and covers the vagina and anterior cervix. The vesicouterine space can be entered by incising the vesicouterine serosa in the midline just below its point of reflection on the uterus. The point of peritoneal reflection typically is 2 to 3 cm above the actual dome of the bladder. This approach allows a visualized dissection of the bladder and

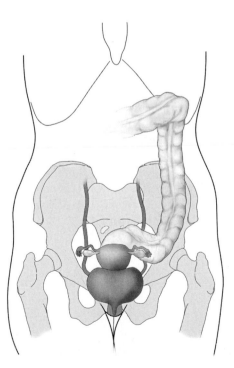

Fig. 1. Pelvic anatomy (anterior to posterior).

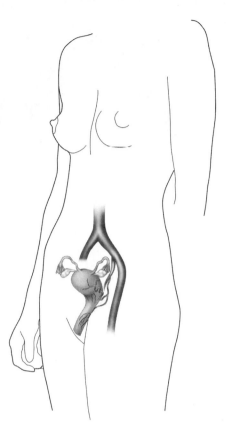

Fig. 2. Pelvic anatomy (lateral).

identification of the pubocervical fascia, the endopelvic fascia between the bladder and cervix. Opening either the vesicouterine and/or rectovaginal spaces may help the laparoscopic surgeon perform pelvic operations safely by restoring pelvic anatomy.

The uterine artery is the primary blood supply to the uterus. It originates as a branch of the anterior division of the internal iliac artery (see Fig. 3). The uterine artery travels through the cardinal ligament and spirals up the cervix to its anastomosis with the ovarian artery in the utero-ovarian ligament. There are small arteriole branches to the uterus throughout its course. The fallopian tubes originate at the lateral fundus of the uterus. The tubes extend laterally along the broad ligament toward the ovary. The tube terminates at the fimbria. Common tubal pathology (infection, endometriosis, previous ectopic pregnancy) can lead to luminal occlusion and pyo- or hydrosalpinx. Both can be a source of chronic pelvic pain.

The ovaries normally rest on the pelvic sidewall, suspended medially by the utero-ovarian ligament and laterally by the infundibulopelvic (IP) or

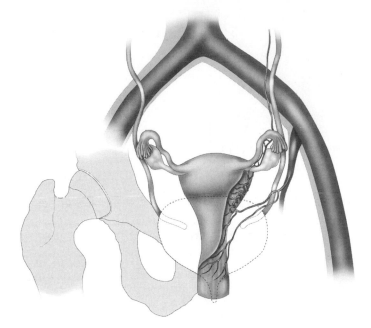

Fig. 3. Uterine and ovarian arterial supply with relation to ureter.

suspensory ligament. A normal, premenopausal ovary ranges from 2 to 4 cm in greatest dimension with a volume (length × width × height × 0.523) not exceeding 20 mL$^3$ [2]. A normal postmenopausal ovary is 1 to 3 cm in greatest dimension with a volume not exceeding 10 mL$^3$. The ovary receives its blood supply from the ovarian artery, which originates from the abdominal aorta. The ovarian veins often are multiple and drain into the inferior vena cava on the right and the renal vein on the left. The ovary should be free of adhesions, mobile on its pedicle, and easily visualized on all surfaces.

Operations in the pelvis are best performed with an understanding of the retroperitoneal space, with specific attention to the blood vessels and the course of the pelvic ureter. The peritoneum is draped over the IP ligament, forming part of the broad ligament. The cardinal ligament is at the base of the broad ligament, adjacent to the uterine cervix. The uterine artery courses through the cardinal ligament. Safe access to the retroperitoneal space is achieved by elevating and incising the peritoneum near the round ligament and lateral to the ovarian vessels. When this incision is extended parallel to the IP ligament toward the pelvic brim, the psoas muscle, external and internal iliac vessels, and ureter can be identified. Visualizing the course of the ureter is essential for the laparoscopic pelvic surgeon. The ureter courses through the retroperitoneum over the common iliac artery at the pelvic brim and continues along the medial leaf of the broad ligament. It travels under the uterine artery approximately 1.2 cm lateral to the cervix and inserts into the posterior bladder base at the trigone (see Fig. 3). It often is possible to visualize the ureter indirectly through the peritoneum without entering the retroperitoneal space; however, direct visualization is preferred, especially when the pelvic anatomy is distorted.

## General approach to gynecologic laparoscopy

### Preparation, positioning, procedures

In preparation for surgery, patients should be given a mechanical bowel regimen (magnesium citrate or Golytely [Braintree Laboratories, Inc., Braintree, Massachusetts]) the day before surgery. General anesthesia is required, and the stomach is emptied with an orogastric tube before placement of ports. The patient's arms should be padded and carefully tucked to the side. Once the patient has been anesthetized and intubated, the patient is positioned in low lithotomy with Allen stirrups (Allen Medical Systems, Inc., Acton, Massachusetts). The patients' thighs should be abducted slightly and parallel to the floor to allow the surgeon a full range of motion. An abdominal and vaginal preparation is performed, and a Foley catheter is placed before the procedure. At this time, a uterine manipulator should be placed with sterile technique. Commonly used uterine manipulators include the Cohen cannula (Richard Wolf Medical Instruments, Inc., Vernon Hills, Illinois), the Kronner cannula, and the ZUMI cannula (Artisan Medical, Inc., Medford, New Jersey). A sponge stick can be placed in the vagina if the patient previously has had a hysterectomy. A laparoscopic drape with leg covers and separate abdominal and pelvic openings is preferred for operative laparoscopy.

Most gynecologic surgeons begin with an intra- or infraumbilical incision. The choice of laparoscope (10 mm, 5 mm, or 2 mm; 30° or 0°) depends on surgeon's preference and the requirements of the surgery. Peritoneal access can be obtained with optical-access trocars such as the Xcel trocar (Ethicon Endo-Surgery, Inc., Cincinnati, Ohio), with or without establishing a pneumoperitoneum with a Veress needle before insertion of the trocar. Types of trocars and placement methods are widely variable and are well described in both academic and industry literature. The authors favor a Veress needle for insufflation followed by an optical-access trocar for patients without previous abdominal surgery. Open laparoscopy using a Hasson [3] trocar is recommended for patients who have had prior abdominal surgery and provides safe and easy access to the peritoneal cavity with minimal complications (0.5%). Some laparoscopic surgeons routinely perform open laparoscopy. After gaining access, the laparoscope is placed immediately and is used to inspect visually for insertional trauma. Fogging of the camera can be prevented by commercially available liquids or by warming the camera before insertion.

Once an umbilical trocar has been inserted and its position confirmed visually with the laparoscope, the peritoneum is insufflated with $CO_2$ gas. Three accessory ports are placed for most operative laparoscopic surgeries: two lateral 5-mm or 10/12-mm ports and one 5-mm suprapubic port (Fig. 4). The suprapubic port should be placed 3 to 4 cm above the symphysis pubis to avoid bladder injury. The lower quadrant ports should be placed at the level of the iliac crest lateral to both the rectus muscle and inferior epigastric vessels, which are visible with the laparoscope through the peritoneum. This diamond configuration allows the assisting surgeon to retract in the field of surgery with a lateral or suprapubic port while exposing the field with the camera (umbilical port). Many pelvic surgeons prefer to operate on adnexal structures contralateral to their table position. A laparoscopic procedure is not complete until all port incisions larger than 5 mm have been closed.

Patient selection depends on the laparoscopic procedure; however, there are some general rules of exclusion. Previous abdominal surgery is the most common reason to exclude a laparoscopic approach. The pelvis is the most dependent portion of the abdomen, so a previous abscess, bleeding, or surgical procedure may involve the pelvic structures primarily or secondarily. The adhesions can be thin, avascular, and easily separated, or thick, vascular, and surgically challenging. Dense pelvic adhesions markedly increase

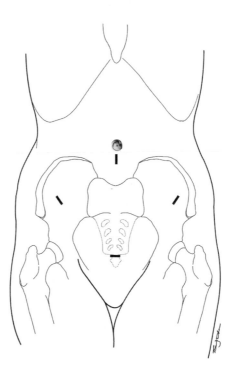

Fig. 4. Laparoscopic port placement.

the difficulty of any procedure, including the length of surgery and its com-plications. Pelvic inflammatory disease, appendicitis, and ruptured tubal pregnancies or ovarian cysts all increase the likelihood of pelvic adhesions. Morbid obesity (body mass index > 45) is a relative contraindication to lap-aroscopic surgery. The increase in adipose tissue requires longer ports and instruments and can complicate initial access to the peritoneal cavity. The obese patient will have greater peak airway pressures and often cannot sus-tain prolonged Trendelenberg position. In addition, the small and large bowel is of greater size, which may further limit visualization of pelvic struc-tures. Although laparoscopic surgery can be performed on the morbidly obese, each operation should be evaluated carefully for the feasibility of suc-cess and potential risk.

## Instrumentation

The tools of a laparoscopic surgeon are diverse and best categorized ac-cording to function. For tissue handling, atraumatic graspers are preferred when manipulating small bowel, colon, or adnexal structures. Maryland for-ceps have a fine tip that is useful for delicate procedures, and a Babcock clamp is ideal for grasping the adnexae. For a more secure hold, an Allis or alligator clamp is available. A blunt probe is useful for many gynecologic procedures because it can move small bowel out of the operative field safely and can ma-nipulate the uterus and ovaries. Some blunt probes allow irrigation or aspira-tion of pelvic fluid, which may be helpful for evacuating clot, evaluating pelvic inflammatory disease or endometriosis, or obtaining washings.

Instruments that cut or cauterize tissue are the mainstay of laparoscopic surgery. Basic Metzenbaum scissors are useful for almost all pelvic proce-dures. They can be used with monopolar cautery to aid in hemostasis. Monopolar cutting current can be useful in dissection or desiccation; how-ever, coagulation current should be avoided near bowel, bladder, or ureter because of the possibility of lateral thermal injury. Bipolar cautery is a safer method of cauterizing tissue. Electrical current is passed directly between the two arms of the instrument, minimizing lateral thermal injury. It is used suc-cessfully to occlude fallopian tubes and to provide hemostasis during lapa-roscopic hysterectomy (LH) and adnexal surgery. Finally, a tripolar instrument combines a bipolar grasper with a retractable cutting blade. This time-saving device allows the surgeon to cauterize and divide tissue without exchanging instruments.

New technologies are replacing monopolar and bipolar cautery. The Harmonic Scalpel (Ethicon Endo-Surgery, Inc.) is a tissue dissector that works through ultrasonic vibration: one arm of the instrument oscillates at 70,000 rpm against a second fixed arm. This high-speed oscillation dis-sects and seals tissue at the same time. It can provide hemostasis to vessels as large as 8 mm in diameter and has very little lateral thermal injury. The dependent mechanical portion of the instrument is located in its handle; the independent shaft can be interchanged between different instruments (hook, spatula, and grasper). LigaSure (ValleyLab, Inc., Boulder, Colorado) is another thermal device that seals the tissue through pressure and thermal energy. Lateral thermal spread is minimal, and it is capable of providing hemostasis to vessels as large as 7 mm. Endoscopic staplers are another method of managing vascular pedicles. The Endopath endoscopic linear cutter (Ethicon Endo-Surgery, Inc.) is a 45-mm stapler that can divide the IP ligaments and its arterial and venous supply safely. This device is easy to use and often can remove one ovary with as few as two staple loads. Last, the $CO_2$ laser is a common choice to ablate endometriosis. It is precise and has minimal lateral thermal injury. The depth of dissection is controlled and can ablate lesions as small as 0.1 mm adequately.

The gynecologic literature currently is devoid of comparative instrument studies, but the surgical literature has some pertinent information. One study compared electrothermal bipolar vessel sealing to ultrasonic coagulation shears for laparoscopic colectomy. There was no difference in mean operating time or length of hospital stay; but there was a significant difference in estimated blood loss favoring electrothermal bipolar vessel sealing over ultrasonic coagulation shears [4]. Another study compared the Harmonic Scalpel and bipolar current. There was no difference in operative time, estimated blood loss, postoperative pain, or hospital stay [5]. A comparative study of the Harmonic Scalpel versus endoscopic stapling also showed no difference between operative time and estimated blood loss [6]. With the exception of blood loss in one of the studies mentioned [4], endoscopic staplers, the Harmonic Scalpel, and bipolar current seem to be comparable.

Suturing for laparoscopic procedures can be performed with standard or self-righting needle holders. Once the tissue is sutured, intra- or extracorporeal knots are tied. After LH, the vaginal cuff must be sutured closed. Most surgeons close with interrupted sutures and extracorporeal ties, but new instruments like the Endostitch (AutoSuture, US Surgical Inc., Norwalk, Connecticut) allow faster closures. The Endostitch passes a straight needle (with suture) back and forth between two arms creating a continuous, running closure. Each end of the suture is secured with a bead to prevent slipping of the suture. This technique reduces surgical time by avoiding knot tying.

## Common gynecologic procedures

### Tubal ligation

It is estimated that 600,000 tubal ligations are performed in the United States each year, with most performed by laparoscopy [7]. The model candidate for tubal sterilization is married, older than 30 years, and finished with child bearing. Tubal reversal is possible but costly and carries a low fertility rate. Laparoscopic tubal ligation is an outpatient surgery that generally requires a 2-day recovery. Two ports are recommended for this procedure, one umbilical and one suprapubic. A single umbilical port can be used with an operating laparoscope. Once a pneumoperitoneum is established, the surgeon elevates the uterus with the uterine manipulator and identifies each tube at its origin in the uterine fundus. Each tube must be followed to its fimbriated end to avoid mistaking the round ligament for a fallopian tube. Methods for ligating the fallopian tube include Falope-ring band, Hulka Clip, bipolar current, monopolar current, or resection with suture ligation. The failure rate for tubal ligation is 0.55 per 100 women in 1 year, 1.31 per 100 women in 5 years, and 1.85 per 100 women in 10 years [7]. Tubal ligation using bipolar current in young women had the highest failure rate; monopolar current and postpartum (mini-laparotomy) tubal ligation had the highest success rate in preventing pregnancy [8,9]. Electrosurgery was more likely to cause hydrosalpinx and adhesion formation [8]. Complications from laparoscopic tubal ligation range from 0.1% to 4.6% [8–12]. The most common complication is hemorrhage from the fallopian tube or mesosalpinx. Major complications, which are rare (0.6%), include bowel perforation, vascular injury, and genitourinary perforation.

## Diagnostic laparoscopy

Laparoscopy is used for evaluation of many pelvic problems. Pain is the most common indication and may result from adhesions, endometriosis, pelvic inflammatory disease, or bowel or bladder pathology. Pelvic adhesive disease is managed best with dissecting scissors and electrosurgery or $CO_2$ laser. Care with thermal ablation always is required when bowel, bladder, or ureters are in close proximity. Both diagnosis and treatment of endometriosis can be accomplished through the laparoscope. Endometriosis is a pathologic diagnosis that requires any two of the following on histologic review: hemosiderin, endometrial glands, or endometrial stroma. Treatment for early disease requires either surgical resection or fulguration with electrosurgery or $CO_2$ laser. A lateralizing endometrioma should be excised completely (ovarian cystectomy or oophorectomy). Advanced disease is treated with hysterectomy and bilateral salpingo-oophorectomy. Pelvic inflammatory disease is diagnosed by visualization of purulent discharge from the fimbria. In chronic pelvic inflammatory disease, the fimbria is agglutinated, and the tubes frequently are occluded. Chromopertubation can be performed to evaluate tubal patency. Dilute methylene blue or indigo carmine dye is introduced with a syringe through the lumen of the uterine manipulator. Tubal patency is confirmed by visualization of dye effluent from the fimbria. A thorough inspection of the pelvis should include the sigmoid colon, appendix, and bladder surface.

## Adnexal surgery

The adnexae consist of ovaries and fallopian tubes. A multitude of adnexal pathology may contribute to pelvic pain, pressure or fullness, urinary or gastrointestinal frequency and urgency, or malignancy. A preoperative evaluation should include imaging (ultrasound, CT scan), a bimanual examination, laboratory testing (biomarkers, complete blood cell count), and a pregnancy test when relevant. Unfortunately, even the most thorough of evaluations may not answer the question of malignancy. The risk of ovarian biopsy is unknown but in a malignant ovary may create the potential for peritoneal or needle track dissemination, altering both stage and treatment. The mainstay of treatment remains careful surgical removal.

Salpingostomy or salpingectomy may be required for treatment of an ectopic pregnancy. Ideally, a linear salpingostomy performed over the dilated segment of the fallopian tube will allow complete extraction of the ectopic gestation with forceps and irrigation. The tube does not need to be closed surgically. Occasionally, salpingectomy may be necessary for complete removal of the abnormal pregnancy. If possible, the blood should be aspirated completely from the pelvis using an irrigator-aspirator instrument.

Ovarian cystectomy is indicated for a benign cyst (hemorrhagic corpus luteum, cystadenoma, teratoma, endometrioma) in a cycling woman. The cyst typically can be distinguished from ovarian parenchyma with close inspection. Electrosurgery and sharp dissection are used to separate the cyst wall from the ovary. The dissection is facilitated by careful traction on both cyst and ovary. Electrosurgery is used for hemostasis. The ovarian capsule rarely is closed after laparoscopic cystectomy, but a 4-0 absorbable suture can be used for closure if desired.

In some carefully selected patients, ovarian aspiration and biopsy can be considered. Candidates for this procedure have a persistent ($> 6$ months) unilocular ovarian cyst on ultrasound and desire both ovarian preservation and immediate return to daily activities. This minimally invasive diagnostic procedure utilizes a 2-mm laparoscope (Bioview, Santa Ana, California) through a 2-mm MiniPort (US Surgical, Inc.). The MiniPort is introduced as a Veress needle, and the abdomen is insufflated. The 2-mm laparoscope then can be introduced directly through the port. The abdomen, pelvis, and ovarian cyst are inspected carefully for signs of malignancy. If the appearance is benign, a long 18-gauge needle is introduced through the midline abdominal wall and directed into the ovarian cyst. The cyst is aspirated completely, and the fluid is sent for cytology. Ovarian biopsy can be performed with a spring-loaded true-cut biopsy instrument. If all gas is removed from the abdomen, most patients are healthy in 1 to 2 days. Narcotic use is infrequent following the procedure. If cancer is discovered by the procedure, patients should receive surgical staging within 5 to 7 days.

Laparoscopy is an excellent choice for salpingo-oophorectomy when the ovary is cystic, mobile, and smaller than 10 cm. Depending on anatomy and the difficulty of the procedure, three or four ports are used. The ovary is elevated with an atraumatic forcep or Babcock clamp, and the peritoneum is incised lateral to the ovary from the round ligament to the pelvic brim. The ureter is visualized, and the IP ligament is ligated and divided. The remainder of the broad ligament is dissected to the utero-ovarian ligament, which is ligated securely (Fig. 5). The specimen is placed in an Endo Catch pouch (AutoSuture, US Surgical, Inc.) to facilitate aspiration and minimize spill. The primary challenge with laparoscopic salpingo-oophorectomy is removal of the ovary, because most ovarian tumors cannot be removed through a port. A cystic ovary smaller than 5 cm can be placed in a pouch, pulled to the abdominal wall, and aspirated with a large-bore spinal needle and syringe. If the remaining ovary still is too large for removal, the fascial incision is enlarged (mini-laparotomy), incorporating the suprapubic port site to accommodate safe removal of tumor and pouch. Before the fascial incision is enlarged, all pedicles are inspected, and the primary surgery is completed, because the pneumoperitoneum will be difficult to re-establish without complete closure of the incision. Cystic ovarian tumors too large to fit in a pouch can be aspirated directly, but only if the risk of malignancy is thought to be low. Ovarian tumors larger than 10 cm, solid tumors larger than 5 cm, or tumors at high risk for malignancy are managed best with laparotomy.

Most of the studies comparing laparoscopic salpingo-oophorectomy and open salpingo-oophorectomy were conducted in the 1990s. One large, nonrandomized study by Mettler and colleagues [13] compared 493 laparoscopic salpingo-oophorectomies and 138 open procedures. The laparoscopic surgeries removed smaller ovaries (mean, 4.5 cm versus 8.2 cm) with less blood loss (193 mL versus 431 mL) and shorter operative time (75 minutes versus 126

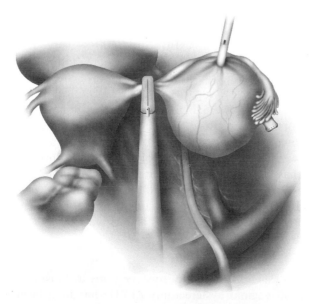

Fig. 5. Laparoscopic resection of an ovarian tumor.

minutes). Twelve cases were converted to laparotomy for adhesive disease (6 cases) or the suspicion of malignancy (6 cases/4 ovarian carcinomas). Laparotomy and laparoscopy are reported to have similar complication rates; laparoscopy increases surgical costs and operative times but shortens hospitalization and reduces blood loss [14–17].

## Myomectomy

Laparoscopic myomectomy is gaining popularity. Pedunculated uterine myomata usually are removed safely with either electrosurgery or the Harmonic Scalpel. Excision of subserosal and intramural fibroids is more challenging. Use of a vasoconstricting agent (20 U vasopressin in 100 mL normal saline) is reported in the literature and has been utilized for decades but can result in cardiac dysrhythmias and should be used with caution. The uterine incision is made with electrosurgery, and the myoma capsule is dissected in its entirety. A laparoscopic myoma screw (5 or 11 mm) may be helpful in providing traction during the dissection. Electrosurgery, sharp dissection, and laser have been used successfully for myomectomy. The irrigator-aspirator may be used for aquadissection and to maintain a clear surgical field. Multiple myomata should be removed through a single uterine incision, if possible. Venous bleeding can be managed with fulguration. The Argon beam coagulator can be used for persistent bleeding. A defocused $CO_2$ laser and Kleppinger bipolar current are available for arterial hemostasis. The myometrium should be closed with 0 or 2-0 absorbable suture; the serosa is closed with 4-0 suture. The irrigator-aspirator often is useful in providing a clear surgical field during laparoscopic myomectomy. For removal, small myomata can be fragmented surgically (in the anterior cul-de-sac) and removed directly through the large ports. Larger fibroids can be pulverized with an endoscopic morcellator (Ethicon Endo-Surgery, Inc., Cincinnati, Ohio) or removed through a colpotomy incision. Indigo carmine dye can be injected into the endometrial cavity to evaluate its integrity after myomectomy. Contraindications to laparoscopic myomectomy include diffuse disease, multiple myomata exceeding 5 cm, uterine size larger than 16 weeks, or a single myoma larger than 15 cm. The safety of pregnancy following laparoscopic myomectomy is still unknown when myomectomy has been extensive, or following the removal of deeply embedded fibroids or when the myometrium has not been reapproximated. Thermal injury to the uterus always should be minimized, particularly if future pregnancy is a consideration. Postoperative bowel adhesions to the uterine fundus have been reported to cause small bowel obstruction, but this is a rare occurrence.

## Hysterectomy

Laparoscopy was first utilized for hysterectomy to assist with vaginal hysterectomy. Total vaginal hysterectomy (TVH) has long been an accepted route to remove the uterus and ovaries safely without the need for a laparotomy. The problem with vaginal hysterectomy is the limited visualization of the upper pelvis. Large ovaries, a bulky uterus, or pelvic adhesions made TVH a difficult operation. Laparoscopy is used to visualize the upper pelvis, safely restore pelvic anatomy, and divide the IP ligaments. The surgeon then completes the procedure with vaginal removal of the uterus. This combination of laparoscopy and vaginal hysterectomy is called "laparoscopic-assisted vaginal hysterectomy" (LAVH).

The LAVH begins with laparoscopy. Four ports are introduced (one 10/12-mm camera port and three 5-mm ports). With the uterus displaced anteriorly, the retroperitoneal space is entered, the ureter is identified, and the IP ligaments are ligated and divided. The remainder of the broad and round ligaments is divided to the level of the cardinal ligament. The pneumoperitoneum is released, but the ports remain in situ for a final inspection after completion of the LAVH. Once the specimen is removed and the vagina is closed, the abdomen is re-insufflated, and the pelvis is visualized. Historically, ablation of the uterine artery was thought to be unsafe; thus the laparoscopic portion of the surgery ended at the cardinal ligament. With the advent of new coagulation technologies (eg, Harmonic Scalpel and LigaSure), the common procedure now is to divide the uterine artery with laparoscopic instrumentation.

Two Italian prospective, randomized, multicenter studies have documented the efficacy and safety of LAVH compared with total abdominal hysterectomy (TAH) [18,19]. Marana and colleagues [18] reported a statistical reduction in blood loss, postoperative pain, and hospital stay with LAVH. There was no difference between the two groups in regards to age, parity, uterine weight, operative time, or operative complications. Muzii and colleagues [19] showed fewer operative complications with LAVH than with TAH.

Improved thermal technologies have given the laparoscopic surgeon additional options for hysterectomy. The laparoscopic supracervical hysterectomy (LSH) involves amputation of the uterine fundus at the internal cervical os (Fig. 6). In this procedure, the vesicouterine space is developed, and the bladder is mobilized from the anterior portion of the uterus. Uterine artery ablation is performed safely with electrosurgery (Harmonic Scalpel, LigaSure, or bipolar cautery) immediately adjacent to the cervix to avoid the course of the ureter. Then the cardinal ligament is dissected further to the level of the internal cervical os. Electrosurgery is used to amputate the uterine fundus. The uterus is reduced in size to allow its removal through the 10/12-mm port using a tissue morcellator (Ethicon Endo-Surgery, Inc.). The morcellator is placed through a lateral 10/12-mm port. Spinning blades pulverize the tissue (the uterus and ovaries) and expel it from the operative field through the 10/12-mm port. Surgeons should use considerable caution with this device. There are multiple reports of inadvertent morcellation of colon, small bowel, bladder, ureter, and even iliac vessels.

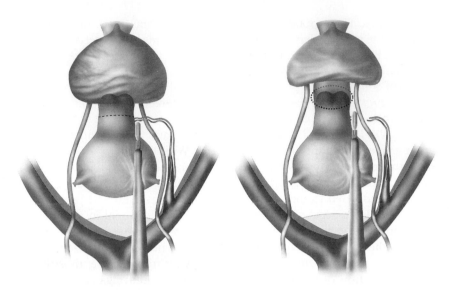

Fig. 6. Laparoscopic hysterectomy. (*Left*) Laparoscopic supracervical hysterectomy. (*Right*) Total laparoscopic hysterectomy.

The LSH literature includes both retrospective case-based and cohort studies. One study reported on their complication rate of 1706 cases. The authors had five intraoperative injuries (0.03%): three bladder, one ureter, and one hemorrhage. There were 20 postoperative complications (1.2%) [20]. Data from three cohort studies show that LSH has a significantly shorter operative time than LAVH or TAH; two studies also reported fewer complications and shorter hospital stays [21–23]. From these limited data, LSH seems to be at least comparable to LAVH. The private sector has endorsed LSH as the hysterectomy of choice for most patients who have benign gynecologic diseases. The surgery can be performed quickly (1 hour), has few complications, a short hospital stay, and a prompt return to normal activity (2 weeks). To be considered for LSH, patients should have normal cervical cytology and understand that continued cervical cancer screening is recommended after surgery.

Inevitably, gynecologic surgeons began to perform a complete hysterectomy (uterus, cervix, tubes, and ovaries) or total laparoscopic hysterectomy (TLH). The technique is similar to LSH, but the surgeon continues the dissection below the cervix to the level of the vagina (see Fig. 6). A colpotomizer is used to facilitate the vaginal incision. This device, which is placed at the beginning of the surgery, encircles the cervix and provides a clear line of demarcation between the vagina and cervix when visualized laparoscopically. The device also provides a stable surface on which to perform the colpotomy. Once the surface of the colpotomizer is visualized through a 2-cm colpotomy, the incision is continued circumferentially until the cervix is amputated completely from the vagina. Colpotomy generally is performed with a thermal device (Harmonic Scalpel or monopolar cautery) to maintain hemostasis. The specimen is extracted through the vagina, and the vagina is closed with continuous, running or interrupted absorbable suture. Large specimens (> 10 cm) may require morcellation before vaginal removal.

The TLH literature also consists predominantly of case-based and cohort studies. The average TLH in experienced hands is a 1- to 2-hour operation, with a mean blood loss of 130 mL, and a 1-day hospital stay. The conversion rate to laparotomy is 2% with a 2% to 5% complication rate (Table 1) [24–29]. TLH takes longer to perform than TAH but involves less blood loss and a shorter hospital stay. The complication rates between the two hysterectomies are equivalent [27]. TLH and LAVH are equivalent, except that TLH has a reduced operating time [29].

Laparoscopic hysterectomy has been evaluated carefully by the Cochrane Database, which analyzed the differences between TAH, TVH, and LH. LH included LAVH, LSH, and TLH. Twenty-seven randomized trials (3643 patients) were reviewed. The meta-analysis compared LH with TAH and found that the benefits of LH included reduced blood loss, smaller decline in postoperative hemoglobin levels, shorter hospital stay, more rapid return to normal activity, fewer infections, and fewer wound infections. LH consistently had longer operating times and more frequent urologic injuries (ureter and bladder) [30]. There was no difference between TVH and LH except that LH took longer to perform. In summary, for benign gynecological indications, LH has a number of advantages over abdominal hysterectomy, although patients should be cautioned that urologic injury is more common.

## Cancer procedures

In the early 1990's, Nezhat and colleagues [31] reported the first laparoscopic radical hysterectomy with pelvic and para-aortic lymphadenectomy. There were additional reports of surgical staging procedures for endometrial cancer [32]. These early reports outlined the potential advantages of laparoscopy in patients who had gynecologic malignancies; these advantages included reduced time of hospitalization, reduced postoperative pain, low incidence of postoperative wound complications, and a presumed accelerated return to normal daily activities. Today, many of the common pelvic cancers (early-stage ovarian, endometrial, and cervical) are amenable to laparoscopic surgery. Vulvar carcinoma is an extracorporeal disease, and advanced ovarian cancer frequently is associated with carcinomatosis, small bowel adhesions, and bulky disease; both vulvar carcinoma and advanced ovarian cancer are managed inadequately through the laparoscope.

### Lymphadenectomy

Lymphadenectomy, or a selective lymph node sampling, is an important technique for early cervical, ovarian, and endometrial cancer staging

Table 1
Total laparoscopic hysterectomy

| Author [reference #] | N | Operative time (minutes) | Mean uterine weight (g) | Mean estimated blood loss (mL) | Conversion rate (%) | Complications (%)[a] | Mean hospital stay (days) |
|---|---|---|---|---|---|---|---|
| Cheung, et al [24] | 175 | 108.2 ± 29.6 range 60–199 | 292.2 range 50–1126 | n/a | n/a | 6.9 | 1.2 |
| O'Hanlan, et al [25] | 830 | 132 ± 55 range 28–355 | 239 range 50–3131 | 130 | 0.6 | 10 | 1.4 |
| Ng, et al [26] | 427 | 136 range 40–257 | n/a | 313 | 1.8 | 4.8 | 2.7 |
| Hoffman, et al [27] | 108 | 131 range 70–300 | 144 range 49–900 | 50 range 10–400 | n/a | 21.3 | 1.25 |
| Vaisbuch, et al [28] | 79 | 145 ± 37 no range | 169.8 ± 107.3 | n/a | 1.8 | 17.7 | 3.5 |
| Ghezzi, et al [29] | 35 | 184 ± 46 | n/a | 100 range 50–500 | 0 | 17.1 | n/a |

*Abbreviation:* n/a, not available.

[a] Intraoperative and postoperative complications.

procedures. Utilizing four ports, arranged in the previously described diamond configuration, the surgeon operates contralateral to table position and removes the common iliac, external and internal iliac, and obturator lymph nodes. The boundaries of an adequate pelvic lymph node dissection include the deep circumflex iliac vein as it crosses the external iliac artery (inferior), the genitofemoral nerve (lateral), the ureter (medial), and the bifurcation of the aorta (superior). Resection of the para-aortic lymph nodes is required for deeply invasive uterine tumors, for early ovarian cancers, and in all patients known to have positive pelvic lymph nodes. The peritoneum is incised over the common iliac artery and extended superiorly to the level of the inferior mesenteric artery. The peritoneum and right ureter are retracted laterally. The lymph nodes are removed with electrosurgery, the Harmonic Scalpel, or with a combination of dissecting scissors and titanium clips. It is common to find small perforating veins between the vena cava and the lymph nodes. These veins should be clipped or cauterized before nodal removal. Once harvested, the lymph nodes can be removed vaginally or with an Endo Catch pouch. Unresectable lymph nodes should be biopsied with fine-needle aspiration.

## Endometrial cancer

Endometrial cancer is staged surgically and involves removal of the uterus, cervix, tubes, ovaries, and pelvic and para-aortic lymph nodes. The surgery is both diagnostic (staging) and therapeutic (80% cure). With the advent of LAVH and TLH, it was not long before laparoscopic surgery was being performed for endometrial carcinomas. For endometrial cancers, laparoscopic pelvic and para-aortic lymph node sampling and pelvic cytology are added to the previously described hysterectomy procedures. Several retrospective cohort studies and a few prospective, randomized publications have compared staging with LAVH or TLH and TAH (Table 2) [33–39]. As expected, the laparoscopic approach is a longer operation but involves less blood loss, a shorter hospitalization, and fewer intraoperative and postoperative complications. The most common postoperative complication with laparotomy is related to the abdominal wall (seroma, wound separation, or infection). To date, most studies have shown similar recurrence and overall survival rates. Results from the large, randomized LAP2 trial comparing laparotomy and laparoscopy by the Gynecologic Oncology Group are expected in 2008. LAP2 compared LAVH (n = 1696) and TAH (n = 920) for the definitive treatment of early-stage endometrial cancer.

## Cervical cancer

Cervical cancer is staged clinically by examination, but early cancers are treated by radical abdominal hysterectomy and pelvic lymphadenectomy (RAH). Advanced cancers of the cervix (stages II–IV) are treated with

Table 2
Laparoscopy versus laparotomy for endometrial carcinoma

| Author [reference #] | Study type | N | | Operative time (minutes) | | Mean estimated bloodloss (mL) | | Mean hospital stay (days) | | Total complication rate (%)[a] | | Recurrence rate (%) | | Survival rate (%) | |
|---|---|---|---|---|---|---|---|---|---|---|---|---|---|---|---|
| | | LAVH | TAH | LAVH | TAH | LAVH | TAH | LAVH | TAH | LAVH | TAH | LAVH | TAH | LAVH | TAH |
| Kalogiannidis, et al [33] | Prospective, cohort | 69 | 100 | 172 | 137 | 300 | 355 | 5 | 8 | 7 | 8 | 8.7 | 15 | 92 | 87 |
| Tollund, et al [34] | Retrospective, cohort | 28 | 58 | 91 | 92 | 184 | 379 | 2.7 | 5.4 | 7 | 14 | 7.1 | 10.3 | — | — |
| Zapicc, et al [35] | Retrospective, cohort | 38 | 37 | 165 | 129 | — | — | 5 | 7 | 32 | 57 | 5.4 | 5.3 | 81.1 | 81.6 |
| Eltabbahk [36] | Retrospective, cohort | 100 | 86 | — | — | 200 | 250 | 2 | 5 | 11 | 18.6 | 7 | 10.5 | 98 | 96 |
| Obermair, et al [37] | Retrospective, cohort | 42 | 36 | 139 | 126 | 278 | 320 | 4.4 | 7.9 | 24 | 50 | 4.7 | 5.5 | — | — |
| Malur, et al [38] | Prospective, randomized | 37 | 33 | 176 | 166 | 229 | 594 | 8.6 | 11.7 | 29.7 | 39.3 | 2.7 | 3.0 | 83.9 | 90.9 |
| Tozzi, et al [39] | Prospective, randomized | 63 | 59 | — | — | 241 | 586 | 7.8 | 11.4 | 12 | 34 | 12.6 | 8.5 | 82.7 | 86.5 |

*Abbreviations:* LAVH, laparoscopic-assisted vaginal hysterectomy; TAH, total abdominal hysterectomy.
[a] Intraoperative and postoperative complications.

chemoradiation. There are two primary distinctions between RAH and TAH. First, RAH removes the lymphatic tissue (parametria) lateral to the uterus, requiring a meticulous dissection of the pelvic ureter as it courses through the cardinal ligament. Mobilizing the ureter enables the surgeon to reposition it safely before removing the parametrial tissue. Second, a complete pelvic lymphadenectomy is performed with RAH, including the common iliac, external and internal iliac, and obturator lymph nodes. The operative time for a RAH ranges from 2 to 4 hours and typically is performed through a midline or Maylard incision.

There are a few published reports of laparoscopic radical hysterectomy and lymphadenectomy (LRH). Most studies are retrospective with a small number of patients. Similar to endometrial cancer and benign laparoscopic hysterectomies, reports of LRH found less blood loss, fewer complications, and a shorter hospital stay than with RAH. For inexperienced surgeons, however, the operative time for LRH often exceeds 8 hours. Even for experienced surgeons, the mean operating time is 344 minutes (6 hours). There was no reported difference between RAH and LRH in the number of lymph nodes removed, amount of parametrial tissue resected, recurrence, or overall survival [40–42].

*Ovarian cancer*

Malignant ovarian tumors may be encountered during laparoscopy. Ovarian cancer staging includes removal of the affected ovary and fallopian tube, pelvic and para-aortic lymph nodes, infracolic omentectomy, pelvic and subdiaphragmatic washings, and multiple peritoneal biopsies (anterior, posterior, right, and left pelvis; right and left para-colic spaces; beneath the diaphragm; and any suspicious areas). Patients who have ovarian cancer who desire fertility-sparing surgery can preserve the uninvolved uterus and opposite ovary provided they have stage IA to IC disease. All others should have a hysterectomy and bilateral salpingo-oophorectomy in addition to the complete staging procedure. Although laparoscopic staging of early ovarian cancer is possible, most gynecologic oncologists prefer midline laparotomy for the staging ovarian cancer.

Reassessment laparoscopy can be considered in patients who have a history of ovarian cancer who have a moderate elevation in the biomarker (CA-125 = 50–100) but have no clinical evidence of recurrence (normal CT scan). In this setting, proof of recurrence can facilitate chemotherapy treatment planning. The procedure requires a thorough inspection of the abdominal cavity. Any free fluid should be sampled, pelvic and upper abdominal washings obtained, and multiple peritoneal biopsies performed. The entire peritoneal surface is at risk for recurrence; however, the omental bed, the undersurface of the diaphragm, and the pelvis should receive the majority of the surgeon's attention in looking for microscopic recurrence.

## Training

Training for laparoscopic surgery in gynecologic oncology takes place at most fellowship programs and is a point of emphasis with the American Board of Obstetrics and Gynecology. Dry labs can provide familiarity with instrumentation, practice with pelvic simulators, and, sometimes, realistic teaching with advanced computerized simulators. Porcine labs may allow novice surgeons an opportunity to train and learn to manage surgical complications with the laparoscope. As with most surgical procedures, confidence is gained through mentorship, careful patient selection, and repetition. Laparoscopic techniques are gaining popularity and probably will become the standard of care for endometrial cancer, because the newly trained gynecologic oncologists are well versed in these techniques.

## Robotics

No discussion about laparoscopy would be complete without mention of the most recent robotic platform, da Vinci (Intuitive Surgical, Inc., Sunnyvale, California). The da Vinci robotic system consists of a patient cart, which houses the three or four robotic arms, and the surgeon console through which the surgeon controls the robotic arms. Access to the abdominal cavity is gained by traditional techniques. Once the robotic trocars are placed, the robotic arms are docked to their respective trocars. Instruments are attached to the robotic arms and placed through the trocars. The surgeon then leaves the operative field for the console.

The advantages of the da Vinci robotic system over conventional laparoscopy are improved optics and wristed instruments. At the console, the surgeon has a three-dimensional view of the abdominal cavity. This view is achieved by the da Vinci optics system, which employs two cameras (right and left) and blends the images together for a three-dimensional view. The computer processor also can magnify images with greater precision than traditional laparoscopy. Instruments for the da Vinci are wristed. They can move more than 180° and closely mimic the natural movement of a surgeon's hand. These refinements make intracorporeal knot tying much easier with the da Vinci system.

Any gynecologic procedure performed with laparoscopy can be performed with the da Vinci robot [43–45]. Besides hysterectomy, the best applications for robotic surgery are in gynecologic oncology. Lymphadenectomy and ureteral dissection are easier to perform with the robotic system (especially for novice surgeons). The wristed instruments make the surgeon more adept at complicated or delicate dissection. Surgeons who find laparoscopic surgery difficult often are more facile with robotic surgery.

The main disadvantage of robotic surgery is the cost to both institution and patient. The initial investment for a robotic platform is about $1.5 million. In addition, the instruments are disposable (each is limited to 10 uses) and need to be replaced periodically ($2000–3000). Intuitive Surgical, Inc. updates the robotic platform every 3 to 4 years, which requires the purchase of a new machine. To offset the cost of capital equipment, patients or third-party payors are likely to be charged more for robotic procedures than for laparoscopic or traditional procedures. Currently, the charges for these procedures are ill defined, because there are no Current Procedural Terminology codes for any robotic procedure. Most surgeons code the procedure with standard laparoscopic codes.

One has to ask "Is it worth it?" The honest answer is that it is too early to tell. If, because of improved optics and instrument ergonomics, the technology evolves as the safest route for minimally invasive surgery, the industry probably will bear the cost. If robotic surgery continues to march in parallel with laparoscopy (ie, without any clear advantage in safety, hospital stay, blood loss, or other considerations), the cost of robotics surgery eventually will lead to its disuse. For now, robotic surgery is the bright new star in minimally invasive surgery.

## Summary

Laparoscopic gynecologic surgery has undergone a rapid evolution in the past 2 decades. Industry, partnered with surgical pioneers, has been primarily responsible for the advances. Today, laparoscopy is integrated fully into pelvic surgery and is essential to the gynecologic surgeon. Laparoscopy is a learned technique, with a unique set of skills and necessities that are not necessarily transferable to the seasoned surgeon trained before the advent of laparoscopy. The novel instrumentation, challenges of exposure, reliance on electrosurgery, and nominal tactile feedback require a distinct surgical expertise. During the past 20 years, it has become clear that laparoscopy is well suited to the female patient. Many procedures are accomplished with less blood loss, fewer wound complications, and shorter hospitalizations. It is a near certainty that with the next generation of pelvic surgeons, both the operative times and the incidence urologic injuries will decline. It also is likely that technological innovations (tactile feedback, greater articulating freedom, and a more universally accepted three-dimensional platform) will eliminate some of the present challenges of laparoscopy.

## References

[1] Hulka JF. Current status of elective sterilizations in the United States. Fertil Steril 1977;28: 515–20.
[2] Pavlik EJ, DePriest PD, Gallion HH, et al. Ovarian volume related to age. Gynecol Oncol 2000;77:410–2.
[3] Hasson HM, Rotman C, Rana N, et al. Open laparoscopy: 29-year experience. Obstet Gynecol 2000;96:763–6.

 [4] Campagnacci R, de Sanctis A, Baldarelli M, et al. Electrothermal bipolar vessel sealing device vs. ultrasonic coagulating shears in laparoscopic colectomies: a comparative study. Surg Endosc 2007;21:1526–31.
 [5] Chung CC, Ha JP, Tai YP, et al. Double-blind, randomized trial comparing Harmonic Scalpel hemorrhoidectomy, bipolar scissors hemorrhoidectomy and scissors excision: ligation technique. Dis Colon Rectum 2002;45:789–94.
 [6] Chung CC, Cheung HY, Chan ES, et al. Stapled hemorrhoidopexy vs. Harmonic Scalpel hemorrhoidectomy: a randomized trial. Dis Colon Rectum 2005;48:1213–9.
 [7] Schwartz DB, Wingo PA, Antarsh L, et al. Female sterilization in the United States, 1987. Fam Plann Perspect 1989;21:209–12.
 [8] Peterson HB, Xia Z, Hughes JM, et al. The risk of pregnancy after tubal sterilization: findings from the U.S. Collaborative Review of Sterilization. Am J Obstet Gynecol 1996;174: 1161–8.
 [9] Peterson HB, Xia Z, Wilcox L, et al. Pregnancy after tubal sterilization with bipolar electrocoagulation. Obstet Gynecol 1999;94:163–7.
[10] Huber AW, Mueller MD, Ghezzi F, et al. Tubal sterilization: complications of laparoscopy and minilaparotomy. Eur J Obstet Gynecol Reprod Biol 2007;134:105–9.
[11] Chaovisitsaree S, Piyamongkol W, Pongsatha S, et al. Immediate complications of laparoscopic tubal sterilization: 11 years of experience. J Med Assoc Thai 2004;87:1147–50.
[12] Jamieson DJ, Hillis SD, Duerr A, et al. Complications of interval laparoscopic tubal sterilization: findings from the United States collaborative review of sterilization. Obstet Gynecol 2000;96:997–1002.
[13] Mettler L, Jacobs V, Brandenburg K, et al. Laparoscopic management of 641 adnexal tumors in Kiel, Germany. J Am Assoc Gynecol Laparosc 2001;8:74–82.
[14] Papasakeleriou C, Saunders D, De La Rosa A. Comparative study of laparoscopic oophorectomy. J Am Assoc Gynecol Laparosc 1995;2:407–10.
[15] Leetanaporn R, Tintara H. A comparative study of outcome of laparoscopic salpingo-oophorectomy versus open salpingo-oophorectomy. J Obstet Gynaecol Res 1996;22:79–83.
[16] Reich H, Johns DA, Davis G, et al. Laparoscopic oophorectomy. J Reprod Med 1993;38: 497–501.
[17] Sadik S, Onoglu AS, Gokdeniz R, et al. Laparoscopic management of selected adnexal masses. J Am Assoc Gynecol Laparosc 1999;6:313–6.
[18] Marana R, Busacca M, Zupi E, et al. Laparoscopically assisted vaginal hysterectomy versus total abdominal hysterectomy: a prospective, randomized, multicenter study. Am J Obstet Gynecol 1999;180:270–5.
[19] Muzii L, Basile S, Zupi E, et al. Laparoscopic-assisted vaginal hysterectomy versus minilaparotomy hysterectomy: a prospective, randomized, multicenter study. J Minim Invasive Gynecol 2007;14:610–5.
[20] Bojahr R, Raatz D, Schonleber G, et al. Perioperative complications in 1706 patients after a standardized laparoscopic supracervical hysterectomy technique. J Minim Invasive Gynecol 2006;13:183–9.
[21] Milad MP, Morrison K, Sokol A, et al. A comparison of laparoscopic supracervical hysterectomy versus laparoscopic assisted vaginal hysterectomy. Surg Endosc 2001;15:286–8.
[22] El-Mowafi D, Madkour W, Lall C, et al. Laparoscopic supracervical hysterectomy versus laparoscopic vaginal hysterectomy. J Am Assoc Gynecol Laparosc 2004;11:175–80.
[23] Sarmini OR, Lefholz K, Froeschke HP. A comparison of laparoscopic supracervical hysterectomy and total abdominal hysterectomy outcomes. J Minim Invasive Gynecol 2005;12: 121–4.
[24] Cheung VY, Rosenthal DM, Morton M, et al. Total laparoscopic hysterectomy: a five-year experience. J Obstet Gynaecol Can 2007;29:337–43.
[25] O'Hanlan KA, Dibble SL, Garnier AC, et al. Total laparoscopic hysterectomy: technique and complications of 830 cases. JSLS 2007;11:45–53.

[26] Ng CC, Chern BS, Siow AY. Retrospective study of the success rates and complications associated with total laparoscopic hysterectomy. J Obstet Gynaecol Res 2007;33:512–8.

[27] Hoffman CP, Kennedy J, Borschel L, et al. Laparoscopic hysterectomy: the Kaiser Permanente San Diego experience. J Minim Invasive Gynecol 2005;12:16–24.

[28] Vaisbuch E, Goldchmit C, Ofer D, et al. Laparoscopic hysterectomy versus total abdominal hysterectomy: a comparative study. Eur J Obstet Gynecol Reprod Biol 2006;126:234–8.

[29] Ghezzi F, Cromi A, Bergamini V, et al. Laparoscopic-assisted vaginal hysterectomy versus total laparoscopic hysterectomy for the management of endometrial cancer: a randomized clinical trial. J Minim Invasive Gynecol 2006;13:114–20.

[30] Johnson N, Barlow D, Lethaby A, et al. Surgical approach to hysterectomy for benign gynaecological disease. Cochrane Database Syst Rev 2005;(1):CD003677.

[31] Nezhat CR, Burrell MO, Nezhat FR, et al. Laparoscopic radical hysterectomy with para-aortic and pelvic node dissection. Am J Obstet Gynecol 1992;166:864–5.

[32] Childers JM, Surwit EA. Combined laparoscopic and vaginal surgery for the management of two cases of stage I endometrial cancer. Gynecol Oncol 1992;45:46–51.

[33] Kalogiannidis I, Lambrechts S, Amant F, et al. Laparoscopy-assisted vaginal hysterectomy compared with abdominal hysterectomy in clinical stage I endometrial cancer: safety, recurrence and long-term outcome. Am J Obstet Gynecol 2007;196:248.e1–8.

[34] Tollund L, Hansen B, Kjer J. Laparoscopic-assisted vaginal vs. abdominal surgery in patients with endometrial cancer stage 1. Acta Obstet Gynecol Scand 2006;85:1138–41.

[35] Zapico A, Fuentes P, Grassa A, et al. Laparoscopic-assisted vaginal hysterectomy versus abdominal hysterectomy in stages I and II endometrial cancer: operating data, follow up and survival. Gynecol Oncol 2005;98:222–7.

[36] Eltabbahk GH. Analysis of survival after laparoscopy in women with endometrial carcinoma. Cancer 2002;95:1894–901.

[37] Obermair A, Manolitsas TP, Leung Y, et al. Total laparoscopic hysterectomy versus total abdominal hysterectomy for obese women with endometrial cancer. Int J Gynecol Cancer 2005;15:319–24.

[38] Malur S, Possover M, Michels W, et al. Laparoscopic-assisted vaginal versus abdominal surgery in patients with endometrial cancer- a prospective randomized trial. Gynecol Oncol 2001;80:239–44.

[39] Tozzi R, Malur S, Koehler C, et al. Laparoscopy versus laparotomy in endometrial cancer: first analysis of survival of a randomized prospective study. J Minim Invasive Gynecol 2005; 12:130–6.

[40] Frumovitz M, Reis R, Sun C, et al. Comparison of total laparoscopic and abdominal hysterectomy for patients with early-stage cervical cancer. Obstet Gynecol 2007;110:96–102.

[41] Ghezzi F, Cromi A, Ciravolo G, et al. Surgicopathologic outcome of laparoscopic versus open radical hysterectomy. Gynecol Oncol 2007;106:502–6.

[42] Ramirez P, Slomovitz BM, Soliman PT, et al. Total laparoscopic radical hysterectomy and lymphadenectomy: the M.D. Anderson Cancer Center experience. Gynecol Oncol 2006;102: 252–5.

[43] Fiorentino RP, Zepeda MA, Goldstein BH, et al. Pilot study assessing robotic laparoscopic hysterectomy and patient outcomes. J Minim Invasive Gynecol 2006;13:60–3.

[44] Beste TM, Nelson KH, Daucher JA. Total laparoscopic hysterectomy utilizing a robotic surgical system. JSLS 2005;9:13–5.

[45] Nezhat C, Saberi N, Shahmohamady B, et al. Robotic-assisted laparoscopy in gynecologic surgery. JSLS 2006;10:317–20.

ELSEVIER
SAUNDERS

SURGICAL
CLINICS OF
NORTH AMERICA

Surg Clin N Am 88 (2008) 343–359

# Complications of Gynecologic Surgery

Michael P. Stany, MD[a], John H. Farley, MD[b],*

[a]Division of Gynecologic Oncology, Walter Reed Army Medical Center,
6900 Georgia Avenue, NW, Washington, DC 20307, USA
[b]Department of Obstetrics and Gynecology, Uniformed Services University
of the Health Sciences, 4301 Jones Bridge Road, Bethesda, MD 20814, USA

Within the last several decades, many advances have been made in the field of gynecologic surgery. Specifically, both laparoscopy and hysteroscopy have provided patients with minimally invasive procedures for treatment of conditions previously thought to require laparotomy. Regardless of the nature of the procedure, the proximity of the female reproductive tract to the urinary tract, bowel, nerves, and pelvic vasculature places these structures at risk for injury during surgery. This article presents the intraoperative and postoperative complications most commonly encountered during gynecologic surgery and reviews strategies for both prevention and management.

## Intraoperative complications

### Urinary tract injury

The urinary tract is at risk for injury during gynecologic surgery because of its proximity to the blood supply of the uterus and ovaries. The overall incidence of urinary tract injury during pelvic surgery is between 0.33% and 4.8% [1,2]. Bladder injury is more common than ureteral injury, representing 80% of urinary tract injuries [1]. Risk factors for urinary tract injury include pelvic adhesions, malignant tumor, and history of previous irradiation [1,3]. In a prospective study by Vakili and colleagues [2] that employed universal cystoscopy after hysterectomy, the incidence of urinary tract injury was found to be 4.8%. Bladder injury (3.6%) occurred more frequently than ureteral injury (1.7%). Interestingly, only 12.5% of ureteral injuries and 35.3%

The opinion or assertions contained herein are the private views of the authors and are not to be construed as official or as reflecting the views of the Department of the Army or the Department of Defense.
* Corresponding author.
E-mail address: jfarley@usuhs.mil (J.H. Farley).

of bladder injuries were detected before cystoscopy. Early recognition of urinary tract injury lowers the risk of patients needing re-operation for these complications [1]. Any time a surgeon suspects urinary tract injury, he or she is obligated to investigate and prove the suspicion to be unwarranted.

*Ureteral injury*

Ureteral injury most commonly occurs proximally at the pelvic brim during ligation of the infundibulopelvic ligament and distally during ligation of the uterine artery during hysterectomy [1,4,5]. A review of total laparoscopic hysterectomies found a 0.3% incidence of ureteral injury, with all injuries occurring at the distal ureter at the level of the uterine artery/uterosacral ligament [6]. Up to 50% of cases of unilateral ureteral injury are asymptomatic postoperatively [7].

The best way to prevent ureteral injury is to identify the ureter before clamping critical pedicles. If injury occurs, however, management depends on the location and mechanism of injury.

If the ureter is ligated with suture, the suture should be removed and the ureter assessed for viability. If it is deemed viable, a stent should be placed. This procedure can be performed by cystoscopy or by performing a cystotomy and then placing a stent [5].

If there is a partial transection injury, a ureteral stent should be placed in the ureterotomy, and the defect closed with 5-0 polyglycolic acid suture [5]. Repair of a complete transection ureteral injury depends on the location. If the injury occurs in the upper or middle third of the ureter, a ureteroureterostomy can be performed [5]. This method, however, is successful only if there is adequate length to allow a tension-free repair and sometimes requires mobilizing the kidney. A ureteroureterostomy is performed by trimming and spatulating the proximal and distal ends of the ureter, with the spatulation on opposite sides of the segments. The ends are sutured together with fine absorbable suture. The spatulation allows a larger lumen and a watertight seal.

If transection occurs within 6 cm of the ureterovesical junction, a ureteroureterostomy should not be performed because of the risk of compromising the vascularity to this distal segment [5]. In such situations, a ureteroneocystotomy with psoas hitch can be performed [5]. With this procedure, the distal segment first is ligated with permanent suture. The bladder then is mobilized from its attachment in the retropubic space. A cystotomy then is performed on the ventral surface of the bladder with the incision running in the direction of the ureteroneocystotomy so as to elongate the bladder. The bladder then is attached to the psoas tendon with two 3-0 nylon sutures. The ureter then is sutured to the bladder over a stent.

*Bladder injury*

Patients who have a history of prior surgery and malignancy are at a higher risk of bladder injury during hysterectomy [3,8]. A history of cesarean section specifically increases the risk of unintentional cystotomy, probably because of the prior scarring between the bladder base and pubo-vesicocervical fascia [9,10]. A history of cesarean section is not necessarily a contraindication for vaginal hysterectomy, because in patients who have a history of a cesarean section the rates of unintentional cystotomy are similar for hysterectomies performed by the abdominal and vaginal routes [9]. During abdominal hysterectomy, the bladder is at risk for injury during the creation of the bladder flap, when the the bladder dome is dissected from the lower uterine segment. Most of the bladder injuries that occur during vaginal hysterectomy occur during dissection of the bladder from the vaginal wall and can involve the trigone [3]. The surgeon must be cognizant of the location of the ureteral orifices when an injury occurs during a vaginal hysterectomy.

When a cystotomy is recognized intraoperatively, the surgeon should complete the hysterectomy before repairing the bladder. Removing the uterus provides optimal visualization during the bladder repair. Bladder injury at the time of vaginal hysterectomy can be repaired successfully from the vaginal route with adequate mobilization and a tension-free, layered repair [3].

A cystotomy should be closed in two layers. The urothelium can be closed with 2-0 chromic suture, and the detrusor muscle is closed with 2-0 polyglycolic acid suture in a running Lembert technique [5]. The bladder then should be catheterized for 5 to 7 days to allowing healing.

*Bowel injury*

The incidence of bowel injury during hysterectomy is low, approximately 0.3% [11]. Bowel injury can occur during adhesiolysis or during dissection in the posterior cul-de-sac. There is a higher rate of bowel injury with abdominal hysterectomy than with vaginal hysterectomy [12].

If less than 50% of the circumference of the bowel wall is injured, a suture repair may be performed in a direction perpendicular to the lumen to avoid narrowing. Larger defects, multiple defects, thermal injuries, or injuries involving the vasculature require resection of the affected bowel segments.

When there is concern about a rectal injury, but an actual defect is not obvious, the surgeon should perform a bubble test [12]. This test consists of insufflating air into the anus through a 22-Fr Foley catheter or sigmoidoscope after the pelvis is irrigated with saline solution. The presence of bubbles confirms a rectal injury. This test can be performed during laparotomy or laparoscopy.

Although uncommon, bowel injury can occur with laparoscopy, specifically with the insertion of the Veress needle and the initial trocar insertion. A meta-analysis evaluating the risk of bowel injury with major operative laparoscopy found the incidence to be 0.33% [13]. Injuries can occur at various locations along the bowel, and patients who have a history of previous abdominal surgery are at a greater risk for such injuries. Although uncommon, gastric injury can occur during Veress needle insertion. The risk can be decreased by gastric decompression before entry. Should an injury occur, it usually heals spontaneously if it is hemostatic and is smaller than 5 mm [5]. Larger injuries often can be repaired laparoscopically, depending on the extent of the defect.

Unrecognized thermal bowel injury during laparoscopy can have a disastrous outcome. Tissue necrosis and then perforation of the affected bowel can occur 72 to 96 hours after surgery. One must have a high index of suspicion for such an injury in patients presenting with fever and abdominal pain several days after an operative laparoscopy [5]. Up to 15% of bowel injuries are not noted at the time of laparoscopy. One study found that one in five cases of delayed diagnosis of bowel injury resulted in death [13].

*Vascular injuries*

When bleeding occurs, the surgeon must use knowledge of pelvic anatomy to achieve hemostasis safely. Blindly clamping areas of bleeding can lead to ureteral injury or worsen the ongoing bleeding. Basic surgical techniques such as pressure, the use of the electrosurgical unit, or vessel ligation should be employed first. If these measures fail to control bleeding, the surgeon needs to employ other measures to achieve hemostasis. The literature has described a range of techniques that have been successful in the face of pelvic hemorrhage.

One such modality is the use of tissue sealants [14]. Several manufacturers make a fibrin sealant that contains both fibrinogen and thrombin (eg, Tisseel, Baxter Healthcare, Deerfield, Illinois; Evicel, OMRIX Biopharmaceuticals Ltd, Israel). These agents contain a supraphysiologic concentration of fibrinogen that, when mixed with thrombin, augments the terminal stage of the coagulation cascade. These compounds rapidly form a clot. Gelatin matrix solutions (eg, FloSeal, Baxter Healthcare) are another option for achieving hemostasis. These solutions contain only thrombin and require contact with the fibrinogen in blood to form a fibrin polymer clot. Gelatin matrix solutions are a pure hemostatic agent.

Another technique that can be used is bilateral hypogastric artery ligation. After incising the peritoneum overlying the common iliac artery, the surgeon identifies the bifurcation of the hypogastric artery and external iliac artery [5]. A dissection is performed between the hypogastric artery and vein, at least 2 cm from the bifurcation. This dissection should be performed in a lateral-to-medial direction to avoid injury to the hypogastric vein. Furthermore, the artery should be ligated at least 2 cm from the bifurcation to avoid ligation of the posterior division of the internal iliac artery, which can lead to ischemia of the skin and subcutaneous tissue of the gluteus.

Papp and colleagues [15] reported a series of 80 gynecologic cases of intractable pelvic hemorrhage, 41 of which were controlled successfully with bilateral hypogastric artery ligation. Although no ureter or bowel complications were noted, one hypogastric vein injury was managed by clamping and ligating.

Acute pelvic hemorrhage has been treated successfully using pelvic vessel arterial embolization [16]. This procedure can identify the bleeding vessel by angiography and occlude it with various materials. This method, however, may be more effective for acute arterial bleeding than for venous bleeding.

When all measures fail, it sometimes is necessary simply to pack the area that is bleeding, especially in the face of a coagulopathy. Multiple laparotomy sponges are packed into a bag over the concerning area to tamponade the bleeding [17]. The abdomen is closed and re-explored approximately 48 hours later. When packing, the surgeon must avoid excessive pressure on the inferior vena cava so to avoid comprising renal function.

## Specific circumstances

### Laparoscopic trocar–related injury

The most common complication of laparoscopic surgery is injury of the superficial or inferior epigastric vessels [18]. This injury is diagnosed by bleeding from the trocar site. Injury to the inferior epigastric vessel can cause retroperitoneal or intraperitoneal bleeding, and injury to the superficial epigastric vessels can cause subcutaneous or intramuscular bleeding. Many techniques for controlling epigastric vessel bleeding have been described. These techniques include compression with a 12-Fr Foley catheter inserted through the trocar sleeve, passing suture through the abdominal wall caudad and cephalad to the trocar to ligate the injured vessel, or bipolar coagulation of the vessel through the peritoneum [18].

Vascular injury in the abdominal wall can be avoided by understanding the course of these vessels and by identifying them before trocar placement. Both transillumination and direct visualization have been advocated for identifying the superficial and inferior epigastric vessels, respectively, before lateral trocar placement. Transillumination, however, has been found to be effective in identifying the superficial epigastric vessels only 64% of the time, and this technique is less effective in patients who have dark skin and a body mass index greater than 25 kg/m$^2$ [19]. Laparoscopic visualization of the inferior epigastric vessels is successful in more than 80% of patients. Because visualization or transillumination is not always possible, knowledge of the course of the epigastric vessels sometimes is helpful. Saber and colleagues [20] performed CT mapping of the inferior and superficial epigastric vessels and found that these vessels usually are located between 4 and 8 cm from midline. They are most lateral at the level of the pubis and are most medial at the midpoint between the pubis and umbilicus [20].

Vascular and bowel complications from laparoscopy can occur during creation of the pneumoperitoneum and placement of the initial trocar.

Dixon and Carrillo [21] described a series of seven iliac vascular injuries that occurred during initial trocar/needle insertion with closed laparoscopy. Right-sided iliac injuries were more common, and the right common iliac vein was the most common site of injury. Interestingly, the common factor for all injuries was the level of surgeon experience. All injuries occurred with surgeons who had performed less than 20 laparoscopies.

Once a vascular injury is recognized during laparoscopy, immediate conversion to exploratory laparotomy and application of the appropriate vascular surgical procedures are required to minimize morbidity and mortality.

In a retrospective comparison of open laparoscopy and closed laparoscopy (Veress needle or blind insertion of first trocar), Bonjer and colleagues [22] found the rates of vascular injury to be 0.075% with closed laparoscopy and 0% with open laparoscopy. Visceral injury rates were 0.083% and 0.048%, respectively [22]. Although the differences in this study were statistically significant, the overall risk for both techniques is low. In fact, a meta-analysis analyzing various entry techniques found no evidence that open laparoscopy is superior or inferior to other entry techniques [23].

## Hysteroscopy

### Uterine perforation during hysteroscopy

Uterine perforation is a complication of approximately 1.5% of hysteroscopic procedures [24]. Uterine perforation must be suspected if the uterine sound can be passed further than the known size of the uterus, if there is difficulty in maintaining distension of the uterine cavity, or if bowel is visualized [18]. Measures used to minimize the risk of uterine perforation include preoperative bimanual examination to determine the size and position of the uterus and the use of transabdominal ultrasound during passage of the cervical dilators to confirm intrauterine location.

The location and method of perforation dictate further management. A uterine fundal perforation usually can be managed expectantly if it is made with a uterine sound or narrow dilator. If there is no evidence of bleeding from the uterus, conservative management with or without a short course of antibiotics may be considered [25]. If there is evidence of bleeding, or if the perforation was made with a sharp instrument, abdominal exploration with laparoscopy and possibly laparotomy may be indicated.

Anterior or posterior wall uterine perforations can occur in patients who have an extremely anteverted or retroverted uterus. Because the bladder and rectum are in these respective locations, one must consider further evaluation with cystoscopy or laparoscopy if there is a concern for bladder or bowel injury.

Lateral uterine wall perforations should be followed by prompt laparoscopy because of the concern for vascular injury. Perforations in these locations can damage the uterine vessels, and a broad ligament hematoma may be seen during laparoscopy [26].

### Complications caused by hysteroscopic distension media

High-viscosity (eg, dextran 70), low-viscosity/electrolyte-poor (eg, glycine and sorbitol), and low-viscosity/electrolyte-containing (eg, normal saline and lactated Ringer's solution) medias are commonly used for distension of the uterus during hysteroscopy. The use and safety profiles of these medias vary, however.

Dextran 70 is used because of its excellent visibility, but the manufacturer recommends that no more than 250 mL be absorbed because of the concern for pulmonary edema. Anaphylactic reactions and coagulopathy also are rare complications that have been described [25].

Glycine and sorbitol allow the use of monopolar cautery during operative hysteroscopy. Large volume deficits have been associated with hyponatremic hypervolemia, however. After intravasation, glycine and sorbitol are metabolized, leaving free water [25]. This free water accumulates in the brain and increases intracranial pressure. When fluid deficits reach 1000 to 1500 mL, the procedure should be terminated, and the patient's serum electrolytes should be assessed. Patients who have excessive intravasation experience headache, nausea, vomiting, and agitation [27]. This manifestation can progress to pulmonary and cerebral edema. These patients require close monitoring and diuretic administration.

Unlike glycine and sorbitol, normal saline and lactated Ringer's solution have physiologic osmolarity and contain sodium. Although excessive intravasation does not lead to hyponatremia, it can lead to volume overload. Media deficits of greater than 2500 mL should prompt conclusion of the procedure, and the patient's electrolytes should be assessed [28].

Several fluid-management systems are available to monitor closely the amount of distension media lost during hysteroscopy. The amount of media intravasation can be lessened by using the minimum intrauterine pressure needed to perform the hysteroscopy, and by minimizing operating time. The physician must be aware that certain procedures such as endometrial ablation and resection of myomas open vascular channels and place the patient at increased risk for fluid overload [25].

## Postoperative complications

### Ileus and bowel obstruction

Postoperative ileus is characterized by abdominal distension, nausea, vomiting, abdominal pain, and delayed passage of flatus [29]. The stomach and small intestine usually resume normal activity 8 hours after surgery. The large bowel usually is the last segment to regain function after surgery, taking 48 to 72 hours after surgery. Factors predisposing patients to postoperative ileus include bowel manipulation and extensive adhesiolysis. Longer operating times also are associated with longer time to return of bowel function [29]. The incidence of postoperative ileus has been found to be 3% among patients undergoing total abdominal hysterectomy [29]. The mean time to first flatus among abdominal hysterectomy patients has been found to be 53 hours [29]. Several studies evaluating the safety of early feeding after major gynecologic surgery did not find an increased incidence of ileus [30,31].

Bowel obstruction can present similarly to postoperative ileus with the symptoms of nausea, vomiting, and abdominal pain. Bowel obstruction, however, will have a more delayed onset, with most patients having an initial period of normal bowel function. When there is a concern for ileus or bowel obstruction, management includes having the patient take nothing by mouth and administering intravenous fluid hydration, electrolyte repletion, and naso-gastric decompression. Small bowel obstruction can be managed conservatively as long as there is no evidence of bowel necrosis or strangulation. Fever, tachycardia, leukocytosis, and metabolic acidosis may be signs of bowel strangulation.

Studies evaluating the etiology of bowel obstruction have found that adhesions are the most common cause of bowel obstruction [32]. Among gynecologic procedures, total abdominal hysterectomy has been found to be the most common adhesion-related cause of bowel obstruction, with an incidence of 13.6 per 1000 procedures [32]. Adhesions to the previous laparotomy site were found in 75% of cases of bowel obstruction. The median time from surgery to presentation with bowel obstruction was 4 years.

Postoperative bowel complications occur less frequently with laparoscopy, probably because there is less bowel manipulation than with laparotomy. In fact, the combined rate of postoperative ileus and small bowel obstruction after operative laparoscopy is 0.036% [33]. Less invasive procedures also are associated with lower rates of bowel obstruction. Al-Sunaidi and Tulandi [32] did not find any greater incidence of bowel obstruction among patients who underwent laparoscopic supracervical hysterectomy than in patients who underwent abdominal hysterectomy.

*Incisional hernia*

The incidence of ventral hernia in patients who have undergone a vertical midline incision is 10% to 16% [34,35]. In an effort to determine if surgical technique can affect the rate of hernia, a prospective study compared a non-locking continuous technique with the interrupted, Smead Jones technique for closure of a vertical midline laparotomy using looped polyglycolic suture [34]. With follow-up of up to 3 years, the authors found no significant difference in the incidence of hernia between the two techniques. Almost 90% of hernias were diagnosed within the first year after surgery [34]. Risk factors for hernia include a body mass index greater than 27 kg/m$^2$, diabetes, and wound infection [35]. Unlike vertical midline incisions, patients who have a history of only one Pfannenstiel incision have a very low incidence of hernia [36].

Incisional hernias after laparoscopy are rare events, especially with the increasing use of smaller, bladeless trocars. When bladed trocars have been used, trocar-site hernias have been found to occur in 0.23% of the sites where 10-mm trocars were used and in 3.1% of the sites where 12-mm trocars were used [37]. Given these higher rates of hernia, it is recommended that the fascia be closed at sites where bladed trocars 10-mm and larger are placed. There are data, however, suggesting that the newer nonbladed trocars do not cause as much fascial trauma and do not require fascial closure. Prospective studies have evaluated the incidence of hernia at lateral port sites above the arcuate line where 10-mm and 12-mm nonbladed trocars were used and no fascial closure was performed. The rates of trocar site hernia ranged from 0% to 0.2% [38,39]. This lower rate of trocar-site hernia is thought to result from the smaller residual fascial defect after the these trocars are removed, which has been found to be 6 to 8 mm after removal of 10-mm and 12-mm bladeless trocars [38].

## Infection

The risk of postoperative infection after hysterectomy, including wound infections and pelvic abscesses, has been found to be between 3% and 10%. Most pelvic and incisional infections are polymicrobial [5]. Abdominal hysterectomy is associated with a higher risk of infection than vaginal hysterectomy [40,41]. Measures to decrease the risk of infection include a preoperative antiseptic shower the night before surgery, appropriate skin preparation, and prophylactic antibiotics. Although antiseptic showers have not been shown definitely to decrease the rate of infection, the Centers for Disease Control and Prevention strongly recommends this practice, because it decreases the skin microbial count [42]. Commonly used preoperative skin preparations include povidone-iodine and chlorhexidine. Although a recent study has shown lower bacterial colony counts with the use of chlorhexidine, prospective studies evaluating its efficacy in prevention of post-hysterectomy infection are lacking [43]. One measure that has been proven to decrease postoperative infection is the use of prophylactic antibiotics. Administration of intravenous antibiotics 1 hour before hysterectomy has been shown to decrease postoperative infections by 25% to 30% [40,44]. Broad-spectrum antibiotics are used for prophylaxis. Cefazolin (1 g) is the most commonly used antibiotic because of its relatively long half-life and low cost [45]. Among gynecologic procedures, prophylactic antibiotics are indicated only for hysterectomies [45]. Laparoscopy, hysteroscopy, and laparotomy without hysterectomy do not require prophylactic antibiotics.

## Wound complications

The incidence of wound infection complicating abdominal hysterectomy has been found to be 3% to 8% [46]. Most wound complications, such as infection, hematoma, and seroma, result in an open wound. These incisions should be opened, irrigated, and débrided as necessary. After they are open, the wounds can heal either by secondary intention or by reclosure with surgical re-approximation. Complete healing by secondary intention can take between 2 and 8 weeks [46]. In a meta-analysis by Wechter and colleagues [46] of disrupted laparotomy wounds, reclosure resulted in faster healing times, 16 to 23 days, versus 61 to 72 days for secondary intention. Generally, reclosure should be performed around 4 days after wound opening. Both en bloc mass techniques, incorporating 3 cm of tissue on each side of the incision, and vertical mattress suture techniques have been described for closure. Vertical mattress closures, however, may make reclosure in the office more practical, because reclosure can be done easily with local anesthesia. Various suture materials have been used successfully. The sutures usually are removed around 10 days after placement.

Obesity has been found to be an independent risk factor for wound complications [41]. Unfortunately, several studies evaluating the efficacy of drain placement or subcutaneous tissue reapproximation have shown no decrease in the rate of wound complications in obese patients [47,48].

## Vaginal cuff abscess

Patients who have a vaginal cuff abscess typically present with fever and pelvic pain after hysterectomy. Management includes intravenous antibiotics and drainage. It may be reasonable, based on the clinical scenario, to treat the patient first with antibiotics. Recommended regimens include imipenem-cilastin, clindamycin/gentamicin, or the addition of metronidazole if there is a suspicion for anaerobes [5]. If there is no clinical improvement, surgical drainage is recommended.

## Vaginal cuff dehiscence

Vaginal cuff dehiscence can present with either abdominal pain or a report of a vaginal bulge. Vaginal cuff dehiscence has been found to occur between 4 weeks and more than a year after surgery [49]. A history of recent intercourse frequently precedes presentation [49]. If there is no bowel injury, a vaginal cuff dehiscence can be repaired vaginally in most instances.

Hur and colleagues [49] evaluated the incidence of vaginal cuff dehiscence after hysterectomy by mode of hysterectomy. They found a significant increase in vaginal cuff dehiscence in patients who underwent total laparoscopic hysterectomy (4.9%) when compared with abdominal (0.12%) and vaginal hysterectomy (0.29%). The authors postulated that this finding might result from the effect of thermal energy on the vaginal cuff when it is transected from the cervix.

## Neuropathy

The lumbosacral plexus supplies many nerves that travel through the pelvis and therefore are at risk for injury during gynecologic surgery. A review of the literature identified improper placement of self-retaining or fixed retractors, improper positioning of patients in the lithotomy position preoperatively, and radical surgical dissection to be three major predisposing risk factors for neurologic injury at the time of gynecologic surgery [50]. In a review of 1210 patients undergoing major pelvic surgery, Cardosi and colleagues [51] found that 1.9% of patients suffered a postoperative neuropathy. The range of injuries included surgical trauma, stretch, suture entrapment, and retractor-related injuries. With physiotherapy and medical or surgical treatment, 73% of patients experienced complete resolution of symptoms [51].

### Femoral nerve injury

Iatrogenic femoral nerve injury occurs in up to 11% of abdominal hysterectomies [52]. The femoral nerve is at risk from injury by direct compression from a retractor or from stretch from incorrect high-lithotomy positioning. In the former case, compression of a retractor blade on the iliopsoas muscle in which the nerve runs can result in injury. In the latter case, excessive hip flexion and abduction with external hip rotation results in extreme angulation of the femoral nerve beneath the inguinal ligament. Femoral nerve injury presents with weakness or inability to flex the hip or extend the knee or with paresthesia over the anterior and medial thigh [50].

In a prospective evaluation comparing self-retaining retractors and handheld retractors, 7.5% of patients in the self-retaining retractor group experienced a femoral neuropathy, compared with 0.7% in the group without self-retaining retractors [53].

### Lateral femoral cutaneous nerve injury

The lateral femoral cutaneous nerve is at risk for injury from compression by a self-retaining retractor. Injury to this nerve presents postoperatively with pain and paresthesia in the anterior and posterior lateral thigh [50].

### Genitofemoral nerve injury

The genitofemoral nerve runs along the ventral surface of the psoas muscle. It is most at risk during external iliac lymph node dissections. Transection of this nerve results in paresthesia of the ipsilateral mons, labia majora, and skin overlying the femoral triangle [50].

*Obturator nerve injury*

The obturator nerve lies among the nodal tissue in the obturator space, predisposing it to injury during lymph node dissections. Injury to this nerve can result in sensory loss in the upper thigh or weakness in the hip adductors [50]. If this nerve is injured, it should be repaired immediately to preserve motor function. The epineural sheaths should be aligned with care to avoid misalignment of the neural fascicles. The nerve endings then should be re-approximated with 8-0 and 10-0 nylon. Repair followed by physical therapy usually results in complete recovery.

*Common peroneal nerve*

The common peroneal nerve runs superficially across the lateral head of the fibula and descends down the lateral calf. Because of its superficial position, this nerve is at risk for compression injury, especially when a patient's lateral knee rests on the boot in low-lithotomy stirrups. The calf must be supported appropriately to avoid injury. Injury to this nerve can cause foot drop and lateral lower-extremity paresthesia [50].

## Incisional pain

Approximately 1% to 4% of patients who undergo a Pfannenstiel incision experience postoperative suprapubic or groin pain [36,54]. This pain usually is from an injury to the ilioinguinal or iliohypogastric nerves. These nerves are most at risk when the incision extends lateral to the rectus muscle and into the internal oblique muscle. Injury to the ilioinguinal and iliohypogastric nerves from laparoscopic trocar insertion also has been described [51].

Often, pain can result from a neuroma. A neuroma occurs when a peripheral nerve is damaged or becomes engulfed in scar tissue. A neuroma should be suspected in patients who have pain lasting more than 6 months that has not responded to nonsteroidal anti-inflammatory drugs, gabapentin, or scar message. Clinical features suggestive of a neuroma include delayed onset of postoperative pain, hyperesthesia around the incision, numbness, referred pain, and reproduction of the pain with point percussion (Tinel's sign). Both diagnostic nerve blocks and electromyography have been described for diagnosing neuromas. Treatment of a neuroma includes resection followed by implantation of the proximal nerve stump into muscle to avoid recurrence. This technique has been found to be very effective in the treatment of patients known to have a postoperative neuroma [55].

## Deep venous thromboembolism/pulmonary emboli

The incidence of deep venous thromboembolism (DVT) among patients undergoing major gynecologic surgery is 7% to 47% depending on the associated risk factors [56]. Although the incidence of pulmonary embolism

(PE) among patients who have benign findings is 0.3%, in gynecologic oncology patients undergoing major abdominal surgery the incidence of PE within 7 weeks of surgery is 4.1% [57].

Multiple risk factors for formation of DVT have been identified, including obesity, malignancy, pelvic surgery, smoking, age greater than 40 years, history of DVT/PE, diabetes, and thrombophilias [57,58]. Early intervention with prophylaxis is imperative, because 50% of all perioperative DVTs form during the operation, and an additional 25% form within 72 hours of surgery [59].

Strategies to prevent DVT include early ambulation, the use of pneumatic compression devices, and various anticoagulants. Maxwell and colleagues [60] found low molecular weight heparin and external compression to be equally effective in postoperative prophylaxis of DVT among patients who had a gynecologic malignancy. There were no statistically significant increases in bleeding complications in patients treated with low molecular weight heparin when compared with patients treated with external pneumatic compression. Table 1 lists various prophylactic measures.

## Cardiac complications

Perioperative myocardial infarction occurs in about 3% of patients undergoing noncardiac surgery, but this rate varies with different risk factors [61]. Myocardial infarction often is a difficult diagnosis to make, because only 14% of patients who are found to have a myocardial infarction

Table 1
Recommendations for deep vein thrombosis prophylaxis for gynecologic surgery

| Procedure | Additional risk factors | Intervention |
| --- | --- | --- |
| Gynecologic procedure < 30 minutes | None | None |
| Gynecologic laparoscopic procedures | Present | LDUH, LMWH, IPC, or GCS |
| Major gynecologic surgery for benign disease | None | IPC started just before surgery, or LDUH, 5000 units bid, or once-daily LMWH |
| Major gynecologic surgery for benign disease | Present | LDUH, 5000 units tid; higher dose of LMW; consider combination with IPC or GCS |
| Major gynecologic surgery for malignancy | Present or absent | LDUH, 5000 units tid; higher dose of LMWH; consider combination with IPC or GCS |

*Abbreviations:* bid, twice daily; GCS, graduated compression stockings; IPC, intermittent pneumatic compression; LDUH, low-dose unfractionated heparin; LMWH, low molecular weight heparin; tid, three times daily.

*Data from* Geerts WH, Pineo GF, Heit JA, et al. Prevention of venous thromboembolism: the Seventh ACCP Conference on Antithrombotic and Thrombolytic Therapy. Chest 2004; 126(Suppl 3):338S–400S.

complain of chest pain. A rise in troponin and ECG changes most commonly lead to the diagnosis of a perioperative myocardial infarction.

Surgery predisposes patients to myocardial ischemia. Large volume shifts, blood loss, heart rate elevations, and increased postoperative platelet reactivity all place patients, especially those who have underlying coronary disease, at risk for cardiac events. Preoperatively, patients at high cardiac risk should be identified so that appropriate testing and therapeutic measures can minimize risk. This preoperative evaluation determines risk by assessing patient-specific variables, exercise capacity, and the surgery-specific risk [62]. Following the American College of Cardiology and the American Heart Association evaluation and management guidelines can optimize a patient's preoperative medical management and provide a low rate of perioperative cardiac complications [63].

## Summary

The gynecologic surgeon must be knowledgeable about common intraoperative and postoperative complications to decrease the risk of patient morbidity. Any time there is a concern for a urinary tract injury or bowel injury, the surgeon should perform a thorough investigation to determine the location of the defect or to rule out the occurrence of an injury. Pelvic hemorrhage should be managed with sound surgical technique, always being cognizant of the location of the ureter. Additional measures such as the use of tissue sealants and bilateral hypogastric artery ligation sometimes are needed to achieve hemostasis. The incidence of postoperative infection is decreased with the proper administration of prophylactic antibiotics before hysterectomy. Wound complications that require reopening the incision can be closed by secondary intention or with reclosure. Neuropathies can be avoided with proper patient positioning, retractor placement, and attention to anatomy. The risks of postoperative DVT/PE can be lowered with the appropriate prophylaxis, and the risks of postoperative myocardial infarction can be lowered with the appropriate preoperative evaluation and medical management.

## References

[1] Bai SW, Huh EH, Jung da J, et al. Urinary tract injuries during pelvic surgery: incidence rates and predisposing factors. Int Urogynecol J Pelvic Floor Dysfunct 2006;17:360–4.
[2] Vakili B, Chesson RR, Kyle BL, et al. The incidence of urinary tract injury during hysterectomy: a prospective analysis based on universal cystoscopy. Am J Obstet Gynecol 2005;192: 1599–604.
[3] Dorairajan G, Rani PR, Habeebullah S, et al. Urological injuries during hysterectomies: a 6-year review. J Obstet Gynaecol Res 2004;30:430–5.
[4] Liapis A, Bakas P, Giannopoulos V, et al. Ureteral injuries during gynecological surgery. Int Urogynecol J Pelvic Floor Dysfunct 2001;12:391–3.

[5] Rock J, Jones H. TeLinde's operative gynecology. 9th edition. Philadelphia: Lippincott Williams and Wilkins; 2003.

[6] Leonard F, Fotso A, Borghese B, et al. Ureteral complications from laparoscopic hysterectomy indicated for benign uterine pathologies: a 13-year experience in a continuous series of 1300 patients. Hum Reprod 2007;22:2006–11.

[7] Nezhat FNC, Nezhat CR. Averting complications of laparoscopy: pearls from 5 patients. OBG Management 2007;19:69.

[8] Rooney CM, Crawford AT, Vassallo BJ, et al. Is previous cesarean section a risk for incidental cystotomy at the time of hysterectomy? A case-controlled study. Am J Obstet Gynecol 2005;193:2041–4.

[9] Carley ME, McIntire D, Carley JM, et al. Incidence, risk factors and morbidity of unintended bladder or ureter injury during hysterectomy. Int Urogynecol J Pelvic Floor Dysfunct 2002;13:18–21.

[10] Boukerrou M, Lambaudie E, Collinet P, et al. A history of cesareans is a risk factor in vaginal hysterectomies. Acta Obstet Gynecol Scand 2003;82:1135–9.

[11] Kafy S, Huang JY, Al-Sunaidi M, et al. Audit of morbidity and mortality rates of 1792 hysterectomies. J Minim Invasive Gynecol 2006;13:55–9.

[12] Cosson M, Lambaudie E, Boukerrou M, et al. Vaginal, laparoscopic, or abdominal hysterectomies for benign disorders: immediate and early postoperative complications. Eur J Obstet Gynecol Reprod Biol 2001;98:231–6.

[13] Brosens I, Gordon A, Campo R, et al. Bowel injury in gynecologic laparoscopy. J Am Assoc Gynecol Laparosc 2003;10:9–13.

[14] Pursifull NF, Morey AF. Tissue glues and nonsuturing techniques. Curr Opin Urol 2007;17: 396–401.

[15] Papp Z, Toth-Pal E, Papp C, et al. Hypogastric artery ligation for intractable pelvic hemorrhage. Int J Gynaecol Obstet 2006;92:27–31.

[16] Mokrzycki ML, Hampton BS. Pelvic arterial embolization in the setting of acute hemorrhage as a result of the anterior Prolift procedure. Int Urogynecol J Pelvic Floor Dysfunct 2007;18:813–5.

[17] Wydra D, Emerich J, Ciach K, et al. Surgical pelvic packing as a means of controlling massive intraoperative bleeding during pelvic posterior exenteration—a case report and review of the literature. Int J Gynecol Cancer 2004;14:1050–4.

[18] Donnez J, Nisolle M. An atlas of operative laparoscopy and hysteroscopy. 2nd edition. New York: The Parthenon Publishing Group Inc.; 2001.

[19] Hurd WW, Amesse LS, Gruber JS, et al. Visualization of the epigastric vessels and bladder before laparoscopic trocar placement. Fertil Steril 2003;80:209–12.

[20] Saber AA, Meslemani AM, Davis R, et al. Safety zones for anterior abdominal wall entry during laparoscopy: a CT scan mapping of epigastric vessels. Ann Surg 2004;239:182–5.

[21] Dixon M, Carrillo EH. Iliac vascular injuries during elective laparoscopic surgery. Surg Endosc 1999;13:1230–3.

[22] Bonjer HJ, Hazebroek EJ, Kazemier G, et al. Open versus closed establishment of pneumoperitoneum in laparoscopic surgery. Br J Surg 1997;84:599–602.

[23] Vilos GA, Ternamian A, Dempster J, et al. Laparoscopic entry: a review of techniques, technologies, and complications. J Obstet Gynaecol Can 2007;29:434–65.

[24] Overton C, Hargreaves J, Maresh M. A national survey of the complications of endometrial destruction for menstrual disorders: the MISTLETOE study. Minimally Invasive Surgical Techniques–Laser, EndoThermal or Endorescetion. Br J Obstet Gynaecol 1997;104:1351–9.

[25] Cooper JM, Brady RM. Intraoperative and early postoperative complications of operative hysteroscopy. Obstet Gynecol Clin North Am 2000;27:347–66.

[26] Isaacson KB. Complications of hysteroscopy. Obstet Gynecol Clin North Am 1999;26: 39–51.

[27] Witz CA, Silverberg KM, Burns WN, et al. Complications associated with the absorption of hysteroscopic fluid media. Fertil Steril 1993;60:745–56.

[28] American College of Obstetricians and Gynecologists. Hysteroscopy. Obstet Gynecol 2005; 106:439–92.

[29] Wolff BG, Viscusi ER, Delaney CP, et al. Patterns of gastrointestinal recovery after bowel resection and total abdominal hysterectomy: pooled results from the placebo arms of alvimopan phase III North American clinical trials. J Am Coll Surg 2007;205:43–51.

[30] MacMillan SL, Kammerer-Doak D, Rogers RG, et al. Early feeding and the incidence of gastrointestinal symptoms after major gynecologic surgery. Obstet Gynecol 2000;96:604–8.

[31] Schilder JM, Hurteau JA, Look KY, et al. A prospective controlled trial of early postoperative oral intake following major abdominal gynecologic surgery. Gynecol Oncol 1997;67: 235–40.

[32] Al-Sunaidi M, Tulandi T. Adhesion-related bowel obstruction after hysterectomy for benign conditions. Obstet Gynecol 2006;108:1162–6.

[33] Milad MP, Escobar JC, Sanders W. Partial small bowel obstruction and ileus following gynecologic laparoscopy. J Minim Invasive Gynecol 2007;14:64–7.

[34] Colombo M, Maggioni A, Parma G, et al. A randomized comparison of continuous versus interrupted mass closure of midline incisions in patients with gynecologic cancer. Obstet Gynecol 1997;89:684–9.

[35] Franchi M, Ghezzi F, Buttarelli M, et al. Incisional hernia in gynecologic oncology patients: a 10-year study. Obstet Gynecol 2001;97:696–700.

[36] Luijendijk RW, Jeekel J, Storm RK, et al. The low transverse Pfannenstiel incision and the prevalence of incisional hernia and nerve entrapment. Ann Surg 1997;225:365–9.

[37] Kadar N, Reich H, Liu CY, et al. Incisional hernias after major laparoscopic gynecologic procedures. Am J Obstet Gynecol 1993;168:1493–5.

[38] Liu CD, McFadden DW. Laparoscopic port sites do not require fascial closure when non-bladed trocars are used. Am Surg 2000;66:853–4.

[39] Rosenthal RJ, Szomstein S, Kennedy CI, et al. Direct visual insertion of primary trocar and avoidance of fascial closure with laparoscopic roux-en-Y gastric bypass. Surg Endosc 2007; 21:124–8.

[40] Lofgren M, Poromaa IS, Stjerndahl JH, et al. Postoperative infections and antibiotic prophylaxis for hysterectomy in Sweden: a study by the Swedish National Register for Gynecologic Surgery. Acta Obstet Gynecol Scand 2004;83:1202–7.

[41] Molina-Cabrillana J, Valle-Morales L, Hernandez-Vera J, et al. Surveillance and risk factors on hysterectomy wound infection rate in Gran Canaria, Spain. Eur J Obstet Gynecol Reprod Biol 2007;136:232–8.

[42] Mangram AJ, Horan TC, Pearson ML, et al. Guideline for prevention of surgical site infection, 1999. Hospital Infection Control Practices Advisory Committee. Infect Control Hosp Epidemiol 1999;20:250–78.

[43] Culligan PJ, Kubik K, Murphy M, et al. A randomized trial that compared povidone iodine and chlorhexidine as antiseptics for vaginal hysterectomy. Am J Obstet Gynecol 2005;192: 422–5.

[44] Ledger WJ. Prophylactic antibiotics in obstetrics-gynecology: a current asset, a future liability? Expert Rev Anti Infect Ther 2006;4:957–64.

[45] American College of Obstetricians and Gynecologists. ACOG practice bulletin no. 74. Antibiotic prophylaxis for gynecologic procedures. Obstet Gynecol 2006;108:225–34.

[46] Wechter ME, Pearlman MD, Hartmann KE. Reclosure of the disrupted laparotomy wound: a systematic review. Obstet Gynecol 2005;106:376–83.

[47] Cardosi RJ, Drake J, Holmes S, et al. Subcutaneous management of vertical incisions with 3 or more centimeters of subcutaneous fat. Am J Obstet Gynecol 2006;195:607–14.

[48] Ramsey PS, White AM, Guinn DA, et al. Subcutaneous tissue reapproximation, alone or in combination with drain, in obese women undergoing cesarean delivery. Obstet Gynecol 2005;105:967–73.

[49] Hur HC, Guido RS, Mansuria SM, et al. Incidence and patient characteristics of vaginal cuff dehiscence after different modes of hysterectomies. J Minim Invasive Gynecol 2007;14: 311–7.

[50] Irvin W, Andersen W, Taylor P, et al. Minimizing the risk of neurologic injury in gynecologic surgery. Obstet Gynecol 2004;103:374–82.

[51] Cardosi RJ, Cox CS, Hoffman MS. Postoperative neuropathies after major pelvic surgery. Obstet Gynecol 2002;100:240–4.

[52] Morgan K, Thomas EJ. Nerve injury at abdominal hysterectomy. Br J Obstet Gynaecol 1995;102:665–6.

[53] Goldman JA, Feldberg D, Dicker D, et al. Femoral neuropathy subsequent to abdominal hysterectomy. A comparative study. Eur J Obstet Gynecol Reprod Biol 1985;20:385–92.

[54] Kisielinski K, Conze J, Murken AH, et al. The Pfannenstiel or so called "bikini cut": still effective more than 100 years after first description. Hernia 2004;8:177–81.

[55] Ducic I, Moxley M, Al-Attar A. Algorithm for treatment of postoperative incisional groin pain after cesarean delivery or hysterectomy. Obstet Gynecol 2006;108:27–31.

[56] Oates-Whitehead RM, D'Angelo A, Mol B. WITHDRAWN: anticoagulant and aspirin prophylaxis for preventing thromboembolism after major gynaecological surgery. Cochrane Database Syst Rev 2007;4:CD003679.

[57] Martino MA, Borges E, Williamson E, et al. Pulmonary embolism after major abdominal surgery in gynecologic oncology. Obstet Gynecol 2006;107:666–71.

[58] Krivak TC, Zorn KK. Venous thromboembolism in obstetrics and gynecology. Obstet Gynecol 2007;109:761–77.

[59] Davis JD. Prevention, diagnosis, and treatment of venous thromboembolic complications of gynecologic surgery. Am J Obstet Gynecol 2001;184:759–75.

[60] Maxwell GL, Synan I, Dodge R, et al. Pneumatic compression versus low molecular weight heparin in gynecologic oncology surgery: a randomized trial. Obstet Gynecol 2001;98: 989–95.

[61] Devereaux PJ, Goldman L, Yusuf S, et al. Surveillance and prevention of major perioperative ischemic cardiac events in patients undergoing noncardiac surgery: a review. CMAJ 2005;173:779–88.

[62] Eagle KA, Berger PB, Calkins H, et al. ACC/AHA guideline update for perioperative cardiovascular evaluation for noncardiac surgery–executive summary: a report of the American College of Cardiology/American Heart Association Task Force on Practice Guidelines (Committee to Update the 1996 Guidelines on Perioperative Cardiovascular Evaluation for Noncardiac Surgery). J Am Coll Cardiol 2002;39:542–53.

[63] Cinello M, Nucifora G, Bertolissi M, et al. American College of Cardiology/American Heart Association perioperative assessment guidelines for noncardiac surgery reduces cardiologic resource utilization preserving a favourable clinical outcome. J Cardiovasc Med (Hagerstown) 2007;8:882–8.

ELSEVIER
SAUNDERS

SURGICAL
CLINICS OF
NORTH AMERICA

Surg Clin N Am 88 (2008) 361–390

# CT, MRI, PET, PET/CT, and Ultrasound in the Evaluation of Obstetric and Gynecologic Patients

Andrew C. Gjelsteen, MD*, Brian H. Ching, DO,
Mark W. Meyermann, DO, Douglas A. Prager, MD,
Thomas F. Murphy, MD, Bryan D. Berkey, MD,
Lex A. Mitchell, MD

*Department of Radiology, Tripler Army Medical Center,
1 Jarrett White Road, Honolulu, HI 96859-5000, USA*

Ectopic pregnancy has increased concurrently with a correlative rise in risk factors over the past 3 decades. Some of the risk factors associated with ectopic pregnancy include a history of pelvic inflammatory disease or endometriosis, prior tubal ligation or tuboplasty, the use of an intrauterine device, and pregnancies achieved through in vitro fertilization [1]. The good news is that despite the increase in the prevalence of ectopic pregnancy, the mortality rate (related most often to massive intraperitoneal hemorrhage) has decreased secondary to earlier detection and increased awareness [2].

Endovaginal ultrasound is the imaging modality widely accepted as the standard of care in evaluating the patient in whom an ectopic pregnancy is suspected. Indeed, endovaginal ultrasound gives exquisite visualization of the uterus and usually of the adnexae without harmful ionizing radiation exposure. The authors ensure that a current quantitative beta-human chorionic gonadotropin ($\beta$-hCG) (quant) is available or has been drawn before performing the study. Our laboratory uses the World Health Organization 3rd International Standard (ADVIA Centaur Total hCG Assay, Siemens Healthcare, Tarrytown, New York). The approach described herein is extremely helpful. Before performing endovaginal ultrasound, three possible clinical/imaging

Disclosure statement: The views expressed herein are of the authors and do not reflect the official policy of the Department of the Army, Department of Defense, or the US Government.

* Corresponding author.

*E-mail address:* andrew.gjelsteen@us.army.mil (A.C. Gjelsteen).

scenarios are considered: (1) an intrauterine pregnancy, either normal or abnormal; (2) an ectopic pregnancy; or (3) an "empty uterus."

An intrauterine pregnancy is confirmed by identifying a gestational sac with a yolk sac in the uterus (Fig. 1). In an early pregnancy (less than 5 weeks gestational age), only a small anechoic "cyst" is identified in the endometrium, preventing definitive positive identification of a gestational sac. This isolated finding could be confused with an incidental endometrial cyst or "pseudogestational sac," which is really blood in the central cavity; therefore, correlation with the quant is needed. As a rule of thumb, one should expect to see via endovaginal ultrasound a gestational sac with a quant of 1000 mIU/mL, a yolk sac with a quant of approximately 7000 mIU/mL, and an embryo with a quant of approximately 11,000 mIU/mL. This pattern is referred to as the 1/7/11 rule [3]. A normal intrauterine pregnancy should always be seen in the endometrium, eccentric to, and not in the central cavity of the uterus (Fig. 2). The central cavity is often visible as a specular reflection (caused by the reflective interface of each layer of endometrium). A normal intrauterine pregnancy will be eccentric to this specular reflection, burrowed into the wall of the endometrium.

Although extremely reassuring, identifying an intrauterine pregnancy does not exclude a coexisting ectopic pregnancy (defined as a heterotopic pregnancy). This type of pregnancy is rare, with an incidence at most of 1:5000 [4], increasing with assisted fertility and pelvic inflammatory disease. When an intrauterine pregnancy is identified, the authors attempt to get an accurate estimate of the gestational age using ultrasound criteria. Very early in a pregnancy, such attempts are accurate to within ±3 days and may eliminate problems associated with less accurate dating performed during subsequent obstetric ultrasounds or by relying on an often unreliable last menstrual

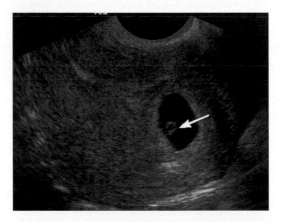

Fig. 1. Gestation sac in uterus with yolk sac (*tiny circle*) confirming an intrauterine pregnancy. On closer examination, some thickening on the yolk sac is visible (*arrow*), representing a tiny embryo consistent with a 6 week 0 day gestational age by endovaginal ultrasound. The patient's last menstrual period was exactly 6 weeks before examination.

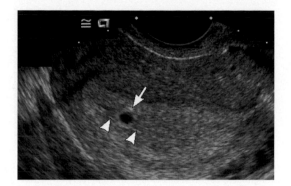

Fig. 2. Eccentric gestation sac. Note the specular reflection (*arrowheads*) seen as a thin echo-genic line. The specular reflection is the central cavity of the uterus. Note the eccentric gesta-tional sac (*arrow*) with an echogenic wall burrowed into the endometrium. Because only a gestational sac was seen measuring 5 mm, the date by ultrasound is 5 weeks 0 days.

period. The "Rule of Benson and Doubilet" is useful for normal gestations and states that if a 5-mm gestational sac is identified by endovaginal ultra-sound, it will be at 5 weeks gestational age; if a gestational sac plus yolk sac are seen, it will be at 5.5 weeks gestational age; and if a gestational sac plus yolk sac plus tiny embryo are seen, it will be at 6 weeks gestational age [5] (see Figs. 1 and 2). This rule should be accurate to within ±3 days. When an embryo is identified that is large enough to measure, the authors allow the ul-trasound machine to calculate the ultrasound date based on established tables in the software. Accurately dating the gestation is a beneficial byproduct of a first trimester ultrasound once ectopic pregnancy has been excluded.

An ectopic pregnancy is often visualized as a round echogenic mass usu-ally located between the uterus and ovary; however, it is also important to consider the rare cervical or interstitial (located in the corneal portion of the uterus) ectopic pregnancy. In most cases, the ectopic pregnancy is within the fallopian tube and will be appear as a rounded mass, usually with some peripheral flow representing the vascular supply (Figs. 3–5). Occasionally, an embryo with a heartbeat can be identified. Echogenic free fluid in the pelvis is a sign of rupture (Fig. 6). About 2% of ectopic pregnancies are located in the interstitial portion of the fallopian tube where it passes through the smooth muscle wall of the uterus and into the endometrium. These pregnancies may appear initially as intrauterine; however, a closer look will reveal a paucity of surrounding myometrium. There should be at least 5 mm of myometrium surrounding the gestational sac on all imaging planes (Fig. 7) [6]. In uncertain cases, an MRI should be obtained.

An "empty uterus" presents the greatest challenge. The three possibilities are (1) an intrauterine pregnancy that is too small to see (too early to tell) [6], (2) a spontaneous abortion, or (3) an occult ectopic pregnancy.

The authors would consider the finding of an intrauterine pregnancy that is too small to see with endovaginal ultrasound if the quant is less than

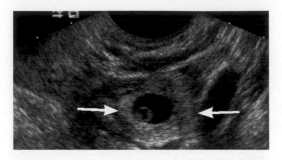

Fig. 3. Ectopic pregnancy in adnexae. Note the echogenic ring (*arrows*) with an inner yolk sac. An absent surrounding uterus confirms an ectopic pregnancy. A tiny embryo can be seen which appears to be on the yolk sac.

1000 mIU/mL. The quant is expected to double every 48 hours; however, some variability is allowed. For a normal intrauterine pregnancy that is too early to see, one would expect an increase every 48 hours of at least 60% to 70%. An endovaginal ultrasound is not pointless with very low quants, such as in the 100 to 200 range. Certainly, before modern times, not all women with ectopic pregnancies died of intraperitoneal hemorrhage. A percentage of these gestations must have died before rupture, most likely from the poor blood supply and environment of the fallopian tube. These ectopic gestations would be resorbed, and, at some point, the quant would return to normal. If these patients are imaged on the downward slope of a declining quant, there may be an advanced ectopic pregnancy with a very low quant. The key to recognizing this is that the gestational age based on the last menstrual period will be much farther along than the quant would suggest, likely past 7 to 8 weeks. A spontaneous abortion is likely given the passage of tissue. With a completed spontaneous abortion, the quant should drop quickly. Often, this can be confirmed with a subsequent quant a few hours later, which should show a definite decline. In

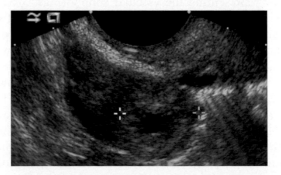

Fig. 4. This round mass was initially thought to be a corpus luteum in the ovary, a normal finding; however, by pushing on the probe, the mass was found to move independently of the ovary, confirming an ectopic pregnancy. A normal corpus luteum should not have been so echogenic.

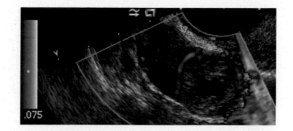

Fig. 5. Same patient and region shown in Fig. 4. Power Doppler images demonstrate a "ring of fire" classically seen in ectopic pregnancies. The bright red region in the lower right is flash artifact caused when the sensitivity is turned up.

approximately one third of all ectopic pregnancies, the actual ectopic is never seen on imaging studies. The diagnosis is made with a high quant and the ultrasound findings of an empty uterus. Although one would expect to see at least a gestational sac in the uterus with a quant of 1000 mIU/mL, this number is not an absolute cutoff, and a gray area exists. An empty uterus with a quant of 1000 mIU/mL or greater significantly raises our suspicion for an ectopic pregnancy.

## Imaging during pregnancy

The use of diagnostic imaging in the United States has grown considerably over the past years, and it is clear the growth will continue. Approximately 3 million CT scans were performed in 1980, and this number increased to approximately 60 million scans by 2005 [7]. Invariably, requests for imaging in women who are pregnant to evaluate acute pelvic pain have

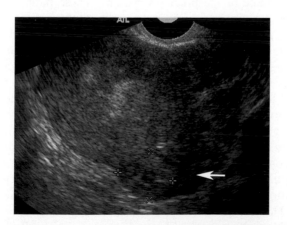

Fig. 6. The echogenic ring at the bottom of the image is an ectopic pregnancy. Note the slightly lesser echogenic mass partially surrounding the ectopic and outlining the uterus (*arrow*), consistent with hemorrhage, highly suggestive of rupture.

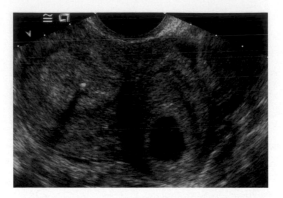

Fig. 7. Coronal endovaginal ultrasound image of uterus with shadowing intrauterine device centered in endometrium. Note the gestational sac at the periphery of the uterus, with less than 5 mm of surrounding myometrium, consistent with an interstitial (cornual) ectopic. Because there is generally a good blood supply, these ectopic pregnancies can progress to term with disastrous consequences.

paralleled this increase. The number of pregnant women exposed to ionizing radiation has more than doubled in the past decade [8]. The largest increase in imaging was with CT scans (25%), with approximately one third of the CT scans being performed in an evaluation for appendicitis.

Although the etiology of acute pelvic pain in a pregnant female may be other than acute appendicitis, this disease complicates approximately 1 in 1500 pregnancies and is the most common nonobstetric surgical emergency in pregnancy [9]. Acute appendicitis in pregnant women has been associated with premature labor as well as fetal and maternal death, especially when peritonitis from perforation occurs [10]. The diagnosis of acute appendicitis is difficult to make in the pregnant patient. These patients rarely present with the classic symptoms such as anorexia, fever, nausea, vomiting, and periumbilical pain localizing to the right lower abdominal quadrant. An elevated white count or elevated sedimentation rate is an unreliable parameter during pregnancy [11]. The location of the appendix is variable. During pregnancy as the uterus enlarges, the appendix commonly moves upward and outward toward the flank; therefore, the pain and tenderness may not be localized to the right lower abdominal quadrant (Fig. 8) [12].

Diagnostic imaging during pregnancy carries the risk of ionizing radiation exposure to the fetus. The human body absorbs approximately 90% of the diagnostic radiation to which it is exposed [13]. The radiation dose absorbed by a person (that is, the amount of energy deposited in human tissue by radiation) is measured using the conventional unit Rad or the SI unit Gray (Gy). The biologic risk of exposure to radiation is measured using the conventional unit Rem or the SI unit Sievert (Sv). The Rad, which stands for "radiation absorbed dose," was the conventional unit of measurement, but it has been replaced by the Gy.

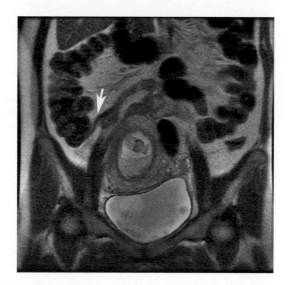

Fig. 8. MRI of the abdomen in a 31-year-old woman at 11 weeks gestation demonstrating a normal appendix (*arrow*).

A person's biologic risk (ie, the risk that a person will sustain health effects from an exposure to radiation) is measured using the conventional unit Rem or the SI unit Sievert [14]. Table 1 shows the relative radiation level designations along with common examples for each classification. The relative radiation level is included for each imaging examination to help assess potential adverse health effects associated with radiation exposure.

The primary risk associated with exposure to ionizing radiation is cancer. It is estimated that approximately 1 in 1000 individuals will develop cancer from an exposure of 10 mSv [15]. The developing fetus is sensitive to radiation exposure. Organogenesis occurs predominantly between weeks 2 to 15 during gestation. During this time period, the fetus is most susceptible to the teratogenic effects of ionizing radiation. These effects include microcephaly, microphthalmia, mental retardation, growth retardation, behavioral defects, and cataracts. Teratogenic effects are extremely unlikely before 2 weeks and after 15 weeks gestation [16]. Guidelines for exposure limits are recommended by the National Council on Radiation Protection and Measurements (NRCP). The recommended maximum permissible radiation dose by the NRCP dose for a fetus throughout pregnancy is 5 mSv [17].

The carcinogenic potential of radiation has been studied for more than 50 years based on atomic bomb survivors. Although the correlation between prenatal radiation exposure and carcinogenesis is not well established, radiation doses from CT scans of the pelvis could potentially double the risk of developing childhood cancer [18]. In light of the teratogenic and carcinogenic risks from ionizing radiation, ultrasonography and MRI should be used as alternative imaging modalities whenever possible in the

Table 1
American College of Radiology appropriateness criteria, relative radiation level information

| Relative radiation level | Effective dose estimate range | Example examinations |
|---|---|---|
| None | 0 | Ultrasound, MRI |
| Minimal | <1 mSv | Chest radiographs, hand radiographs |
| Low | 1–5 mSv | Head CT, lumbar spine radiographs |
| Medium | 5–10 mSv | Abdomen CT, barium enema, nuclear medicine bone scan |
| High | >10 mSv | Abdomen CT without and with contrast, whole body PET |

Reprinted with permission of the American College of Radiology. No other representation of this material is authorized without express, written permission from the American College of Radiology, www.acr.org/ac.

evaluation of acute appendicitis (Fig. 9). Ultrasonography has demonstrated sensitivity of 100%, specificity of 96%, and accuracy of 98% [19]. MRI has demonstrated sensitivity of 100%, specificity of 93.6%, and accuracy of 94% [20]. The algorithm shown in Fig. 10 is used at the authors' center.

The pregnancy status of a female of childbearing age should be established before performing any imaging procedure that uses ionizing radiation. Other disease processes may result in the necessity for diagnostic imaging, such as trauma, pulmonary embolism, renal colic, and biliary disease. Ultrasonography and MRI should be employed when possible to avoid radiation exposure to the fetus, especially in the first trimester. If a CT scan is ultimately needed, the patient should be informed of the risks and benefits of the examination, and the radiation dose to the fetus should be kept as low as possible by using low dose techniques.

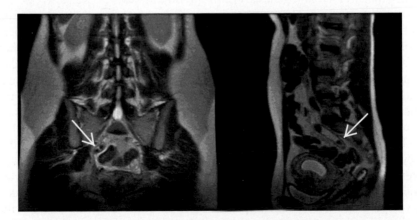

Fig. 9. MRI of the abdomen in a 22-year-old woman at 9 weeks gestation with pathology proven appendicitis and two fecaliths (*arrows*).

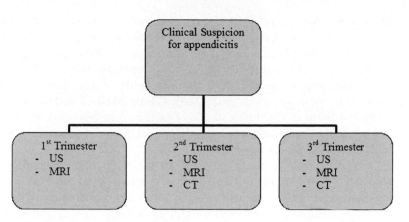

Fig. 10. Algorithm for imaging during pregnancy with suspected appendicitis.

*Imaging adnexal masses*

Endovaginal ultrasound is the imaging modality of choice in the initial evaluation of adnexal masses. There is always a trade-off between high frequency and low frequency scanning. High frequency scanning gives high quality images yet has poor penetration. The flexible vagina allows the tip of the endovaginal transducer to be placed within 1 to 2 cm of the area of interest, allowing a high scanning frequency and giving exquisite imaging. On occasion, the abnormality is too far from the probe on endovaginal ultrasound to obtain good images, which is why the authors always start with a transabdominal examination with a full bladder. This examination allows relatively unimpeded sound to reach deep into the pelvis, albeit, with a low frequency transducer yielding poorer quality images but a large field of view. We then have the patient empty her bladder and obtain an endovaginal ultrasound. Ultrasound also allows real-time imaging. If it is unclear whether a mass is connected to the ovary, one can push on the endovaginal probe. If the mass moves with the ovary, it is likely of ovarian origin. If the mass moves separately, it is almost certainly not of ovarian origin. Color flow Doppler and its variant, power Doppler, are useful in determining whether the mass is vascular; however, several reports have demonstrated that malignant lesions can demonstrate absence of flow [21,22]. Although the presence of flow indicates a much more suspicious lesion, the reverse is not always true. When flow is present, ultrasonography can analyze the waveforms. Malignant lesions tend to have different waveform characteristics than benign lesions, but there is enough overlap that waveform analysis is not a useful discriminator between malignant and benign lesions. In current practice, the best evaluation of an adnexal mass consists of gray scale morphologic assessment with Doppler imaging used to confirm the initial gray scale diagnosis. With future improvements on the horizon this may change.

Ultrasonography is a relatively inexpensive imaging modality. A normal endovaginal ultrasound has a high negative predictive value for gynecologic pathology. Ultrasound does have several drawbacks. First, it cannot adequately image bowel because the air in bowel corrupts the signal. A loop of bowel overlying a mass may also obscure the mass. Second, it has a poor field of view when compared with CT or MRI. Third, it provides poor contrast between dissimilar tissues. For these reasons, once an abnormality is identified, subsequent CT or MRI is often useful to see the full extent of the abnormality.

The typical pathology of adnexal masses varies radically depending on the menstrual status of the patient. The vast majority of adnexal masses in premenopausal patients are not neoplastic. In a postmenopausal patient, a solid adnexal mass is a much more ominous finding. A common adnexal mass in a premenopausal patient is a hemorrhagic ovarian cyst in which there is hemorrhage into the mature follicle, usually at the midcycle of menses. This hemorrhage expands the follicle, causing acute onset of pain, often at night, and occasionally a trip to the emergency room. Its appearance depends on how the blood clots in the cyst. It typically has a reticulated or fish net appearance on gray scale imaging. Occasionally, it can mimic a solid neoplasm. The key point in the diagnosis is the absence of internal flow, which confirms the gray scale finding (Figs. 11 and 12). Internal flow suggests a solid mass in any age group, a finding that needs to be explained, often by surgical means (Figs. 13 and 14).

An endometrioma is another common finding in a premenopausal patient. This lesion usually appears as a uniform hypoechoic mass on or adjacent to the ovary. Color flow Doppler is important in demonstrating the absence of internal flow (Figs. 15 and 16). Another common finding is a fluid-filled dilated tubular structure, commonly diagnosed as a hydrosalpinx. These structures are often bilateral and the product of pelvic inflammatory disease scarring, which obstructs the fallopian tubes. One of the most commonly imaged ovarian neoplasms in a premenopausal female is

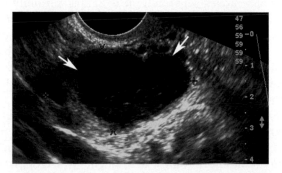

Fig. 11. Endovaginal ultrasound demonstrating the typical appearance of a hemorrhagic ovarian cyst (*arrows*) in a 38-year-old woman 2 weeks after menses.

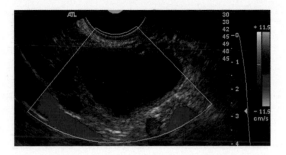

Fig. 12. Same patient shown in Fig. 11. Note the absence of internal flow on color flow Doppler imaging.

a dermoid cyst, also known as a mature cystic teratoma. These neoplasms usually form hair, teeth, sebaceous material, as well as other products, giving them a variety of appearances on ultrasound (Fig. 17). The presence of fat is diagnostic (Fig. 18). The most commonly imaged ovarian mass in a premenopausal female is a unilocular ovarian cyst, which is defined as having a thin wall, with or without hemorrhage, but without complicating features such as septations, mural nodules, hyperechoic lines or dots, irregular wall thickening, or shadowing densities. Based on previously published recommendations [23], the authors classify unilocular cysts of 3 cm in diameter or less as functional cysts requiring no additional follow-up. When these unilocular cysts are greater than 3 cm in diameter, although the possibility they could represent an epithelial ovarian neoplasm is remote, we re image the patient in 6 to 8 weeks, preferable after one complete menstrual cycle and early in the next. In the vast majority of cases, the unilocular cyst resolves on the follow-up examination. Persistent cysts are removed. If any cysts are complicated by the features discussed previously and the appearance is not typical of a benign entity, such as an endometrioma or dermoid cyst, one 6- to 8-week follow-up is allowed before removal [21].

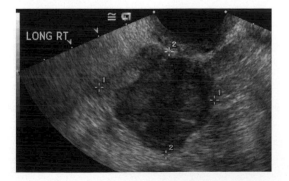

Fig. 13. Hypoechoic mass somewhat similar to appearance of hemorrhagic ovarian cyst in Fig. 11 except for irregular margins in a 68-year-old woman.

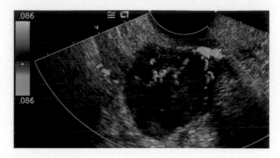

Fig. 14. Same patient shown in Fig. 13. Note internal flow consistent with a solid tumor. The final diagnosis was a poorly differentiated adenocarcinoma of unknown primary.

In postmenopausal patients any complex cystic mass is usually removed, because lesions are much more likely to represent neoplastic disease (Figs. 19 and 20). Statistically, benign epithelial neoplasms such as cystadenomas are more common than malignant neoplasms such as cystadenocarcinomas [24].

## MRI staging of pelvic malignancies

The three major gynecologic malignancies (endometrial, ovarian, and cervical cancers) have typical patterns of spread within the pelvis and have set guidelines regarding their staging. Preoperative contrast-enhanced MRI has been shown to be effective in showing the extent of local invasion and in determining nodal involvement to different degrees. The following sections discuss how each of these three diseases can be staged using MRI, including what to look for.

### Endometrial cancer

MRI has proved to be very important in the staging of endometrial cancer. The prognosis of endometrial cancer depends on many factors, some of which can be determined using MRI. These factors include the depth of

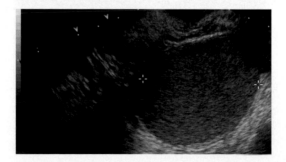

Fig. 15. Typical uniform appearance of an endometrioma in a 32-year-old woman with pelvic pain.

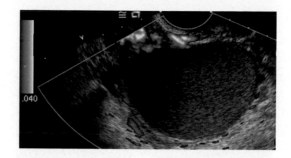

Fig. 16. Same patient shown in Fig. 15. Note the absence of flow on power Doppler imaging. Power Doppler imaging is more sensitive to transverse and slow flow than Color Flow Doppler imaging.

myometrial invasion and nodal status. In most institutions, patients with suspected myometrial invasion are considered for further surgical staging. Because this staging includes pelvic and para-aortic lymphadenectomy, a gynecologic oncologist usually needs to be involved [25]. MRI has been shown to be the best imaging modality for determining the depth of myometrial invasion and is comparable with direct gross visual inspection [26]. The depth of myometrial invasion has been shown to correlate well with pelvic lymph node metastases and tumor recurrence [27].

The most accurate assessment of disease is by surgical staging; the clinical staging criteria of the Cancer Committee of the International Federation of Gynecology and Obstetrics (FIGO) are suboptimal (Table 2) [28]. MRI has been shown to have an accuracy of 92% in staging endometrial cancer, with an accuracy of 82% in assessing the depth of myometrial invasion [28]. Because significant numbers of patients with stage I disease and deep myometrial invasion also have lymph node metastases, MRI, which can reliably demonstrate the depth of myometrial invasion, can assist the surgeon with preoperative counseling on the extent of surgery as well as prognosis [28].

Stage IC disease, or invasion into the outer half of the myometrium, requires further surgical staging by surgical retroperitoneal and pelvic and para-aortic lymph node dissection. For patients with stage IIB disease or

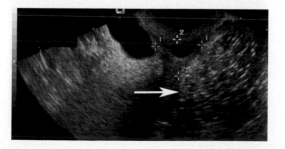

Fig. 17. Ultrasound gray scale image of echogenic mass within ovary (*arrow*) typical of a dermoid. Similar findings were noted on both ovaries.

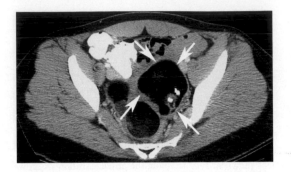

Fig. 18. CT of same patient in Fig. 17 showing three fat containing structures confirming the diagnosis of a dermoid. One structure (*arrows*) contains two small calcifications which were found to be teeth on specimen examination.

invasion of the cervical stroma, a more radical type of hysterectomy is necessary. It is generally agreed upon that grade 2 to 3 tumors and all tumor types for which there is suspected myometrial invasion should be operated on by specialist cancer surgeons trained in lymphadenectomy and staging procedures [29].

Because patients with grade 2 or grade 3 endometrial cancer are at higher risk for deep myometrial invasion, intraoperative frozen sections are obtained or gross inspection of the uterus performed to assess the depth of myometrial invasion. Based on these findings, the surgeon decides whether, at the time of hysterectomy, lymphadenectomy should be performed. If surgery is performed by a general gynecologist who usually does not perform lymphadenectomy, patients with a histopathologic diagnosis of myometrial invasion receive inadequate staging or require a second surgery for lymph node dissection and complete staging [30]. Because the initial treatment in a patient with cancer offers the best opportunity for cure, accurate

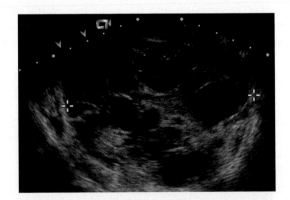

Fig. 19. Gray scale image of a borderline tumor considered to be between clearly malignant and clearly benign. Note the large size with both cystic and solid components. Recommendation for removal could have been easily made based on gray scale imaging alone.

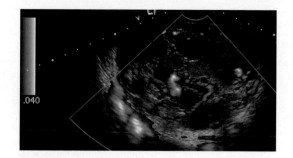

Fig. 20. Color flow images of same patient in Fig. 19. Note the vascular flow within the septations in this complex cystic mass in this postmenopausal patient, confirming the decision based on gray scale imaging.

preoperative assessment of the depth of myometrial invasion will help to se-lect out those patients who should be referred to a subspecialist [30].

The results of meta-analysis and bayesian analysis by Frei and colleagues [30] show that contrast-enhanced MRI is clinically useful for diagnosing deep myometrial invasion. In women with grade 3 endometrial cancer, a pos-itive examination result increases the probability for deep myometrial invasion from 54% to 92%. With this preoperative information, there would be little justification for routinely obtaining frozen sections during surgery. Contrast-enhanced MRI is also clinically useful in reliably exclud-ing deep endometrial invasion in patients with grade 1 or 2 endometrial cancer. In patients with difficult access to a specialist, contrast-enhanced MRI can be an option for treatment stratification [30].

*Ovarian cancer*

In the staging of ovarian cancer, MRI is comparable in accuracy to CT. It is generally used as a problem-solving modality for patients who cannot have contrast-enhanced CT [31]. In a multivariate analysis, the accuracy of MRI with gadolinium enhancement in the diagnosis of ovarian malig-nancy was 93%. MRI is generally recommended in patients with a contrain-dication to the use of iodinated contrast agents, in pregnant patients, and in those who have inconclusive CT findings. It is not generally the first-line imaging modality due to the increased cost over CT, decreased availability, and longer imaging and interpretation times.

Most women with ovarian cancer have advanced disease at the time of presentation; therefore, early detection and improved characterization of ovarian masses are important. Exploratory laparotomy is the typical man-agement for ovarian cancer because it offers both surgicopathologic staging and tumor debulking [32]. Nevertheless, because as many as 40% of patients are understaged at initial laparotomy, cross-sectional imaging can provide staging information that can assist in surgical planning and in selection of treatment options [32].

Table 2
FIGO staging of endometrial carcinoma and corresponding MRI findings

| Stage | Description | MRI findings |
|---|---|---|
| IA | Limited to endometrium | Thickened endometrial stripe with diffuse or focal abnormal signal intensity; endometrial stripe may be normal; intact junctional zone with smooth endometrial-myometrial interface |
| IB | Invasion <50% of myometrium | Signal intensity of tumor extends into myometrium <50%; partial- or full-thickness disruption of junctional zone with irregular endometrial-myometrial interface |
| IC | Invasion >50% of myometrium | Signal intensity of tumor extends into myometrium >50%; full-thickness disruption of junctional zone with intact stripe of normal outer myometrium |
| IIA | Cervical glandular involvement only | Internal os and endocervical canal are widened; low signal of fibrous stroma remains intact |
| IIB | Cervical stromal involvement | Disruption of fibrous stroma |
| IIIA | Involvement of uterine serosa, adnexae, positive peritoneal cytology | Disruption of continuity of outer myometrium; irregular uterine configuration |
| IIIB | Spread to vagina | Segmental loss of hypointense vagina wall |
| IIIC | Metastases to pelvic, para-aortic lymph nodes, or both | Regional lymph nodes >1 cm in diameter |
| IVA | Spread to bladder, rectal mucosa, or both | Tumor signal disrupts normal tissue planes with loss of low signal intensity of bladder or rectal wall |
| IVB | Involvement of bladder, rectal mucosa, or both | Tumor masses in distant organs or anatomic sites |

*Adapted from* Frei KA, Kinkel K. Staging endometrial cancer: role of magnetic resonance imaging. J Magn Reson Imaging 2001;13:851; with permission.

Ovarian cancer most commonly spreads by locoregional extension to the uterus, urinary bladder, sigmoid colon, or pelvic sidewall. The second most common route of spread is via peritoneal and lymphatic pathways. Common sites of peritoneal seeding are the pouch of Douglas, Morison's pouch, right paracolic gutter, subphrenic space, liver surface, porta hepatis, intrahepatic fissure, omentum, and bowel mesentery. Lymphatic spread may occur to retroperitoneal, lateral pelvic, and inguinal nodes. The least most common route of spread is hematogenous. Parenchymal liver or splenic metastases are rare on initial presentation [32].

The goal of imaging is to provide an accurate preoperative assessment of the extent of disease, which is extremely important for management and surgical planning (Table 3) [32]. Imaging can also provide crucial information about areas that are typically difficult to assess surgically (eg, the dome of the diaphragm or retroperitoneum) and can warn the surgeon about

Table 3
Surgical staging of ovarian carcinoma

| Stage | Description |
| --- | --- |
| I | Tumor limited to the ovaries |
| IA | Tumor limited to one ovary; no tumor on the external surface and capsule intact |
| IB | Tumor limited to both ovaries; no tumor on the external surface and capsule intact |
| IC | Stage IA or IB but with tumor on the surface of one or both ovaries, with capsule ruptured or with ascites or peritoneal washings containing malignant cells |
| II | Tumor involving one or both ovaries with pelvic extension or metastases |
| IIA | Extension with or without metastases to uterus, fallopian tubes, or both |
| IIB | Extension to other pelvic tissues |
| IIC | Stage IIA or IIB but with tumor on the surface of one or both ovaries, with capsule ruptured or with ascites or peritoneal washings containing malignant cells |
| III | Histologically confirmed peritoneal metastases outside the pelvis, superficial liver metastases, positive retroperitoneal or inguinal lymph nodes, or tumor limited to the true pelvis but with histologically verified malignant extension to the small intestine or omentum |
| IIIA | Gross tumor limited to the true pelvis with negative lymph nodes but with histologically confirmed microscopic tumor outside pelvis |
| IIIB | Histologically confirmed abdominal peritoneal metastases that extend beyond the pelvis and are <2 cm in diameter and negative lymph nodes |
| IIIC | Abdominal peritoneal metastases that extend beyond the pelvis and are >2 cm in diameter, positive retroperitoneal or inguinal lymph nodes, or both |
| IV | Distant metastases, including parenchymal liver metastases; if pleural effusion is present, cytologic test results must be positive to signify stage IV |

*Adapted from* staging established by the International Federation of Gynecology and Obstetrics and American Joint Committee on Cancer, 1999, 2002, Whitehouse Station (NJ): Merck Manual of Diagnosis and Therapy, 18th edition (online), 2005; section 18, chapter 254. p. 2–3; with permission.

critical findings that would change the surgical plan, such as invasion of the sigmoid colon [32].

The advantages of MRI over CT in the staging of ovarian cancer include the multiplanar capability, superior contrast resolution, and increased sensitivity for detecting uterine invasion, extension to the sigmoid colon or urinary bladder, or spread to the dome of the diaphragm or liver surface. Also, some studies have found MRI to be more sensitive than CT for detection of lymph node metastases [33]. The surgeon can be alerted to the need for assistance from a gynecologic oncologic surgeon or a gastrointestinal oncologic surgeon if a complicated surgical procedure or bowel resection is anticipated [32].

*Cervical cancer*

Contrast-enhanced MRI has been shown to have an accuracy similar to helical CT in the evaluation of pelvic lymph nodes in patients with cervical carcinoma [34]. A study by Yang and colleagues [34] of CT versus MRI compared various criteria for lymph nodes to determine which were predictive of malignancy or benignity. Optimal maximal axial diameter was set at 12 mm and minimal axial diameter at 8 mm. Size was shown to have a positive predictive value of 54%, a negative predictive value of 94%, and an accuracy of 80% when the 12-mm maximal axial diameter size criterion was used. When the minimal axial diameter size was used, the rates were similar, that is, a 54% positive predictive value, 92% negative predictive value, and accuracy of 80%. The shape, signal intensity, contrast enhancement, and central necrosis were also evaluated. Central necrosis had a 100% positive predictive value for metastasis. Shape, signal intensity, and contrast enhancement were not shown to be useful [34]. Others have found a minimum axial diameter using a 1-cm cutoff to be slightly more specific (98%) than a maximal axial dimension (95%) [35]. Some researchers have also found lymph node margins (spiculated or lobulated) to be useful criteria for predicting lymph node metastasis [36].

MRI is the imaging study of choice for tumor visualization, including determination of parametrial invasion [37]. Contrast-enhanced MRI has a relatively high negative predictive value (95%) for stage IIB cervical cancer (which has invaded the parametrium). This characteristic is helpful in identifying patients who may be candidates for surgery [38]. Also, because of its exquisite depiction of tumor size in patients with stage IB cancer, it is useful in deciding among surgery and concurrent chemotherapy and radiotherapy [38].

Tumor staging through MRI parallels the FIGO staging criteria (Table 4). A tumor is classified as stage IB if it is confined to the cervical stroma. This staging occurs when the stroma appears uninvolved on T2-weighted images with low signal intensity. A tumor is considered stage IIA when it extends into the upper two thirds of the vagina. This appearance manifests as loss of the low-intensity signal from the normal vaginal wall. The options for stage I and limited stage IIA disease include surgery, radiotherapy, or both. Stage IIB disease is diagnosed when, in addition to loss of the low-intensity cervical stroma of T2-weighted images, there is diffuse or localized abnormal signal intensity within the parametrial region [38]. Options for stage IIA and greater disease usually consist of radiotherapy only. Stage IIIA disease is seen with replacement of the low-intensity vaginal wall, again on T2-weighted images, by a high-intensity mass extending to the lower third of the vagina. Stage IIIB disease is present if the tumor extends to the pelvic sidewall or causes ureteral obstruction. Pelvic side wall involvement is seen as a loss of low intensity signal on T2-weighted images that correspond to the levator ani, piriformis, or obturator internus muscles. MRI performs well in excluding invasion, with a predictive value of 98% in excluding pelvic sidewall invasion. Stage IVA disease is seen as tumor invasion of the bladder or the rectum. This invasion appears on T2-weighted images as loss of the normally low intensity wall of these organs [38]. MRI is also valuable in

Table 4
FIGO staging of uterine cervical carcinoma and corresponding MRI findings

| Stage | Description | MRI findings |
|---|---|---|
| 0 | Carcinoma in situ | Tumor not seen or tumor confined to cervix |
| IA | Microinvasive carcinoma confined to cervix | Tumor not seen or tumor confined to cervix |
| IB | Clinically invasive carcinoma confined to cervix | Tumor not seen or tumor confined to cervix |
| IIA | Vaginal invasion, upper two thirds | Loss of low signal intensity vaginal wall, upper two thirds |
| IIB | Parametrial invasion | Abnormal signal intensity within parametrial region with obliteration of low signal intensity cervical stroma |
| IIIA | Vaginal invasion, lower third | Loss of low signal intensity vaginal wall extending to lower third |
| IIIB | Pelvic sidewall extension with or without hydronephrosis or nonfunctioning kidney | Same as IIB with extension to pelvic side wall |
| IVA | Spread to bladder or rectum | Loss of low signal intensity of bladder or rectal wall |
| IVB | Spread to distant organs | Evidence of distant metastasis |

*Data from* Kim SH, Choi BI, Han JK, et al. Preoperative staging of uterine cervical carcinoma: comparison of CT and MRI in 99 patients. J Comput Assist Tomogr 1993;17(4):633–40.

identifying concomitant disease, such as leiomyomas or an adnexal mass, which may assist treatment planning. MRI is not necessary in every patient with cervical cancer, such as those who have early stage small lesions, but can be valuable in certain situations [38].

Some have found that the overall staging accuracy of MRI (up to 77%) in cervical cancer is significantly higher than that of CT (up to 69%) [39,40]. MRI has been shown to be cost-effective in the workup of patients with clinical stage IB invasive cervical cancer. Although expensive, it results in a net cost savings because it replaces several less expensive procedures [41]. MRI is now widely accepted as an optimal method for evaluation of tumor volume, uterine corpus involvement, parametrial invasion, and metastatic lymph node involvement [42].

## Fluorodeoxyglucose positron emission tomography imaging of gynecologic malignancies

Positron emission tomography (PET) using the radiolabeled glucose analogue [18]F-fluorodeoxyglucose (FDG) has demonstrated increasing clinical utility in the management of patients with a wide variety of malignancies. This is due to the high sensitivity of the procedure for detecting increased metabolic activity as reflected by greater intracellular glucose utilization by neoplasms in conjunction with its ability to evaluate the entire body in a single examination. The incorporation of CT imaging into a combined hybrid PET/CT scanner has the additional advantages of providing rapid attenuation correction of the PET data and more precise anatomic co-registration of both image data sets to improve the specificity and localization of findings. The current equipment acquisition trend suggests that virtually all clinical PET imaging in the near future will be performed on these hybrid PET/CT systems.

Abdominopelvic imaging with FDG PET can be challenging due to physiologic uptake at sites such as the bowel and ureters as well as in the processes of ovulation and menstruation, which can be confused with areas of tumor involvement [43,44]. Additional benign sources of increased pelvic FDG uptake include endometriosis, uterine fibroids, inflammation, ovarian cysts, teratoma, and schwannoma [45]. Overlap in the relative intensity of FDG uptake, as measured by the standard uptake value (SUV), between these conditions and gynecologic malignancies requires correlation with additional clinical history and ideally, if available, co-registered CT images to assist in determining an etiology for increased metabolic activity.

Data support the use of FDG PET for imaging most gynecologic malignancies, with its efficacy in the staging of cervical cancer as an adjunct to conventional imaging well established as a Medicare-approved indication. The role of PET in the management of these malignancies can be expected to grow as data accumulate supporting its use in staging, restaging, and assessing the therapeutic response of endometrial, cervical, and ovarian cancer. The current status of the role of PET in each of these malignancies as well as its limitations is described in the following sections.

*Endometrial cancer*

Endometrial carcinoma is the most common pelvic malignancy in women, predominantly affecting postmenopausal females, with the most common presenting symptom being dysfunctional uterine bleeding. Tumor dissemination occurs by vascular and lymphatic routes, with the prognosis related to histology, the extent of local invasion, and nodal involvement. Surgical staging with nodal sampling is usually performed, with radiotherapy portals generally determined by nodal sites. Since early reports documenting the diagnosis of endometrial carcinoma with FDG PET [46,47], additional studies establishing its usefulness in the postsurgical monitoring and surveillance for recurrent disease have appeared [48,49]. These studies have demonstrated the value of PET in confirming and localizing recurrent disease (Fig. 21) with improved sensitivities of 96% to 100% and specificities of 78% to 88% when compared with conventional anatomic imaging modalities (CT and MRI) and tumor markers. The FDG PET findings altered patient management in approximately one third of the cases.

Uterine sarcomas are a much less common form of primary uterine malignancy and are typically evaluated with MRI. Nevertheless, FDG PET has demonstrated good sensitivity in the detection of leiomyosarcoma [50,51].

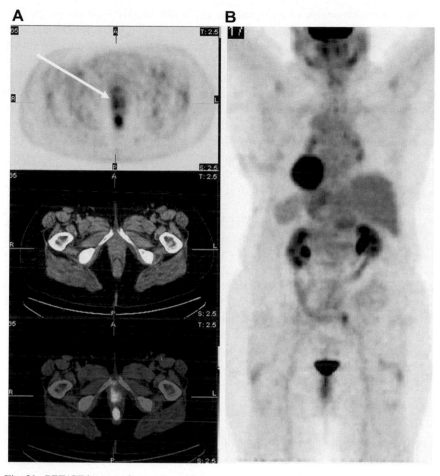

Fig. 21. PET/CT images of a woman with metastatic endometrial cancer. (*A*) Transaxial PET, CT, and fused images in the pelvis show metastasis involving the vagina (*arrow*) with physiologic increased rectal activity posteriorly. (*B*) A posterior maximum intensity projection shows additional small metastatic foci in both hila. (*Courtesy of* Sidney R. Hinds II, MD, Walter Reed Army Medical Center, Washington, DC.)

## Ovarian cancer

As the second most common gynecologic malignancy, ovarian carcinoma accounts for a disproportionate number of deaths related to gynecologic cancer, largely attributable to the vague nature of its early symptoms and the absence of any reliable tumor screening marker, resulting in most cases presenting at advanced stages. Surgical staging with debulking of tumor followed by chemotherapy is the primary treatment. Restaging with second-look laparoscopy or laparotomy can be performed on patients without clinical evidence of disease to assess tumor response, with up to 75% found to have persistent disease.

Because microscopic ovarian cancer often disseminates within the peritoneum, the detection of small volume disease is of great importance. The
inherent spatial limitation of FDG PET imaging (5–7 mm) reduces its ability
to detect this small volume disease following initial treatment and before
a second look. Although some studies have reported low accuracy for
disease detection following a complete clinical response [52], others have
reported sensitivity and specificity as high as 66% and 94%, respectively
[53,54]. A significant decrease in unnecessary invasive second-look staging
procedures and health care costs was associated with the use of FDG
PET for restaging patients with ovarian cancer [55]. A more recent study
identified no significant differences in the progression-free interval between
a second-look laparotomy group and a PET group with a positive predictive
value of 93% [56].

Several studies have shown FDG PET to be superior to CT and MRI in
the detection of recurrent ovarian cancer [57], with a consistently high sensitivity confirmed in a more recent study [58]. A decrease in PET sensitivity
is generally attributable to small lesions less than 5 mm, although there are
no studies assessing the clinical impact of identifying even smaller microscopic disease. A study examining the impact of hybrid FDG PET/CT
imaging (Fig. 22) correlated with histologic findings confirmed a high positive predictive value of 89% for the combined procedure [59]. PET is useful
for localizing sites of disease involvement for biopsy or surgery, especially
when CT or MRI fails to identify disease [60].

*Cervical cancer*

Cervical cancer is the third most common gynecologic malignancy in the
United States. The incidence has declined with the widespread acceptance of
the Papanicolaou smear screening test. Although the international staging
system is clinical, ancillary imaging modalities are routinely used in the
developed world, with surgical sampling of pelvic and aortic lymph nodes
preferred for staging advanced disease. Although CT has high specificity
for nodal metastases, its sensitivity is only 50% [39]. FDG PET has been
approved by the Centers for Medicare and Medicaid Services for the initial
staging of cervical cancer in patients with no evidence of extrapelvic metastatic disease by MRI or CT.

Several studies have demonstrated high sensitivity and specificity of FDG
PET for the initial staging of cervical cancer (Fig. 23), as well as high sensitivity for restaging patients with a role in directing therapy [61–63]. The
excellent performance of MRI in assessing the extent of local involvement
is complemented by the larger imaging area provided by PET, which
improves the evaluation for pelvic and extrapelvic nodal disease as well as
distant metastases. As is true for other malignancies, the detection of small
volume disease is limited by the decreased anatomic resolution of PET,
although this can be mitigated to some extent by an increased metabolic

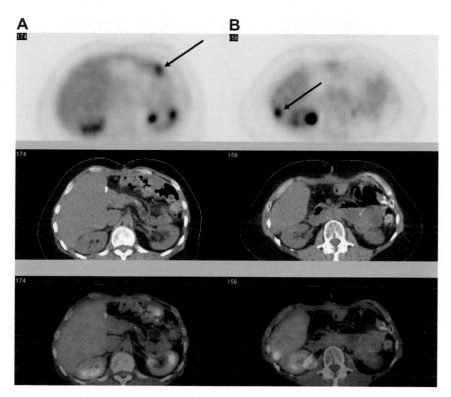

Fig. 22. PET/CT images of a woman with metastatic ovarian cancer. Transaxial PET, CT, and fused images showing metastatic foci (*arrows*) in the (*A*) colon and (*B*) liver with physiologic renal collecting system activity seen in both kidneys. (*Courtesy of* Sidney R. Hinds II, MD, Walter Reed Army Medical Center, Washington, DC.)

activity found in some tumors. A recent meta-analysis of 15 studies examining FDG PET in cervical cancer reported pooled sensitivities of 79% to 84% and combined specificities of 95% to 99% for aortic and pelvic node metastases [64].

Classification of patients into prognostic groups using a scoring system with factors related to poor outcome helped stratify the utility of FDG PET imaging [65]. Patients in the best prognosis group were the most likely to benefit from identification of recurrent disease by PET, which led to a change in management and enhanced survival. The PET findings had an effect on treatment in 65% of all patients. The poorer the prognostic score, the less the impact on management and survival outcome observed due to PET. The clinical management of patients who experience an elevation in their tumor markers following a complete treatment response (with no disease detected using conventional imaging) may be guided by the results of FDG PET [66]. Disease was detected in 94% of these patients, leading to earlier initiation of therapy and a positive impact on survival, with diagnostic accuracy in such clinical situations reported as high as 94% [67].

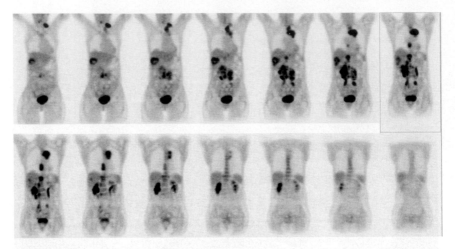

Fig. 23. Coronal PET images of a woman with extensive metastatic cervical cancer involving supraclavicular, mediastinal, and para-aortic lymph nodes with a large hepatic metastasis and obstructive right-sided hydronephrosis. (*Courtesy of* Sidney R. Hinds II, MD, Walter Reed Army Medical Center, Washington, DC.)

The ability of FDG PET imaging to assess nodal status in cervical cancer has prognostic and therapeutic implications. Among patients with more advanced cervical cancer (stage IIIB), there was a direct correlation between the extent of lymph node involvement and mortality [68]. Sites of nodal involvement direct radiation treatment planning. The added co-registered anatomic data obtained with PET/CT can be used to guide intensity modulated radiotherapy, significantly reducing the amount of radiation delivered to surrounding normal structures.

## Imaging the complications of gynecologic surgery

Potential complications of hysterectomy and other gynecologic and obstetric procedures are numerous. These complications include ureteral obstruction or transection, bladder perforation, bowel perforation or obstruction, fistula, bleeding, abscess, retention of surgical instruments or sponges, incisional hernia, and tumor or endometriosis implants in surgical scars. Large retrospective studies of complications following gynecologic surgery have shown the incidence of ureteral injury to range from 0.03% to 1% of all cases, bladder injury 0.03% to 1.7%, and bowel injury 0.06% to 0.5% [69–71].

All of the aforementioned complications can be diagnosed by imaging methods. The available imaging techniques are almost as varied as the problems to be investigated. CT, intravenous urography (IVU), ultrasonography, MRI, gastrointestinal fluoroscopic studies, angiography, and even scintigraphy can be used to diagnose complications. Furthermore, each technique can be optimized to answer a particular question. If the surgeon is looking for a specific complication, the technique should be adjusted to answer that question. The following sections discuss ways to tailor the radiologic search.

## Ureteral injury

CT is most useful for detecting ureteral obstruction or disruption of the ureter and formation of a urinoma. It should be performed before and after the injection of intravenous contrast. Subsequent scanning after a 5- to 20-minute delay improves the sensitivity for urine leakage as the extravasated iodine increases the attenuation of the pooled urine [72].

Alternative tests include IVU, ultrasonography, and MRI. Scintigraphy is useful if direct evidence of urinary tract obstruction or leakage is desired in a patient with a contraindication to iodinated contrast material, such as contrast allergy or renal insufficiency.

## Bladder injury

CT cystography is a technique employing retrograde filling of the bladder by gravity drip of 300 to 400 mL of dilute iodinated contrast, followed by helical CT of the bladder with multiplanar reformations [73]. Its reported sensitivity and specificity for extraperitoneal bladder rupture are 97% and 100% and for intraperitoneal rupture, 78% and 99% [74]. CT cystography can also be used to demonstrate fistulae between the bladder and vagina or intestine [75]. Conventional retrograde cystography is an alternative test.

## Bowel complications

Intestinal perforation is suggested by pneumoperitoneum, detectable on upright abdominal and chest radiographs. Of course, peritoneal air is a normal finding immediately following laparotomy. CT performed with intravenous and oral contrast can also detect peritoneal fluid collections and extravasated enteral contrast [76].

CT is superior to conventional radiography and barium studies in diagnosing small bowel obstruction [77]. When using CT or barium studies to diagnose small bowel obstruction, patience is a virtue; it may take several hours for oral contrast to pass through the small bowel and into the colon, excluding obstruction. Injuries to the colon are better appreciated when a (water-soluble) contrast enema is performed; if this is done in conjunction with CT, the contrast material must be very dilute or beam-hardening artifacts will render the images useless.

## Fluid collections

Even small pockets of fluid can be detected in the abdomen by CT, ultrasonography, or MRI. The problem is to characterize the nature of the collection. Is it an abscess, hematoma, seroma, urinoma, or lymphocele?

CT with intravenous and enteral contrast is more helpful than the alternatives. Gas bubbles in a focal fluid collection are typical of an abscess; however, many abscesses do not have this finding. A fluid pocket that has a capsule that enhances with intravenous contrast is suggestive of an abscess, but noninfected fluid collections can also develop a capsule. A hematoma often has a density equal to or higher than skeletal muscle and may show a fluid-fluid level or "hematocrit," especially if the patient is anticoagulated. Urinomas may fill with excreted contrast material after a delay of several minutes. Lymphoceles are a result of lymph node dissection and are typically seen as water-density fluid collections adjacent to iliac vessels. Useful interpretation of imaging studies which show postoperative abdominal fluid collections is impossible without knowledge of the patient's condition [78]. Many of these cases require percutaneous needle aspiration or catheter drainage guided by CT or ultrasonography [79].

*Retained instruments*

A suspicion that a surgical instrument or sponge has been inadvertently left in the patient should lead to an intraoperative radiograph of the kidneys, ureters, and bladder (KUB). Although the interpretation of the resultant image would seem foolproof, one should recall that the maximal size of the x-ray film or digital receptor is 14 × 17 in and may not cover the entire peritoneal cavity if positioning is careless or the patient large. One should not hesitate to order additional views under these circumstances. Not all surgical sponges include a radio-opaque component; these would be invisible on a KUB. A sponge left in the abdomen may over time acquire a fibrous capsule and simulate a neoplasm, obstruct the intestine, or become a nidus of infection and form an abscess; this condition is called gossypiboma from the Latin *gossypium* (cotton) and the Swahili *boma* (place of concealment) [80].

*Abdominal wall*

Hematoma and abscess are early postoperative complications. If an incisional hernia is suspected, this can be confirmed by ultrasound, which allows real-time assessment of the abdominal wall with a variety of provocative maneuvers [81]. CT provides a clear picture of the contents of the hernia sac. Endometrial tissue may invade a surgical scar, with a superficial mass that causes pain synchronized to the menstrual cycle. Radiologic confirmation of scar endometrioma can be done with any of the cross-sectional imaging modalities [82].

## References

[1] Atri M, Leduc C, Gillett P, et al. Role of endovaginal sonography in the diagnosis and management of ectopic pregnancy. Radiographics 1996;16:755–74 [discussion: 775].

[2] Middleton W, Kurtz A, Hertzburg B. The first trimester and ectopic pregnancy. In: Thrall JH, editor. Requisites in radiology. 2nd edition. St. Louis (MO): Mosby; 2003. p. 357–70.

[3] O'Boyle M. Ectopic pregnancy: an update. Presented at the 29th Annual Spring Diagnostic Ultrasound Conference, Los Angeles. April 23–25, 2004. p. 61–8.

[4] Doubilet P, Benson C. Heterotopic pregnancy. In: The atlas of ultrasound in obstetrics and gynecology: comprehensive otology. 2nd edition. Philadelphia: Lippincott Williams & Wilkins; 2003. p. 327.

[5] Benson C, Doubilet P. Fetal measurements: normal and abnormal fetal growth. In: Rumack C, Wilson S, Charboneau J, editors. Diagnostic ultrasound. 2nd edition. St. Louis (MO): Mosby; 1998. p. 1013–31.

[6] Levine D. Ectopic pregnancy. In: Callen P, editor. Ultrasonography in obstetrics and gynecology. 4th edition. Philadelphia: WB Saunders; 2000. p. 912–34.

[7] IMV 2006 CT Market Summary Report. Des Plains (IL): IMV Medical Information Division; 2006.

[8] Lazarus E, Mayo-Smith W, Spencer P, et al. Utilization of radiological examinations in pregnant women: a ten year review—1997–2006. Chicago: RSNA Meeting; 2007. p. SSJ05–SSJ02.

[9] Wittich AC, DeSantis RA, Lockrow EG. Appendectomy during pregnancy: a survey of two Army medical activities. Mil Med 1999;164:671–4.

[10] Cunningham FG, McCubbin JH. Appendicitis complicating pregnancy. Obstet Gynecol 1975;45:415–20.

[11] Maslovitz S, Gutman G, Lessing JB, et al. The significance of clinical signs and blood indices for the diagnosis of appendicitis during pregnancy. Gynecol Obstet Invest 2003;56:188–91.

[12] Bailey LE, Finley RK Jr, Miller SF, et al. Acute appendicitis during pregnancy. Am Surg 1986;52:218–21.

[13] Weissleder R, Wittenberg J, Harisinghani M. Medical physics. In: Primer of diagnostic imaging. 4th edition. St. Louis (MO): Mosby; 2007. p. 1042–52.

[14] CDC. Fact sheet: radiation emergencies. Available at: http://www.bt.cdc.gov/radiation. Accessed November 25, 2007.

[15] Beir VII: Health Risks from Exposure to Low Levels of Ionizing Radiation, Committee to assess health risks from exposure to low levels of ionizing radiation, Monson R (chairman). The National Academies Report in Brief, Pg 3; National Academies Press, Washington, DC. Available at: http://dels.nas.edu/dels/rpt_briefs/beir_vii_final.pdf.

[16] Wagner L, Lester R, Saladana L. Exposure of the pregnant patient to diagnostic radiations: a guide to medical management. Philadelphia: Lippincott; 1985. p. 61–74.

[17] National Council on Radiation Protection and Measurements (NCRP) Report No. 116. Limitation of Exposure to Ionizing Radiation, Meinhold C, Chairman, Bethesda (MD); 1993.

[18] Hurwitz LM, Yoshizumi T, Reiman RE, et al. Radiation dose to the fetus from body MDCT during early gestation. AJR Am J Roentgenol 2006;186:871–6.

[19] Lim HK, Bae SH, Seo GS. Diagnosis of acute appendicitis in pregnant women: value of sonography. AJR Am J Roentgenol 1992;159:539–42.

[20] Pedrosa I, Levine D, Eyvazzadeh AD, et al. MR imaging evaluation of acute appendicitis in pregnancy. Radiology 2006;238:891–9.

[21] Brown DL, Frates MC, Laing FC, et al. Ovarian masses: can benign and malignant lesions be differentiated with color and pulsed Doppler US? Radiology 1994;190:333–6.

[22] Jain KA. Prospective evaluation of adnexal masses with endovaginal gray-scale and duplex and color Doppler US: correlation with pathologic findings. Radiology 1994;191:63–7.

[23] Dill-Macky M, Atri M. Management of an ovarian mass. In: Callen P, editor. Ultrasonography in obstetrics and gynecology. 4th edition. Philadelphia: WB Saunders; 2000. p. 889–90.

[24] Crum C. Ovarian tumors. In: Robbins S, editor. Pathologic basis of disease. 6th edition. Philadelphia: WB Saunders; 1999. p. 1068.

[25] Frei KA, Kinkel K. Staging endometrial cancer: role of magnetic resonance imaging. J Magn Reson Imaging 2001;13:850–5.

[26] Cunha TM, Felix A, Cabral I. Preoperative assessment of deep myometrial and cervical invasion in endometrial carcinoma: comparison of magnetic resonance imaging and gross visual inspection. Int J Gynecol Cancer 2001;11:130–6.

[27] Cagnazzo G, D'Addario V, Martinelli G, et al. Depth of myometrial invasion in endometrial cancer: preoperative assessment by transvaginal ultrasonography and magnetic resonance imaging. Ultrasound Obstet Gynecol 1992;2:40–3.

[28] Hricak H, Stern JL, Fisher MR, et al. Endometrial carcinoma staging by MR imaging. Radiology 1987;162:297–305.

[29] Swift S. Recurrent endometrial cancer: patterns of recurrent disease and assessment of prognosis. Clin Radiol 2007;62:35–6.

[30] Frei KA, Kinkel K, Bonel HM, et al. Prediction of deep myometrial invasion in patients with endometrial cancer: clinical utility of contrast-enhanced MR imaging—a meta-analysis and Bayesian analysis. Radiology 2000;216:444–9.

[31] Javitt MC, Fleischer AC, Andreotti RF, et al. Expert panel on women's imaging. Staging and follow-up of ovarian cancer. Reston (VA): American College of Radiology (ACR); 2007. p. 1–5. Available at: http://www.guideline.gov/summary/summary.aspx?doc_id=11594.

[32] Forstner R, Hricak H, White S. CT and MRI of ovarian cancer. Abdom Imaging 1995;20: 2–8.

[33] Tempany C, Dou K, Silverman S, et al. Staging of advanced ovarian cancer: comparison of imaging modalities—report from the Radiological Diagnostic Oncology Group. Radiology 2000;215:761–7.

[34] Yang WT, Lam WW, Yu MY, et al. Comparison of dynamic helical CT and dynamic MR imaging in the evaluation of pelvic lymph nodes in cervical carcinoma. AJR Am J Roentgenol 2000;175:759–66.

[35] Kim SH, Kim SC, Choi BI, et al. Uterine cervical carcinoma: evaluation of pelvic lymph node metastasis with MR imaging. Radiology 1994;190:807–11.

[36] Choi HJ, Kim SH, Seo SS, et al. MRI for pretreatment lymph node staging in uterine cervical cancer. AJR Am J Roentgenol 2006;187:W538–43.

[37] Hricak H, Lacey CG, Sandles LG, et al. Invasive cervical carcinoma: comparison of MR imaging and surgical findings. Radiology 1988;166:623–31.

[38] Hricak H, Gatsonis C, Conkley F, et al. Early invasive cervical cancer: CT and MR imaging in preoperative evaluation—ACRIN/GOG comparative study of diagnostic performance and interobserver variability. Radiology 2007;245:491–8.

[39] Kim SH, Choi BI, Han JK, et al. Preoperative staging of uterine cervical carcinoma: comparison of CT and MRI in 99 patients. J Comput Assist Tomogr 1993;17.633–40.

[40] Choi SH, Kim SH, Choi HJ, et al. Preoperative magnetic resonance imaging staging of uterine cervical carcinoma: results of prospective study. J Comput Assist Tomogr 2004;28: 620–7.

[41] Hricak H, Powell CB, Yu KK, et al. Invasive cervical carcinoma: role of MR imaging in pretreatment work-up–cost minimization and diagnostic efficacy analysis. Radiology 1996;198:403–9.

[42] Fischerova D, Cibula D, Stenhova H, et al. Transrectal ultrasound and magnetic resonance imaging in staging of early cervical cancer. Int J Gynecol Cancer 2007, in press.

[43] Subhas N, Patel PV, Pannu HK, et al. Imaging of pelvic malignancies with in-line FDG PET-CT: case examples and common pitfalls of FDG PET. Radiographics 2005;25: 1031–43.

[44] Chander S, Meltzer CC, McCook BM. Physiologic uterine uptake of FDG during menstruation demonstrated with serial combined positron emission tomography and computed tomography. Clin Nucl Med 2002;27:22–4.

[45] Fenchel S, Grab D, Nuessle K, et al. Asymptomatic adnexal masses: correlation of FDG PET and histopathologic findings. Radiology 2002;223:780 8.

[46] Lentz SS. Endometrial carcinoma diagnosed by positron emission tomography: a case report. Gynecol Oncol 2002;86:223–4.

[47] Nakahara T, Fujii H, Ide M, et al. F-18 FDG uptake in endometrial cancer. Clin Nucl Med 2001;26:82–3.

[48] Belhocine T, De Barsy C, Hustinx R, et al. Usefulness of (18)F-FDG PET in the post-therapy surveillance of endometrial carcinoma. Eur J Nucl Med Mol Imaging 2002;29: 1132–9.

[49] Saga T, Higashi T, Ishimori T, et al. Clinical value of FDG-PET in the follow up of postoperative patients with endometrial cancer. Ann Nucl Med 2003;17:197–203.

[50] Umesaki N, Tanaka T, Miyama M, et al. Positron emission tomography using 2-[(18)F] fluoro-2-deoxy-D-glucose in the diagnosis of uterine leiomyosarcoma: a case report. Clin Imaging 2001;25:203–5.

[51] Umesaki N, Tanaka T, Miyama M, et al. Positron emission tomography with (18)F-fluorodeoxyglucose of uterine sarcoma: a comparison with magnetic resonance imaging and power Doppler imaging. Gynecol Oncol 2001;80:372–7.

[52] Rose PG, Faulhaber P, Miraldi F, et al. Positive emission tomography for evaluating a complete clinical response in patients with ovarian or peritoneal carcinoma: correlation with second-look laparotomy. Gynecol Oncol 2001;82:17–21.

[53] Drieskens O, Stroobants S, Gysen M, et al. Positron emission tomography with FDG in the detection of peritoneal and retroperitoneal metastases of ovarian cancer. Gynecol Obstet Invest 2003;55:130–4.

[54] Turlakow A, Yeung HW, Salmon AS, et al. Peritoneal carcinomatosis: role of (18)F-FDG PET. J Nucl Med 2003;44:1407–12.

[55] Smith GT, Hubner KF, McDonald T, et al. Cost analysis of FDG PET for managing patients with ovarian cancer. Clin Positron Imaging 1999;2:63–70.

[56] Kim S, Chung JK, Kang SB, et al. [18F]FDG PET as a substitute for second-look laparotomy in patients with advanced ovarian carcinoma. Eur J Nucl Med Mol Imaging 2004;31: 196–201.

[57] Delbeke D, Martin WH. Positron emission tomography imaging in oncology. Radiol Clin North Am 2001;39:883–917.

[58] Nanni C, Rubello D, Farsad M, et al. (18)F-FDG PET/CT in the evaluation of recurrent ovarian cancer: a prospective study on forty-one patients. Eur J Surg Oncol 2005;31:792–7.

[59] Sironi S, Messa C, Mangili G, et al. Integrated FDG PET/CT in patients with persistent ovarian cancer: correlation with histologic findings. Radiology 2004;233:433–40.

[60] Kubik-Huch RA, Dorffler W, von Schulthess GK, et al. Value of (18F)-FDG positron emission tomography, computed tomography, and magnetic resonance imaging in diagnosing primary and recurrent ovarian carcinoma. Eur Radiol 2000;10:761–7.

[61] Wong TZ, Jones EL, Coleman RE. Positron emission tomography with 2-deoxy-2-[(18)F]fluoro-D-glucose for evaluating local and distant disease in patients with cervical cancer. Mol Imaging Biol 2004;6:55–62.

[62] Weber TM, Sostman HD, Spritzer CE, et al. Cervical carcinoma: determination of recurrent tumor extent versus radiation changes with MR imaging. Radiology 1995;194:135–9.

[63] Havrilesky LJ, Wong TZ, Secord AA, et al. The role of PET scanning in the detection of recurrent cervical cancer. Gynecol Oncol 2003;90:186–90.

[64] Park W, Park YJ, Huh SJ, et al. The usefulness of MRI and PET imaging for the detection of parametrial involvement and lymph node metastasis in patients with cervical cancer. Jpn J Clin Oncol 2005;35:260–4.

[65] Yen TC, See LC, Chang TC, et al. Defining the priority of using 18F-FDG PET for recurrent cervical cancer. J Nucl Med 2004;45:1632–9.

[66] Chang TC, Law KS, Hong JH, et al. Positron emission tomography for unexplained elevation of serum squamous cell carcinoma antigen levels during follow-up for patients with cervical malignancies: a phase II study. Cancer 2004;101:164–71.

[67] Chang WC, Hung YC, Lin CC, et al. Usefulness of FDG-PET to detect recurrent cervical cancer based on asymptomatically elevated tumor marker serum levels: a preliminary report. Cancer Invest 2004;22:180–4.

[68] Singh AK, Grigsby PW, Dehdashti F, et al. FDG-PET lymph node staging and survival of patients with FIGO stage IIIb cervical carcinoma. Int J Radiat Oncol Biol Phys 2003;56: 489–93.

[69] Harkki-Siren P, Kurki T. A nationwide analysis of laparoscopic complications. Obstet Gynecol 1997;89:108–12.

[70] Harkki-Siren P, Sjoberg J, Kurki T. Major complications of laparoscopy: a follow-up Finnish study. Obstet Gynecol 1999;94:94–8.

[71] Mathevet P, Valencia P, Cousin C, et al. Operative injuries during vaginal hysterectomy. Eur J Obstet Gynecol Reprod Biol 2001;97:71–5.

[72] Titton RL, Gervais DA, Hahn PF, et al. Urine leaks and urinomas: diagnosis and imaging-guided intervention. Radiographics 2003;23:1133–47.

[73] Chan DP, Abujudeh HH, Cushing GL Jr, et al. CT cystography with multiplanar reformation for suspected bladder rupture: experience in 234 cases. AJR Am J Roentgenol 2006;187: 1296–302.

[74] Jankowski JT, Spirnak JP. Current recommendations for imaging in the management of urologic traumas. Urol Clin North Am 2006;33:365–76.

[75] Yu NC, Raman SS, Patel M, et al. Fistulas of the genitourinary tract: a radiologic review. Radiographics 2004;24:1331–52.

[76] Pinto A, Scaglione M, Giovine S, et al. Comparison between the site of multislice CT signs of gastrointestinal perforation and the site of perforation detected at surgery in forty perforated patients. Radiol Med (Torino) 2004;108:208–17.

[77] Maglinte DD, Gage SN, Harmon BH, et al. Obstruction of the small intestine: accuracy and role of CT in diagnosis. Radiology 1993;188:61–4.

[78] Antonelli E, Morales MA, Dumps P, et al. Sonographic detection of fluid collections and postoperative morbidity following cesarean section and hysterectomy. Ultrasound Obstet Gynecol 2004;23:388–92.

[79] Heneghan JP, Everts RJ, Nelson RC. Multiple fluid collections: CT- or US-guided aspiration–evaluation of microbiologic results and implications for clinical practice. Radiology 1999;212:669–72.

[80] O'Connor AR, Coakley FV, Meng MV, et al. Imaging of retained surgical sponges in the abdomen and pelvis. AJR Am J Roentgenol 2003;180:481–9.

[81] Aguirre DA, Santosa AC, Casola G, et al. Abdominal wall hernias: imaging features, complications, and diagnostic pitfalls at multi-detector row CT. Radiographics 2005;25: 1501–20.

[82] Hensen JH, Van Breda Vriesman AC, Puylaert JB. Abdominal wall endometriosis: clinical presentation and imaging features with emphasis on sonography. AJR Am J Roentgenol 2006;186:616–20.

ELSEVIER
SAUNDERS

SURGICAL
CLINICS OF
NORTH AMERICA

Surg Clin N Am 88 (2008) 391–401

# Physiologic Changes in Pregnancy

Christina C. Hill, MD[a],*, Jennifer Pickinpaugh, DO[b]

[a]Division of Maternal Fetal Medicine, Department of Obstetrics and Gynecology, Tripler
Army Medical Center, 1 Jarrett White Road, Honolulu, HI 96859-5000, USA
[b]Department of Obstetrics and Gynecology, Tripler Army Medical Center,
1 Jarrett White Road, Honolulu, HI 96859-5000, USA

## Body water homeostasis

Maternal blood volume expands during pregnancy to allow adequate perfusion of vital organs, including the uteroplacental unit and fetus, and to prepare for the blood loss associated with parturition [1,2]. Total body water increases from 6.5 L to 8.5 L by the end of gestation. Changes in osmoregulation and the renin-angiotensin system result in active sodium reabsorption in renal tubules and water retention. The water content of the fetus, placenta, and amniotic fluid accounts for approximately 3.5 L of total body water. The remainder of total body water is comprised of the expansion of maternal blood volume by 1500 mL to 1600 mL, plasma volume of 1200 mL to 1300 mL, and a 20% to 30% increase in erythrocyte volume from 300 mL to 400 mL [2,3]. The pregnant patient can hemorrhage up to 2000 mL of blood before she manifests changes in heart rate or blood pressure. The rapid expansion of blood volume begins at 6 to 8 weeks' gestation and plateaus at approximately 32 to 34 weeks' gestation. The expanded extracellular fluid volume accounts for 6 to 8 kg of weight gain [4]. The larger increase of plasma volume by 1000 mL to 1500 mL relative to erythrocyte volume results in hemodilution and a physiologic anemia.

## Cardiovascular changes

Cardiovascular physiologic adaptations allow optimal oxygen delivery to maternal and fetal tissues [5]. The heart is displaced cephalad and is rotated

---

The views expressed in this article are those of the authors and do not reflect the official policy or position of the Department of the Army, Department of Defense, or the US Government.

* Corresponding author.
E-mail address: christina.hill@amedd.army.mil (C.C. Hill).

0039-6109/08/$ - see front matter. Published by Elsevier Inc.
doi:10.1016/j.suc.2007.12.005                                   surgical.theclinics.com

leftward as a result of the enlarging uterus and elevation of the diaphragm. The heart itself undergoes significant remodeling during pregnancy. All four chambers enlarge, particularly the left atrium [5,6]. Atrial stretching and the increased estrogen of pregnancy lower the threshold for arrhythmias. Valvular annular diameters increase, as does left ventricular volume and wall thickness [6]. Mild pulmonic and tricuspid regurgitation occur in more than 90% of healthy pregnant women, and more than one third manifest clinically insignificant mitral regurgitation [7]. Cardiac volume and mass increase concomitantly so that left ventricular function and ejection fraction remain unchanged. Left ventricular wall thickness returns to prepregnancy measurements approximately 6 months postpartum [8,9].

Cardiac output increases 30% to 50% from 4 L to 6 L/min, particularly during the first two trimesters [10]. This increase is primarily a result of a 20% to 50% increase in stroke volume. Estrogen-mediated increases in myocardial alpha-receptors results in an increase in heart rate of 10 to 20 beats/min [2,4,9]. Cardiac output begins to rise gradually at 8 to 10 weeks' gestation and peaks at approximately 25 to 30 weeks' gestation.

The increase in cardiac output allows increased perfusion to the uterus, maternal kidneys, extremities, breasts, and skin and is at the expense of splanchnic bed and skeletal muscle perfusion. Blood flow through the uterus approaches 450 to 650 mL/min at term and comprises approximately 20% to 25% of maternal cardiac output. Uteroplacental perfusion lacks autoregulation, and therefore perfusion of these organs relies on maternal mean arterial blood pressure. Care should be taken when administering regional anesthesia, because sympathetic blockade may result in hypotension, thereby compromising uterine and fetal perfusion. Patients should be hydrated vigorously with lactated Ringer's solution before establishing conduction anesthesia. Renal blood flow accounts for 20% of maternal cardiac output [11]. Increased blood flow to maternal skin allows dissipation of the heat generated by the fetus [12]. The increased cardiac output speeds delivery of medications administered intravenously, such as induction agents.

Decreased cardiac output resulting from compromised stroke volume may be seen when the parturient is in the supine position [10]. "Maternal supine hypotension syndrome" results when the gravida assumes a supine position, leading to uterine compression of the inferior vena cava and abdominal aorta. Venous blood return to the heart is decreased. The decreased preload reduces stroke volume and may result in a 25% to 30% decrease in cardiac output. Maternal symptoms include pallor, sweating, nausea, vomiting, hypotension, tachycardia, and mental status changes. Symptoms are more pronounced in the third trimester because of the expanding uterus and are alleviated by maintaining a lateral decubitus position and displacing the uterus laterally [10]. During surgical procedures it is imperative to maintain the patient in a left lateral decubitus position to maintain cardiac output. This position can be accomplished by placing a wedge under the patient's right hip.

Cardiac output increases by 50% during labor with increases in blood volume of 300 to 500 mL with each uterine contraction. Fifteen to 20 minutes after delivery cardiac output increases as a result of the loss of diversion of blood flow to the fetus and placenta. This redirection of approximately 500 mL of blood to the maternal circulation is termed "autotransfusion." Autotransfusion and removal of aortocaval compression by evacuation of the uterus result in a 60% to 80% increase in cardiac output. Cardiac output remains elevated for 48 hours after delivery and then gradually returns to nonpregnant values over 2 to 12 weeks [6].

Progesterone acts to vasodilate blood vessels. This vasodilation, in conjunction with the decreased resistance of the placental bed, results in a 15% decrease in systemic vascular resistance and a decreased blood pressure. Systolic and diastolic blood pressure decreases by 5 mm Hg to 15 mm Hg with the nadir occurring at 28 weeks' gestation. Blood pressure then returns to prepregnancy values during the third trimester. Pulmonary vascular resistance is decreased, and pulmonary artery pressure is unchanged in pregnancy [13]. The decreases in systemic vascular resistance and pulmonary vascular resistance maintain central venous pressure within normal parameters. Central venous pressure decreases slightly, from 9 mm Hg to 4 mm Hg, by term. The low-resistance state allows the vasculature to accommodate higher volumes while maintaining pressures consistent with the nonpregnant state [13].

Venous pressure increases progressively during pregnancy, particularly in the lower extremities. Elevated progesterone levels act to increase venous distensibility. These factors, in addition to the compromised venous return from the inferior vena cava, result in dependent edema, varicose veins, hemorrhoids, labial varicosities, and an increased risk of venous thromboembolism [14]. Engorgement of epidural veins narrows the epidural and intrathecal spaces, thereby reducing the volume of medication needed for regional anesthesia [15].

The concentration of plasma proteins, such as albumin, is decreased in pregnancy resulting in a decrease in colloid oncotic pressure [16]. There also is a decrease in the difference between the colloid oncotic pressure and the pulmonary capillary wedge pressure, predisposing the pregnant patient to pulmonary edema in situations of increased cardiac preload or when capillary permeability is compromised. Fluid management in the surgical patient should be meticulous, because aggressive fluid resuscitation may result in extravasation of fluid into extracellular spaces.

Physical examination findings associated with maternal cardiovascular changes include peripheral edema, mild tachycardia, jugular venous distension, and lateral displacement of the left ventricular apex. Components of the first heart sound become louder in the second trimester of pregnancy, and there is an exaggerated splitting. A third heart sound ($S_3$) also is heard in the majority of gravidas. A systolic murmur along the left sternal border may be auscultated in more than 90% of pregnant women and is the result of increased blood flow over the pulmonic and aortic valves [17]. This murmur disappears shortly after delivery.

Continuous murmurs over the breasts in the second to fourth intercostal space also may be heard in the latter part of pregnancy and are referred to as a "mammary souffle." Radiologic findings include an enlarged cardiac silhouette and straightening of the left side of the heart. ECG changes associated with pregnancy include sinus tachycardia, left axis deviation, ectopic beats, inverted or flattened T waves, and a Q wave in lead III and the augmented voltage unipolar left foot lead [18].

## Respiratory changes

The nasal and respiratory tract mucosa become edematous and hyperemic because of the increased estrogen and increased blood volume of pregnancy [19,20]. During pregnancy this change is perceived as congestion and rhinitis. These symptoms resolve within 48 hours following delivery [19]. Because the upper airways are more edematous and friable, the pregnant patient is more prone to nose bleeds and to bleeding with manipulation [21,22]. Laryngoscopy and intubation should be accomplished with care, using sufficient lubricant to minimize trauma.

Difficult endotracheal intubation is a leading cause of maternal morbidity and mortality [23]. Airway edema, breast engorgement, and the generalized weight gain of pregnancy may contribute to airway obstruction and reduced glottic opening [24]. Smaller endotracheal tubes may be required for successful intubation.

As pregnancy progresses, the diaphragm is elevated 4 cm by the enlarging uterus, and the lower ribcage circumference expands by 5 cm [19,25,26]. The increased relaxin levels of pregnancy allow the ligamentous attachments of the ribcage to relax, increasing the ribcage subcostal angle from 68° to 103° [19,21]. Respiratory muscle function remains unaffected in pregnancy, as do the maximum inspiratory and expiratory pressures [27].

Lung volumes change as a result of changes in the configuration of the chest wall and the position of the diaphragm. The enlarging uterus displaces the intra-abdominal contents upward and elevates the diaphragm. This elevation, with the decrement in chest wall compliance, reduces the volume of the lungs in the resting state, resulting in a 5% decrease in total lung capacity and a 10% to 25% decrease in functional residual capacity, (ie, the volume of air remaining after quite exhalation) [19,28,29]. Functional residual capacity is the sum of expiratory reserve and residual volumes, both of which are decreased [30]. Of note, functional residual capacity in the supine parturient is 70% of that in the upright parturient [28].

Minute ventilation is the amount of air moved in and out of the lungs in 1 minute. It is the product of tidal volume and respiratory rate and increases by approximately 30% to 50% with pregnancy [31]. The increase is primarily a result of tidal volume, which increases by 40%, because the respiratory rate remains fairly constant [28,32]. The increase in respiratory drive is believed to result from increased levels of progesterone, which acts as a respiratory stimulant [33]. The increased serum progesterone levels in the first trimester of pregnancy stimulate the medullary respiratory centers in the brain and increase respiratory depth, thereby increasing alveolar ventilation [19,28,32,34]. Changes occur early in pregnancy then remain fairly constant throughout [35].

The increase in minute ventilation coupled with increased erythrocyte production works to increase oxygen-carrying capacity. After delivery, as progesterone levels fall, the respiratory drive returns to normal.

Oxygen consumption increases by 30% to 60% (30–40 mL/min) during the course of pregnancy as a result of the increased metabolic demands of maternal organs, placenta, and fetus [25,28,32]. The increased oxygen consumption coupled with a decreased functional residual capacity decreases maternal oxygen reserve and predisposes the parturient to hypoxemia and hypocapnia during periods of respiratory depression or apnea [36,37]. As such, there is limited time to intubate the pregnant patient safely. Preoxygenation and denitrogenation with 100% oxygen is critical, maximizing oxygen tension within the functional residual capacity and thereby allowing more time before maternal oxygen desaturation [38].

Arterial $PCO_2$ decreases from 40 mm Hg in the nonpregnant state to 32 mm Hg to 34 mm Hg in pregnancy as a result of the increased minute ventilation [34,39]. The patient therefore exists in a state of respiratory alkalosis that is compensated by renal excretion of bicarbonate. Maternal arterial pH is maintained at 7.40 to 7.45 as bicarbonate is excreted to achieve serum bicarbonate levels of 15 mEq/L to 20 mEq/L [19,26,29]. This decrease in buffering capacity renders the pregnant patient susceptible to metabolic acidosis, as occurs in diabetic ketoacidosis. The respiratory alkalosis also shifts the oxyhemoglobin dissociation curve rightward, thereby favoring removal of oxygen to the periphery and facilitating oxygen transfer across the placenta [40]. Maternal oxygen saturation should be maintained at 95% to maintain a $Pao_2$ greater than 70 mm Hg, thereby optimizing oxygen diffusion across the placenta. Fetal oxygenation is maintained when maternal $Pao_2$ remains above 60 mm Hg to 70 mm Hg. When it falls below this level, fetal oxygenation is compromised immediately.

Carbon dioxide diffuses rapidly between maternal and fetal circulations. The lower maternal baseline $PCO_2$ favors transplacental transfer of carbon dioxide from the fetus to the maternal circulation for removal.

Maternal $Pao_2$ increases slightly because of the increased minute ventilation and alveolar ventilation and may achieve levels of 100 to 105 mm Hg. This higher pressure facilitates transplacental oxygen transfer [19,34]. Changing from a supine to sitting position increases $Pao_2$ by approximately 13 mm Hg [19,26].

The increase in minute ventilation is perceived by the pregnant woman as shortness of breath, which affects 60% to 76% of women [19]. This physiologic dyspnea is caused by the increase in respiratory drive, increase in pulmonary blood volume, anemia, and nasal congestion. Symptoms typically are mild and do not tend to worsen with advancing pregnancy. Symptoms typically do not prohibit women from performing daily activities and do not occur with rest. These symptoms typically resolve immediately postpartum.

Pulmonary function remains unchanged during pregnancy [41]. The forced expiratory volume in 1 second ($FEV_1$) and the $FEV_1$/forced vital capacity ratio is unchanged in pregnancy, as are peak expiratory flow rates [42,43]. Therefore it is reasonable to use nonpregnant reference values to evaluate lung function in parturients. Normal chest radiographic findings in a pregnant patient include mild cardiomegaly, a widened mediastinum, an increased anterior-posterior diameter, and prominence of the pulmonary vasculature.

## Gastrointestinal changes

As pregnancy advances, the growing uterus displaces the stomach and intestines upwards. These anatomic alterations can confound diagnosis of surgical intra-abdominal processes and may change the location of surgical incisions. Stretching of the peritoneum acts to desensitize it, thereby complicating the abdominal examination.

Nausea and vomiting affect up to 50% of women during pregnancy, primarily in the first trimester [44]. Elevated progesterone levels, mechanical factors, and the enlarging uterus all contribute to delayed gastric emptying and increased stomach volume. Anxiety, pain, and administration of opiates and anticholinergics also are responsible for delayed smooth muscle motility [15]. Gastric motility decreases further during labor and remains delayed during the immediate postpartum period. Delayed gastric motility and prolonged gastrointestinal transit time may lead to constipation and alter the bioavailability of medications [45,46].

Elevated progesterone levels reduce lower esophageal sphincter tone and increase the placental production of gastrin, increasing gastric acidity. These changes combine to increase the incidence of reflux esophagitis and heartburn, affecting between 50% and 80% of parturients [47].

Aspiration may result in significant maternal morbidity and mortality. The pregnant patient is at increased risk for aspiration of gastric contents when sedated after approximately 16 weeks' gestation. The risk of aspiration is even greater in the obese gravid patient [48]. Therefore regional anesthesia should be accomplished quickly when indicated. If general endotracheal anesthesia is required, the patient should have no oral intake for 6 to 8 hours before anesthetic administration, if possible [48]. Administration of a nonparticulate antacid is given to increase gastric pH. An H2 receptor antagonist also is given to decrease gastric acid production [48,49]. Anesthesia should be accomplished with the use of an intravenous rapid sequence induction, with cricoid pressure applied to prevent reflux of gastric contents into the oropharynx. Gastric contents should be suctioned upon securing the airway.

Pregnancy alters some laboratory values relating to the gastrointestinal system. Transaminase and bilirubin levels are decreased slightly in pregnancy, but alkaline phosphatase levels are increased as a result of placental production.

## Urinary tract changes

During pregnancy, the kidneys are displaced cephalad by the enlarging uterus and increase approximately 1 cm in size as a result of increased vasculature, interstitial volume, and dead space [50]. The renal collecting system becomes more dilated as early as the first trimester, leading to hydroureteronephrosis [51]. This condition is noted more often on the right and is thought to be associated with progesterone-mediated smooth muscle relaxation as well as with the mechanical compression from a dextrorotated, enlarging uterus [52]. Compression of the ureters (of the right ureter more than the left) results in urine stasis, thereby predisposing the pregnant woman to urinary tract infections, nephrolithiasis, and pyelonephritis. The bladder loses tone, resulting in frequency, urgency, and incontinence, the last of which is compounded in the third trimester as the fetal head engages in the pelvis [14]. The physiologic dilatation of the upper collecting system should be considered when interpreting radiographic studies evaluating for possible obstruction.

The renal physiology is perhaps the first to be altered during pregnancy. At the onset of pregnancy, systemic vasodilation occurs, probably associated with the hormonal effects of progesterone and relaxin [53]. There first is dilation of renal vasculature, and as a consequence there is a compensatory increase in glomerular filtration rate (GFR) and effective renal plasma flow (RPF) [54]. Studies measuring GFR and RPF by clearance of inulin and para-aminohippurate have demonstrated that by midpregnancy the GFR increases by 40% to 65%, and the RPF increases by 50% to 85% compared with prepregnancy and postpartum values. Because RPF increases typically are greater than GFR increases, the filtration fraction (GFR/RPF) is reduced during pregnancy [10]. Because there is a marked decrease in systemic and renal vascular resistance, the vessels initially are "underfilled." A shunt effect from the dilated maternal renal circulation provokes the initial increase in cardiac output in the first trimester.

The substantial increase in GFR results in alterations of serum levels of analytes. Creatinine clearance increases by 25% early in pregnancy, resulting in a decrease in serum creatinine from approximately 0.8 mg/dL to 0.5 mg/dL. Protein and albumin excretion into urine also increase, complicating the diagnosis and monitoring of renal diseases during pregnancy. An average of 200 mg and a maximum of 300 mg of protein are excreted in a 24-hour period during normal pregnancy [55]. Similarly, 12 mg (and a maximum of 20 mg) of albumin are excreted in 24 hours during pregnancy. This excretion seems to be caused by the increase in the GFR as well as by changes in charge selectivity of the glomerular membrane. Glucose also is excreted in higher amounts during pregnancy, making glucosuria a nonspecific finding in pregnancy and not helpful in the diagnosis of glucose intolerance. Glucose continues to be filtered freely, but the reabsorption that occurs by active transport in the proximal, and to some degree the collecting, tubule is limited because of the rapid tubular flow. Sodium also is retained during pregnancy (900–950 mEq by end of gestation), which helps sustain the plasma expansion in the dilated vasculature. Although more sodium is filtered, reabsorption of sodium by the renal tubule is increased [10]. The increased glomerular filtration may alter clearance of medications that are excreted through the kidney.

## Hematologic changes

Maternal hemoglobin levels are decreased because of the increase in plasma volume relative to erythrocyte volume, resulting in a physiologic dilutional anemia [17]. A normal pregnancy hematocrit is approximately 32% to 34%, which is lower than nonpregnant values [56]. Transfer of iron stores to the fetus contributes further to this physiologic anemia. There is an adrenocorticoid-mediated leukocytosis with pregnancy that increases white blood cell counts up to $14,000/\text{mm}^3$. Counts may reach $30,000/\text{mm}^3$ during labor and the puerperium. The platelet count may be lower in pregnancy because of aggregation, although it still remains within normal range [17].

Plasma protein concentrations, particularly albumin, are decreased during pregnancy. This change may alter the peak plasma concentrations of drugs that are highly protein bound.

Almost all procoagulants, including factors VII, VIII, IX, X, and XII and fibrinogen, are increased during pregnancy. Fibrinogen is increased by 50%, from a mean of 300 mg/dL in the nonpregnant state to a mean of 450 mg/dL in the gravid patient. Prothrombin, factor V, protein C, and antithrombin III levels remain unchanged. Protein S activity decreases, and there is an increase in activated protein C resistance. There is a decrease in the fibrinolytic system activity mediated by an increase in the plasminogen activator inhibitors 1 and 2.

The increase in procoagulants, decreased fibrinolysis, and increased venous stasis, particularly in the lower extremities, explains why the incidence of venous thromboembolic complications is five times greater during pregnancy [56,57]. As the uterus enlarges, venous compression impedes lower body venous return. Pneumatic compression stockings should be placed before induction of anesthesia. This precaution improves venous return and provides protection against thromboembolism.

## Summary

A myriad of physiologic changes occur with pregnancy, and these changes impact virtually every organ system. These adaptations allow the mother to support the metabolic demands of the fetoplacental unit and withstand the hemorrhage associated with delivery. It is crucial for the health care provider to be aware of these changes, because they may mimic disease. They also may alter a patient's response to stress from trauma or surgery and require modifications in standard management protocols.

## References

[1] Whittaker PG, MacPhail S, Lind T. Serial hematologic changes and pregnancy outcome. Obstet Gynecol 1996;88(1):33–9.
[2] Lee W. Cardiorespiratory alterations during normal pregnancy. Crit Care Clin 1991;7(4): 763–75.
[3] Scott DE. Anemia in pregnancy. In: Wynn RM, editor. Obstetrics and gynecology annual. New York: Appleton, Century, Crofts; 1972. p. 219–44.
[4] Brown MA, Gallery EDM. Volume homeostasis in normal pregnancy and pre-eclampsia: physiology and clinical implications. Baillieres Clin Obstet Gynaecol 1994;8(2):287–310.
[5] Duvekot JJ, Cheriex EC, Pieters FA, et al. Early pregnancy changes in hemodynamics and volume homeostasis are consecutive adjustments triggered by a primary fall in systemic vascular tone. Am J Obstet Gynecol 1993;169(6):1382–92.
[6] Fujitani S, Baldisseri MR. Hemodynamic assessment in a pregnant and peripartum patient. Crit Care Med 2005;33(10):S354–61.
[7] Robson SC, Hunter S, Moore M, et al. Haemodynamic changes during the puerperium: a Doppler and M-mode echocardiographic study. Br J Obstet Gynaecol 1987;94(11):1028–39.
[8] Mabie WC, DiSessa TG, Crocker LG, et al. A longitudinal study of cardiac output in normal human pregnancy. Am J Obstet Gynecol 1994;170(3):849–56.
[9] Hunter S, Robson SC. Adaptation of the maternal heart in pregnancy. Br Heart J 1992;68(6): 540–3.
[10] Yeomans ER, Gilstrap LC III. Physiologic changes in pregnancy and their impact on critical care. Crit Care Med 2005;33(10):S256–8.
[11] Metcalfe J, Romney SL, Ramsey LH, et al. Estimation of uterine blood flow in women at term. J Clin Invest 1955;34(11):1632–8.
[12] Ginsburg J, Duncan SL. Peripheral blood flow in normal pregnancy. Cardiovasc Res 1967; 1(2):132–7.
[13] Clark SL, Cotton DB, Lee W, et al. Central hemodynamic assessment of normal term pregnancy. Am J Obstet Gynecol 1989;161(6 pt 1):1439–42.
[14] Diaz J. Perinatal anesthesia and critical care. Philadelphia: Saunders; 1991.
[15] Beilin Y. Anesthesia for nonobstetric surgery during pregnancy. Mt Sinai J Med 1998;65(4): 265–70.
[16] Mendenhall HW. Serum protein concentrations in pregnancy: I. concentrations in maternal serum. Am J Obstet Gynecol 1970;106(3):388–99.
[17] Northcote RJ, Knight PV, Ballantyne D. Systolic murmurs in pregnancy: value of echocardiographic assessment. Clin Cardiol 1985;8(6):327–8.
[18] Pedersen H, Finster M. Anesthetic risk in the pregnant surgical patient. Anesthesiology 1979;51(5):439–51.
[19] Elkus R, Popovich J. Respiratory physiology in pregnancy. Clin Chest Med 1992;13(4): 555–65.
[20] Fishburne JI. Physiology and disease of the respiratory system in pregnancy: a review. J Reprod Med 1979;22(4):177–89.

[21] Bonica JJ. Maternal respiratory changes during pregnancy and parturition. In: Marx GF, editor. Parturition and perinatology. Philadelphia: FA Davis; 1973. p. 2–19.
[22] Camaan WR, Ostheimer GW. Physiological adaptations during pregnancy. Int Anesthesiol Clin 1990;28(1):2–10.
[23] Chadwick HS, Posner K, Caplan R, et al. A comparison of obstetric and nonobstetric anesthesia malpractice claims. Anesthesiology 1991;74(2):242–9.
[24] Lewin SB, Cheek TG, Deutschman GS. Airway management in the obstetric patient. Crit Care Clin 2000;16(3):505–13.
[25] Crapo R. Normal cardiopulmonary physiology during pregnancy. Clin Obstet Gynecol 1996;39:3–16.
[26] Weinberger SE, Weiss ST, Cohen WR, et al. Pregnancy and the lung: state of the art. Am Rev Respir Dis 1980;121(3):559–81.
[27] Gilroy R, Mangua B, Lavietes M. Ribcage displacement and abdominal volume displacement during breathing in pregnancy. Am Rev Respir Dis 1988;137(3):668–72.
[28] Cugell DW, Frank NR, Gaensler EA, et al. Pulmonary function in pregnancy, 1: serial observations in normal women. Am Rev Tuberc 1953;67(5):568–97.
[29] Lapinsky SE, Kruczynski K, Slutsky AS. Critical care in the pregnant patient. Am J Respir Crit Care Med 1995;152(2):427–55.
[30] Gee JBL, Packer BS, Millen JE, et al. Pulmonary mechanics during pregnancy. J Clin Invest 1967;46(6):945–52.
[31] Knuttgen HG, Emerson JRK. Physiologic response to pregnancy at rest and during exercise. J Appl Physiol 1974;36(5):549–53.
[32] Rees GB, Pipkin FB, Symonds EM, et al. A longitudinal study of respiratory changes in normal human pregnancy with cross-sectional data on subjects with pregnancy-induced hypertension. Am J Obstet Gynecol 1990;162(3):826–30.
[33] Contreras G, Gutierrez M, Beroiza T, et al. Ventilatory drive and respiratory muscle function in pregnancy. Am Rev Respir Dis 1991;144(4):837–41.
[34] Templeton A, Kelman GR. Maternal blood gases, $PAO_2$-$PaO_2$, physiological shunt and Vd/Vt in normal pregnancy. Br J Anaesth 1967;48(10):1001–8.
[35] Liberatore SM, Pistelli R, Patalano F, et al. Respiratory function during pregnancy. Respiration 1984;46(2):145–50.
[36] Archer GW, Marx GF. Arterial oxygen tension during apnoea in parturient women. Br J Anaesth 1974;46(5):358–60.
[37] Awe RJ, Nicotra B, Newsom TD, et al. Arterial oxygenation and alveolar-arterial oxygen gradient in term pregnancy. Obstet Gynecol 1979;53(2):182–6.
[38] Goodman S. Anesthesia for nonobstetric surgery in the pregnant patient. Semin Perinatol 2002;26(2):136–45.
[39] Prowse CM, Gaensler EA. Respiratory acid-base changes during pregnancy. Anesthesiology 1965;26:381–92.
[40] Tsai C, De Leeuw NK. Changes in 2,3-diphosphoglycerate during pregnancy and puerperium in normal women and beta-thalassemia heterozygous women. Am J Obstet Gynecol 1982;142(5):520–3.
[41] Goucher D, Rubin A, Russo N. The effect of pregnancy upon pulmonary function in normal women. Am J Obstet Gynecol 1956;72(5):963–9.
[42] Milne JA. The respiratory response to pregnancy. Postgrad Med J 1979;55(643):318–24.
[43] Milne JA, Mills RJ, Howie AD, et al. Large airways function during normal pregnancy. Br J Obstet Gynaecol 1997;84(6):448–51.
[44] Broussard CN, Richter JE. Nausea and vomiting of pregnancy. Gastroenterol Clin North Am 1998;27(1):123–51.
[45] Hunt JN, Murray FA. Gastric function in pregnancy. J Obstet Gynaecol Br Emp 1958;65(1): 78–83.
[46] Parry E, Shields R, Turnball AC. Transit time in the small intestine in pregnancy. J Obstet Gynaecol Br Commonw 1970;77(10):900–1.

[47] Conklin KA. Maternal physiological adaptations during gestation, labor and the puerperium. Semin Anesth 1991;10:221–34.

[48] Glassenberg R. General anesthesia and maternal mortality. Semin Perinatol 1991;15(5): 386–96.

[49] Cheek TG, Gutsch BB. Pulmonary aspiration of gastric content. In: Shneider SM, Levinson G, editors. Anesthesia for obstetrics. 3rd edition. Philadelphia: Williams & Wilkins; 1993.

[50] Gabbe SG, Niebyl JR, Simpson JL. Obstetrics: normal and problem pregnancies. 5th edition. Philadelphia: Churchill Livingston; 2007. p. 70.

[51] Fried A, Woodring J, Thompson D. Hydronephrosis of pregnancy: a prospective sequential study of the course of dilatation. J Ultrasound Med 1983;2(6):225–9.

[52] Hytten F, Lind T. Indices of renal function. In: Hytten FE, Lind T, editors. Diagnostic indices in pregnancy. Basel (Switzerland): Documenta Geigy; 1973. p. 18.

[53] Davison J. The effect of pregnancy on kidney function in renal allograft recipients. Kidney Int 1985;27(1):74–9.

[54] Lindheimer M, Davison J, Katz A. The kidney and hypertension in pregnancy. Twenty exciting years. Semin Nephrol 2001;21(2):173–89.

[55] Higby K, Suiter C, Phelps J, et al. Normal values of urinary albumin and total protein excretion during pregnancy. Am J Obstet Gynecol 1994;171(4):984–9.

[56] Barron WM. Medical evaluation of the pregnant patient requiring nonobstetric surgery. Clin Perinatol 1985;12(3):481–96.

[57] Toglia MR, Weg JG. Venous thromboembolism during pregnancy. N Engl J Med 1996; 335(2):108–14.

SURGICAL
CLINICS OF
NORTH AMERICA

ELSEVIER
SAUNDERS

Surg Clin N Am 88 (2008) 403 419

# Surgical Diseases Presenting in Pregnancy

Charles S. Dietrich III, MD[a],*, Christina C. Hill, MD[b],
Matthew Hueman, MD[c]

[a]Gynecologic Oncology Service, Department of Obstetrics and Gynecology, Tripler Army
Medical Center, 1 Jarrett White Road, Honolulu, HI 96859-5000, USA
[b]Division of Maternal Fetal Medicine, Department of Obstetrics and Gynecology, Tripler
Army Medical Center, 1 Jarrett White Road, Honolulu, HI 96859-5000, USA
[c]General Surgery, Department of Surgery, The Johns Hopkins Hospital, Blalock 665,
600 North Wolfe Street, Baltimore, MD 21287, USA

There are an estimated 6 million pregnancies in the United States each year resulting in more than 4 million live births. It comes as no surprise that nonobstetric surgical diseases frequently arise in this patient cohort. Approximately 1 in 500 pregnant women require general surgery [1,2]. Although the tenets of diagnosis and treatment remain mostly unchanged, there are a few caveats when a coexisting pregnancy is found. This article highlights some of the more common surgical diseases pregnant women may experience, including appendicitis, biliary disease, bowel obstruction, inflammatory bowel disease (IBD), hemorrhoids, and malignancies (Table 1).

In most cases, the pregnant patient presents with the classic signs and symptoms associated with the surgical disease. The decision to operate is relatively straightforward, and quick intervention minimizes maternal and fetal risks. In other cases the diagnosis may be delayed, because mild symptoms may be confused with pregnancy complaints. Close interactions with maternal-fetal specialists help with development of the treatment plan and with postsurgical monitoring of the pregnancy.

## Appendicitis

Appendicitis is the most common nonobstetric surgical complication and the most common gastrointestinal disorder requiring surgery during

---

The views expressed in this article are those of the authors and do not reflect the official policy or position of the Department of the Army, Department of Defense, or the US Government.
* Corresponding author.
*E-mail address:* chuck.dietrich@us.army.mil (C.S. Dietrich III).

0039-6109/08/$ - see front matter. Published by Elsevier Inc.
doi:10.1016/j.suc.2007.12.003

Table 1
Incidence of surgical diseases in pregnancy

| Disease | Incidence |
| --- | --- |
| Appendicitis | 1 in 1500–2000 pregnancies |
| Cholecystitis | 1 in 1600–10,000 pregnancies |
| Bowel obstruction | 1 in 3000 pregnancies |
| Cervical cancer | 1 in 2000–2500 pregnancies |
| Breast cancer | 1 in 3000 pregnancies |
| Melanoma | 2.8 per 1000 births |
| Ovarian cancer | 1 in 20,000–30,000 pregnancies |

pregnancy [3–5]. It accounts for 25% of surgeries for nonobstetric indications in pregnancy and complicates every 1 in 1500 to 2000 pregnancies [3,6,7]. It occurs with equal frequency in each trimester [7,8]. Pregnant women are not at greater risk for developing appendicitis than nonpregnant women, but, because appendicitis is a disease affecting a younger population, it is common for women of reproductive age to be affected. The incidence of perforated appendicitis in pregnant women is 43%, which is greater than the 4% to 19% seen in the nonobstetric population [9,10]. This increased incidence may reflect a reluctance to operate on a pregnant woman and a delay in diagnosis commonly noted with appendicitis in pregnancy.

Maternal and fetal morbidity and mortality correlate with perforation, which usually results from delayed diagnosis, and its associated complications [11]. Uncomplicated appendicitis has a 3% to 5% fetal loss rate with negligible maternal mortality. Appendiceal perforation, however, is associated with a 20% to 35% fetal loss rate and a 4% rate of maternal mortality [8,12–14]. Maternal mortality rates from appendicitis have dropped significantly during the past several years as a result of prompt surgical intervention, improved antibiotic regimens, and surgical techniques. Maternal mortality increases with advancing gestational age, as does the proportion of appendicitis cases with perforation. Preterm contractions caused by uterine irritation from peritonitis are common, occurring in up to 83% of cases, although preterm labor and delivery occur only 5% to 14% of the time. Preterm delivery is more common in the third trimester, with up to a 50% rate [15]. The incidence of preterm delivery and other complications are similar between open procedures and laparoscopy [13]. Mazze and Kallen [6] found the risk for preterm delivery is highest within the first postoperative week, with rates as high as 22% and with 16% delivering on the day of surgery. The authors also found that beyond the first postoperative week preterm delivery rates were not increased. Cohen-Kerem and colleagues [16] reviewed 12,452 obstetric surgical cases and found a miscarriage rate of 5.8%; however, there were no matched controls. The rate of premature labor induced by surgical intervention for appendectomy was 3.5%, a rate statistically higher than that for other medical conditions. Fetal loss associated with appendectomy was 2.6% and increased to 10.9% in the presence of peritonitis.

The fetal loss rate for patients undergoing appendectomy was significantly greater than the fetal loss rate for patients undergoing other surgical procedures during pregnancy. The authors concluded that the effects of appendicitis and surgery somehow were more severe and differed from other acute surgical conditions of pregnancy. The authors also concluded that the risk for major birth defects was not increased over that of the general obstetric population.

In the first trimester the appendix remains in its normal anatomic position. The appendix undergoes progressive displacement cephalad and laterally with advancing pregnancy [17]. After 24 weeks' gestation, the appendix is shifted superiorly above the right iliac crest, and the tip of the appendix is rotated medially toward the uterus [1,18]. By late pregnancy, the appendix may be closer to the gallbladder than McBurney's point, occupying the right upper quadrant [19]. This change may alter the location of the pain, making diagnosis difficult. The commonly held belief that appendix location changed during pregnancy was challenged by Hodjati and Kazerooni [20]. In a prospective study comparing pregnant and nonpregnant women undergoing appendectomy to women undergoing cesarean delivery at term, they found no difference in appendiceal location. As the peritoneum is displaced from the appendix and cecum by the growing uterus, the increased separation of the visceral and parietal peritoneum decreases the somatic sensation of pain and compromises the ability to localize pain on examination [1]. The enlarging uterus may interfere with the ability of the omentum and bowel to wall off the inflamed appendix. Diffuse peritonitis from perforation is facilitated by this inability of the omentum to isolate the infection. The appendix returns to its normal position by the tenth postpartum day [17].

Symptoms of appendicitis often are confused with normal pregnancy-related conditions, particularly in the third trimester. When symptoms occur beyond the first trimester, are sudden in onset, or exacerbate, immediate evaluation is indicated. The most common and reliable symptom of appendicitis is right lower quadrant pain [3,7]. It may start as colicky, epigastric, or periumbilical pain that ultimately localizes to the right lower quadrant [5]. Associated symptoms include anorexia, nausea, and vomiting. These symptoms are common in the first trimester and therefore are not specific or sensitive predictors of pathology. A perforated appendix should be suspected in patients whose pain changes from localized tenderness to pain of a more diffuse nature. A retrocecal appendix may produce symptoms of back or flank pain. The differential diagnosis for appendicitis includes ligamentalgia, ovarian torsion, ovarian cyst, degenerating fibroid, pulmonary embolism, right lower lobe pneumonia, pancreatitis, pyelonephritis, urolithiasis, or biliary tract disease. Obstetric conditions to consider include ectopic pregnancy, placental abruption, or pre-eclampsia with liver involvement. Virtually all patients have right-sided direct abdominal tenderness. Approximately 70% of patients may demonstrate rebound, guarding, and referred tenderness, findings that are not normal in pregnancy [1,3,7,21]. Rebound tenderness and guarding are less specific because of laxity of the abdominal wall muscles and the interposition of the uterus between the appendix and anterior abdominal wall. Abdominal wall muscle rigidity is seen in 50% to 65% of patients [3]. Psoas irritation (psoas sign) is seen less frequently than in nonpregnant patients [22]. Rectal and pelvic tenderness may not be present if the uterus has enlarged to the point that the appendix is displaced cephalad. Fever may be present in 25% of patients. Diagnosis is confounded further, because the leukocytosis that commonly accompanies appendicitis in nonpregnant patients exists in normal pregnant women. The presence of a high granulocyte count suggests infection, however.

Ultrasound may identify an inflamed appendix or periappendiceal abscess and is the imaging study of choice; the specificity of ultrasound is high when an abnormal appendix is identified. An abnormal appendix appears as a tubular, blind-ended, noncompressible structure occupying the right lower quadrant and measuring more than 6 mm in diameter [23]. The diagnostic accuracy of ultrasound is highest in the first and second trimesters and decreases in the third trimester because of the displacement of the appendix. A ruptured appendix is identified less clearly on ultrasound [24]. If the appendix is not identified, or the study is equivocal, MRI is the next-best study and is considered safe in pregnancy [25]. The benefit of MRI is that it avoids exposing the fetus to the ionizing radiation associated with CT. Findings on MRI consistent with appendicitis include an enlarged, fluid-filled appendix measuring more than 7 mm in diameter. CT should be reserved for cases in which ultrasound and MRI imaging are nondiagnostic or unavailable. Although unenhanced, focused, single-detector helical CT has been shown to have sensitivity and specificity similar to those of graded-compression sonography, its documented use in pregnancy is limited to case series. Its advantage over traditional CT imaging is its limited ionizing radiation [24]. CT findings consistent with appendicitis include inflammation and an enlarged, nonfilling tubular structure with or without a fecalith [23].

Despite reluctance to operate on a pregnant patient, immediate surgical intervention is indicated when the diagnosis of appendicitis is made. The choice of surgical procedure is based on uterine size and operator experience. The only indication for delay in surgery is active labor, and in these cases the surgery is performed immediately postpartum. Cesarean delivery is indicated for the usual obstetric indications or if there is appendiceal rupture [26]. Diagnostic and operative laparoscopy is reasonable before 20 weeks' gestation and is as safe as laparotomy [12–14]. When performing laparoscopy, the open (Hasson) technique should be employed to avoid inadvertent trocar or Veress needle entry into the uterus. As the uterus grows and the site of the appendix changes, trocar placement also may need to change [27]. Laparoscopy has been shown to reduce the false-positive appendectomy rate by 15% [12,27]. Laparoscopy is contraindicated when peritonitis is present because of its high complication rate [28]. Beyond the later second trimester, laparoscopy becomes more technically challenging, and laparotomy may be more prudent. When performing laparotomy, a standard muscle-splitting incision is made over the point of maximal tenderness. Incisions also may be a right paramedian or a midline vertical incision; the latter is recommended if there is appendiceal rupture or peritonitis. Care should be taken not to place traction medially on the uterus, because doing so may create uterine irritability. If the appendix has ruptured or if there is peritonitis, copious irrigation is recommended. Placement of a peritoneal drain may be considered to drain any abscesses, although in most cases this precaution is not necessary. The skin is not closed because of the high risk of wound infection. Patients should receive perioperative antibiotics, including a second-generation cephalosporin, extended-spectrum penicillin, or carbapenam. Antibiotics also should include anaerobic coverage, because 95% of patients grow *Bacteroides fragilis* on culture. Dosing may be either a single dose prophylactically or continuous. If the appendix has ruptured, antibiotics are continued until the patient remains afebrile, bowel function has returned to normal, and the leukocytosis has improved [26]. Perioperative tocolytics are indicated only for documented uterine contractions and are not used prophylactically. Appendiceal abscesses may be managed using parenteral antibiotics and percutaneous drainage followed by an interval appendectomy. An open procedure may be indicated if the patient does not respond to this management [1]. Appendicitis is confirmed pathologically in only 36% to 50% of cases. The accuracy of diagnosis in the first trimester is greater, with only 24% of cases demonstrating normal pathology [6,29]. A higher false-positive rate is acceptable in pregnant women, because any delay in diagnosis may compromise maternal or fetal well-being.

## Gallbladder disease

Acute cholecystitis affects approximately 10% of the population in Western societies [30]. More than 90% of cases are caused by cystic duct obstruction with gallstones or biliary sludge. Parasitic infections such as ascariasis also can cause obstruction and are a common reason for cholecystitis in developing countries. Once the cystic duct is obstructed, intraluminal pressure within the gallbladder increases. The resulting trauma to the gallbladder wall induces the release of prostaglandins $I_2$ and $E_2$, which mediate an inflammatory response. Secondary infection with enteric flora such *Escherichia coli, Klebsiella,* or *Streptococcus faecalis* complicates one fifth of cases [30].

Well-defined risk factors for developing gallstones include age, female sex, obesity, and family history [31]. By the end of the first trimester of pregnancy, progesterone causes smooth muscle relaxation and a decrease in gallbladder tone. Weakened contractions and decreased emptying lead to increased gallbladder volume during fasting and after eating. In turn, biliary stasis contributes to cholesterol crystal sequestration, theoretically leading to the formation of sludge and stones. Elevated estrogen levels during pregnancy may further increase the lithogenicity of bile [32]. Lower gallbladder ejection fractions and increasing parity seem to increase the risk of sludge formation [33]. A high prepregnancy body mass index also may increase the risk of sludge formation [34,35]. Despite these physiologic changes, it is unclear if pregnancy increases the incidence of gallstones and cholecystitis [2,23]. In a German population study looking at 1111 females, current pregnancy and the number of prior pregnancies were not associated with an increased risk [31]. On the other hand, Gilat and Konikoff [36] reported a 7% prevalence of gallstones in nulliparous women but an increase to 19% in women who had had two or more pregnancies. Cholelithiasis has been documented in up to 10% of pregnancies, and cholecystitis reportedly affects 0.1% of pregnant patients [37]. Although it affects only 1 in 1600 to 10,000 pregnancies, biliary tract disease is the second most common nonobstetric surgical problem [32].

The clinical presentation of acute cholecystitis in pregnancy mirrors the presentation in the nonpregnant patient. Common symptoms include nausea and vomiting, anorexia, intolerance of fatty foods, dyspepsia, and mid-epigastric or right upper quadrant pain. Murphy's sign may be elicited less frequently in pregnant patients [32]. Patients may have a history of prior biliary colic, but many have been asymptomatic before presentation. In more severe cases, the patient may have mild jaundice or appear septic. Laboratory assessment can reveal elevated direct bilirubin and transaminase levels as well as bilirubinuria. An elevated white blood cell count and serum alkaline phosphatase level also may be associated with acute cholecystitis, but these indices normally are increased during pregnancy and may not be as helpful in assessing the gravid patient [2,32,38]. Elevated lipase and amylase levels may indicate associated pancreatitis. The differential diagnosis for cholecystitis is broad and includes appendicitis, pyelonephritis, right lower lobe pneumonia, the syndrome of hepatitis, acute fatty liver, hemolytic anemia/elevated liver enzymes/low platelet count (HELLP syndrome), pancreatitis, peptic ulcer disease, myocardial infarction, and herpes zoster [1,2,32].

The pregnant patient who has right upper quadrant tenderness should undergo ultrasound evaluation first because it is noninvasive and quickly obtained. Gallstones are detected reliably in 95% to 98% of studies [1,32,38]. Classic ultrasonic findings suggestive of acute cholecystitis also can be seen during pregnancy and include wall edema (>3 mm), pericholecystic fluid, calculi, and sonographic Murphy's sign [32]. Intra- and extrahepatic duct dilation may be noted with associated choledocholithiasis or Mirizzi syndrome. MR cholangiography can be performed safely during pregnancy if extrahepatic ductal stones are suspected but not demonstrated on ultrasound [1].

Symptomatic cholelithiasis often is managed initially with a conservative approach, delaying elective cholecystectomy until after delivery. This treatment includes bowel rest, intravenous hydration, and appropriate analgesia. Antibiotics should be given if no improvement is seen in 12 to 24 hours or if systemic symptoms are noted [30]. A short course of indomethacin can reverse gallbladder inflammation and is safe during the second trimester of pregnancy. If conservative management fails, or if repeated hospitalizations are required, especially in the same trimester, cholecystectomy is indicated. Severe sequelae if intervention is delayed include gangrenous cholecystitis, gallbladder perforation with biliary peritonitis, cholecystoenteric fistulas, choledocholithiasis, ascending cholangitis, and gallstone pancreatitis.

Recently, earlier surgical intervention for biliary tract disease in pregnancy has been advocated [32,39–41]. Lu and colleagues [40] retrospectively reviewed 78 pregnancies complicated by biliary disease and compared the outcomes of patients managed conservatively with the outcomes of patients who underwent surgical intervention. They reported shorter hospital stays and a reduced rate of preterm deliveries in the surgical patients and concluded surgical management of biliary disease is safe during pregnancy. Other proponents of earlier intervention report reduced medication usage and lower rates of life-threatening complications [41].

Undoubtedly, the laparoscopic approach to cholecystectomy has revolutionized the approach to treating biliary disease during pregnancy. A growing body of evidence suggests that it is least as safe, and perhaps is safer, than open cholecystectomy [16,42,43]. In a review of 61 reported cases of laparoscopic cholecystectomy in gravid patients, Barone and colleagues [42] found only three spontaneous abortions and two cases of premature labor. All the spontaneous abortions occurred in one series, and two of these patients had associated gallstone pancreatitis. All the cases of premature labor occurred remote from the time of surgery. Historically, the second trimester has been considered the optimal time to perform surgery, because organogenesis is complete, and the risk of spontaneous abortions is lower. Laparoscopic cholecystectomy has been performed safely in all trimesters, although premature labor is more common when surgery is performed in the third trimester [1,23,39,42]. The use of an open technique for entry, insufflation to 12 mm Hg, and maintaining a left lateral decubitus position minimize risk to the fetus and help maintain adequate placental blood flow during surgery [39].

Patients presenting with acute cholecystitis and symptomatic choledocholithiasis during pregnancy should be considered in a higher risk category. The incidence may approach 1 in 1200 pregnancies [32]. If complications such as cholangitis or gallstone pancreatitis develop, maternal mortality approaches 15%, and fetal loss occurs in 60% of cases [32]. Surgical approaches include open cholecystectomy with choledocotomy or a laparoscopic approach, depending on patient stability and surgeon preference. Although not routinely recommended, intraoperative cholangiography is safe after fetal organogenesis is complete and does not increase the risk of preterm labor or adverse fetal outcomes [44]. Pelvic shielding should be used to protect the uterus during its use. Alternatively (and perhaps more commonly employed), postoperative endoscopic retrograde cholangiopancreatography with sphincterotomy for stone extraction or stent placement also has been shown to be safe during pregnancy [45].

## Bowel obstruction

Bowel obstruction occurs complicates 1 in 3000 pregnancies and is the third most common reason for a nonobstetric laparotomy [1,2,23,32]. Approximately 60% to 0% of cases are caused by adhesions, and 25% are the result of volvulus. By comparison, in nonpregnant patient, only 3% to 5% of obstructions are caused by volvulus [32]. The risk of volvulus is highest during rapid changes in uterine size, usually during the early portions of the second trimester and in the postpartum period. Redundant bowel (usually the cecum) can be rotated around a fixed point causing obstruction during this time. Intussusception accounts for most of the other cases of bowel obstruction [2]. The impact of obstruction can be significant. Perdue and colleagues [46] reported on 66 patients undergoing laparotomy for obstruction. Maternal mortality was 6%, and the fetal loss rate was 26%.

Typical pregnancy symptoms can cause delayed diagnosis of intestinal obstruction. Usual symptoms include crampy abdominal pain, constipation, and nausea/emesis. Most pregnant patients experience some or all of these symptoms, especially in the first trimester. The gravid uterus can mask the abdominal distention seen with obstruction. Severe or persistent vomiting should alert the consulting physician to look for other etiologies, including obstruction. Plain abdominal films can be helpful for diagnosis showing the typical air-fluid levels and dilated bowel loops in 82% of cases [2]. Sensitivity for volvulus is 95% with plain-film radiographs [32]. If plain-film radiographs are normal, and obstruction is still suspected, contrast studies should be obtained, given the high risk of fetal death with delayed treatment.

Treatment for bowel obstruction during pregnancy is the same as for the nonpregnant patient. Conservative measures are used initially, including bowel decompression with nasogastric suctioning, bowel rest, fluid and electrolyte replacement, and enemas as indicated. If conservative measures are unsuccessful, or if the patient develops fever, tachycardia, or peritoneal signs, surgical exploration is mandatory. Colonoscopy has been used successfully in reduction of volvulus and may prevent emergency laparotomies. Definitive surgery after pregnancy is warranted, because the recurrence rate exceeds 50% [32]. Surgical principles at the time of laparotomy do not change in the pregnant patient and include enterolysis and resection of necrotic bowel. Cecopexy can be performed for cases involving volvulus; if cecopexy is technically difficult, resection is recommended [32].

## Inflammatory bowel disease

IBD often develops in women during their reproductive years with a peak incidence in the third or fourth decades [47]. In the past, patients who had either Crohn's disease (CD) or ulcerative colitis were encouraged to avoid pregnancy because of the possibility of disease exacerbation and pregnancy complications. Advances in treatment have led to prolonged remissions, however, prompting many affected patients to consider family planning [48].

Patients who have IBD have fewer children than the general population, perhaps reflecting voluntary choice [49]. Patients who have chronic CD in remission seem to be as fertile as unaffected individuals. Active CD, on the other hand, reduces fertility rates through several mechanisms including tubo-ovarian inflammation, perianal disease causing dyspareunia, and adhesive disease from prior surgeries [47,49]. Women who have ulcerative colitis have rates of fertility similar to those of the general population before surgery. After surgical treatment (including ileal pouch anal anastomosis and proctocolectomy with ileostomy), infertility rates increase significantly, probably from tubal factors [50,51].

Literature reviewing the impact of IBD on pregnancy outcomes is mixed. Several recent studies have concluded that neither CD nor ulcerative colitis has an adverse effect, especially if the disease is quiescent [47,49]. In a meta-analysis of 748 women who had CD, Miller [52] found rates of congenital anomalies and stillbirth similar to those in the general population. Other studies, however, have shown increased rates of spontaneous abortion, preterm birth, low birth rate, intrauterine growth restriction, and stillbirth [48]. Most studies indicate poorer outcomes when active disease is present [49], but some have shown poor outcome independent of disease activity [48]. One study suggests patients who have ulcerative colitis may have a higher incidence of congenital malformations, although these results have not been replicated [51].

Most consultants recommend clinical remission of IBD before conception. If pregnancy occurs during a period of quiescence, the risk of disease relapse is the same as in a nonpregnant woman [49]. Relapse rates range from 10% to 54% [47], and most relapses occur during the first trimester [1]. Most patients who experience a relapse of quiescent disease can be controlled medically and deliver at term [53]. If patients conceive during an active exacerbation, two thirds will have persistent symptoms throughout pregnancy, and of these, two thirds will have deterioration [49]. Initial presentation of IBD during pregnancy is rare. Diagnosis can be difficult, because many nonspecific symptoms also are found in normal pregnancies. In general, outcome is poorer, probably from delayed diagnosis [1].

When evaluating a pregnant patient suspected of having a flare or new onset of IBD, imaging studies should begin with ultrasound. Bowel wall thickening or abscess formations may be evident. Additional studies may be necessary including MRI or CT. The reference standard for diagnosis is endoscopy with biopsy. Both sigmoidoscopy and colonoscopy have been performed on gravid patients with minimal risk to the developing fetus [47,53,54].

Initial management of IBD during pregnancy begins with medical therapy. Multiple options exist, and most treatments are not associated with adverse fetal outcomes. 5-Aminosalicylic acid (5-ASA) medications such as sulfasalazine have the longest track record in pregnancy and usually are the first-line treatment. Folate absorption is inhibited in patients taking sulfasalazine, so supplementation is recommended [53]. Often, prednisone is added to the treatment regimen. Stress-dose steroids are necessary during delivery or surgery in these patients. Short-term use of antibiotics also is common during initial treatment. In patients who do not respond to treatment with 5-ASA and corticosteroids, the use of immunosuppressants such as cyclosporine and anti–tumor necrosis factor-$\alpha$ antibiotics such as infliximab can be considered; both been shown to be safe during pregnancy [49,53]. Medications such as methotrexate or thalidomide should be avoided during pregnancy because of their known teratogenic effects. Input from a gastroenterologist and a maternal fetal specialist should be obtained during treatment planning and follow-up.

Indications for surgery in the treatment of IBD do not change during pregnancy and include obstruction, megacolon, perforation, hemorrhage, abscess formation, and failed medical management [47,49]. Multiple procedures have been described in case reports ranging from loop ileostomy to total proctocolectomy. Loop ileostomy alone usually is insufficient because of the continued risk of colonic perforation. On the other hand, total proctocolectomy may be inappropriate because the operation is complex and long and because the enlarged uterus interferes with pelvic dissection. In the severely ill patient, a Turnbull procedure can be performed. The colon is decompressed via a cutaneous blowhole colostomy, and the bowel is diverted with a loop ileostomy. This procedure can be performed quickly and minimizes iatrogenic perforation of severely diseased colons. The primary disadvantage is that the remaining colon can continue to cause ongoing problems that could require repeated operations [53]. Stable patients can undergo subtotal colectomy and ileostomy. The rectal stump can be oversewn or brought out as a mucous fistula. The ileostomy placement generally should be higher on the abdominal wall, because it will descend in the postpartum period with uterine involution [54]. Definitive treatment with rectal resection and ileal pouch and anastomosis can be considered following delivery, because anastomotic leaks during pregnancy can be catastrophic [49,53]. Concurrent cesarean delivery at the time of colectomy should be based on fetal indications usually after 28 weeks [53,54].

The rate of cesarean delivery is higher in patients who have IBD than in the general population [51], probably reflecting the unknown effects of a vaginal delivery on the disease state or bowel anastomotic sites within the pelvis. In general, vaginal delivery is the standard for patients who have quiescent or mild disease, with cesarean section being reserved for obstetric indications [49]. Patients who have active perianal disease should avoid vaginal delivery, and patients who have an ileal pouch and anastomosis may consider cesarean section to prevent injury to the anal sphincter. Lacerations, especially with extension into the external anal sphincter, should be avoided if possible, because the rate of perianal disease may be increased [49,51]. Episiotomies should be avoided also, but if the risk for extension exists, a mediolateral or J-flap incision can be made to avoid sphincter injury.

## Hemorrhoids

Hemorrhoidal complaints are very prevalent, affecting from 4% to 36% of the population [55]. Hemorrhoids develop from pathologic changes in prolapsed anal cushions. These anal cushions are derived from submucosal tissue lining the anal canal and contain arteriovenous communications. Disruption of the connective tissue supporting the cushions results from age, hard stools, and associated straining. Prolapse results, leading to venous stasis, inflammation, and erosion of the epithelium [55]. First-degree hemorrhoids only bleed. Second-degree hemorrhoids reduce spontaneously. Third-degree hemorrhoids require manual reduction. Fourth-degree hemorrhoids are incarcerated [55]. Internal hemorrhoids are found above the dentate line, whereas external hemorrhoids are found below.

Thrombosed external hemorrhoids are common during pregnancy and the postpartum period. Abramowitz and colleagues [56] reported a prevalence of anal lesions (thrombosed external hemorrhoids or anal fissures) of 9.1% during pregnancy and 35.2% in the postpartum period in his series of 165 patients. Ninety-one percent of the thrombosed hemorrhoids were seen on postpartum day 1. Risk factors for their development included a maternal history of dyschezia, post-date delivery, larger babies, and perineal lacerations. Thirty-two of 33 hemorrhoids were seen in patients delivering vaginally [56].

Treatment of hemorrhoids during pregnancy initially involves a conservative approach. Dietary fiber supplementation helps relieve constipation and reduces straining. Episodes of bleeding and symptoms can be improved, but the degree of prolapse does not change. Often 6 weeks or longer are necessary before improvements are noticed. Anesthetics and steroids can provide short-term relief, but they do not affect the underlying pathologic changes. Surgery for intractable disease should be delayed until fetal viability or until the postpartum period. Rubber-band ligation provides significant improvement for 79% of patients who have second- and third-degree internal hemorrhoids [55]. Hemorrhoidectomy is reserved for patients who have third- and fourth-degree internal hemorrhoids and those in whom banding has been unsuccessful. Acutely strangulated hemorrhoids from thrombus formation require emergency débridement [55].

## Malignancies

Although cancer is the second most common reason for death in women of reproductive age, malignancies, fortunately, are rarely encountered during pregnancy, with an estimated incidence of 1 in 1000 to 1500 live births [57]. Cancer diagnosis during pregnancy often is unanticipated and can overwhelm the patient and physician. A multidisciplinary treatment team is required with input from surgeons, oncologists, radiation oncologists, and maternal-fetal medicine specialists to assess carefully the risks and benefits of treatment modalities. Often, the most critical decision to make when dealing with a malignancy during pregnancy is the timing of treatment. Considerations at the forefront include pregnancy termination, concurrent treatment during pregnancy, and early delivery before treatment versus delayed treatment until fetal lung maturity is documented. The benefit of delaying treatment to achieve fetal maturity must be balanced carefully against the risks of delayed intervention. The patient's desires, after careful education, should weigh heavily in the ultimate plan.

The most common malignancies encountered during pregnancy are cervical cancer, breast cancer, and melanoma. Other less common malignancies include Hodgkin's lymphoma, ovarian cancer, colorectal cancer, and leukemia [57]. This section focuses primarily on breast cancer and melanoma, because they are the malignancies most likely to be encountered by a general surgeon.

### Breast cancer

Breast cancer is the most frequent cancer diagnosed in women in the United States and is the second leading cause of cancer death. In 2007 there were an estimated 178,480 new cases and 40,460 deaths in women [58]. The risk of developing breast cancer by age 39 years is 1 in 210, whereas the lifetime risk is 1 in 8 [58]. Despite this high prevalence, only 1% to 3% of breast cancers are diagnosed during pregnancy [57]. The estimated incidence is 1 in 3000 pregnancies [59].

The histologic subtypes of breast cancer in pregnancy mirror those in the non-pregnant patient. Ductal carcinoma predominates, and lobular carcinomas and inflammatory carcinoma are uncommon. Most cancers are high grade, and lymphovascular invasion is commonly noted. Twenty-eight percent are estrogen receptor positive, 24% are progesterone receptor positive, and the *Her2/neu* expression rate is 28% [59]. Essentially, pregnancy has minimal impact on the histobiologic aspects of the tumor, whereas the age at diagnosis is most important. Stage-for-stage, survival rates for pregnant patients are identical to those of their nonpregnant cohorts. Unfortunately, most pregnant patients are diagnosed with more advanced disease: 42% of pregnant patients are found to have stage III or IV disease [60], perhaps reflecting the difficulty in diagnosing breast cancer during pregnancy.

Breast cancer can be difficult to diagnose during pregnancy. The delay from symptoms to diagnosis averages 5 months [60]. The normal physiologic changes of breast tissue during pregnancy (including hypertrophy and increasing nodularity) make detecting a mass challenging. When a mass is discovered, definitive evaluation should be initiated, which often involves tissue diagnosis. With proper shielding, mammograms can be performed safely during pregnancy and pose minimal risks to the developing fetus. Sensitivity probably is diminished, however, by the increased glandularity of the breasts. Ultrasound also can be used to differentiate solid from cystic lesions. Experience with MRI for breast cancer during pregnancy is limited, so its routine use is not recommended [59]. Fine-needle aspiration of a suspicious lesion can be performed but carries a real risk of both false-negative and false-positive results in pregnancy [60]. Directed core-needle biopsy is the reference standard for diagnosis, with excisional biopsy reserved for cases in which the core is nondiagnostic. Concerns about increased vascularity and edema are warranted, but complications such as hematoma, infection, or milk fistula are rarely encountered [59].

When breast cancer is diagnosed in pregnancy, treatment should conform as closely as possible to standardized protocols. The treatment plan should take into consideration the gestational age and the stage of disease. During the first trimester, pregnancy termination may be considered, but a survival benefit has not been shown with elective abortion [60]. Surgery can be performed safely in all trimesters. Some surgeons may opt to wait until after the twelfth week to minimize the risk of spontaneous abortion. Most pregnant patients who have breast cancer have mastectomies with axillary staging primarily because of the concern regarding radiation treatment [59]. Breast-conserving surgery may be considered for patients diagnosed in the late second and third trimester, with adjuvant radiation given in the postpartum period, usually following adjuvant chemotherapy. Sentinel lymph node biopsy has not been investigated thoroughly in pregnancy although the radiation dose to the fetus from technetium is estimated to be low. Isosulfan blue dye mapping is not recommended, because it has not been approved by the Food and Drug Administration for use during pregnancy [59].

Adjuvant treatment for breast cancer includes radiation, systemic chemotherapy, and hormonal therapy. External beam radiation is contraindicated during pregnancy and should be delayed until the postpartum period. During the preimplantation and early implantation phases (days 0–10), an all-or-none effect is seen. Organogenesis occurs from days 11 to 56, and during this time doses of ionizing radiation as small as 10 cGy cause measurable increases in fetal anomalies. Following organogenesis, larger radiation doses are needed to produce external malformations. Doses exceeding 50 cGy have been shown to cause mental retardation [61]. Likewise, hormonal therapy should be delayed until after delivery. Tamoxifen has been associated with neonatal genital tract defects following in utero exposure [59]. Patients who have locally advanced breast cancer, inflammatory breast cancer, or metastatic disease require systemic chemotherapy. Although few studies have reported on chemotherapy use during pregnancy, the risk of malformations when chemotherapy is used after the period of organogenesis seems to be similar to the baseline population risk of 3% [59]. Growth retardation and hematologic toxicities can be anticipated, however. Chemotherapy should be withheld after 35 weeks to minimize the risk of neonatal neutropenia at birth. 5-Fluorouracil, doxorubicin, and cyclophosphamide have been used with reasonable safety and minimal risk to the fetus [59].

## Melanoma

It has been estimated that 26,030 new cases of melanoma will be found in women in 2007, with 2890 deaths from the disease [58]. Melanoma is the sixth most common malignancy in women. During the past decade, the incidence of melanoma has been increasing by 3% per year [62]. This increase is greater than that of all other solid tumors and also is associated with a decreasing age at presentation [60]. The median age of women diagnosed as having melanoma is 45 years, and melanoma represents 8% of malignancies found during pregnancy. The estimated incidence is between 0.14 and 2.8 cases per 1000 births [57,60,61]. Fortunately, most pregnant patients present with stage I disease [57].

Pregnancy poses some theoretic risks to patients who have melanoma. Melanocyte-stimulating hormone (MSH) levels rise after the second month of pregnancy, and elevated production of adrenocorticotropic hormone further increases MSH activity. Estrogen further modulates melanocyte response [57,61]. As a result, increased pigmentation of the nipple, vulva, linea nigra, and pre-existing nevi is common during pregnancy. It has been postulated that these hormonal changes also could stimulate tumor growth [61]. Furthermore, hyperpigmentation of pregnancy can delay the diagnosis of melanoma. Several reports have documented significantly thicker primary tumors in pregnancy and more unfavorable histopathologic features [57,61,62]. Despite these concerns, in more recent investigations pregnancy has not been an independent factor associated with poorer prognosis. O'Meara and colleagues [62] evaluated 412 pregnant women diagnosed as having melanoma. They found no difference in disease distribution, histologic type, tumor thickness, positive lymph nodes, or survival between pregnant patients and matched controls. Furthermore, pregnancy termination has not been associated with regression of melanoma or improved survival [60].

Clinical signs of melanoma are identical in pregnant and nonpregnant patients. Changes in size, color, or shape of any pigmented lesion should raise suspicions. Bleeding and ulceration are more ominous findings. Any suspicious lesion should undergo excisional biopsy. Surgical staging for melanoma includes assessment of the local tumor site and surrounding tissue as well as the regional lymph nodes. Potential metastatic sites also should be evaluated. Routine lymph node dissection is controversial and has not had a consistent impact on survival [60]. Most patients who have melanoma undergo sentinel node mapping, with formal lymph node dissection if metastatic disease is found. As in breast cancer, however, the role of sentinel node mapping in pregnancy is unknown [57]. Adjuvant therapy in melanoma is largely investigational. The only treatment with proven benefit is high-dose interferon-α2b, and no cases of its use during pregnancy have been reported [57].

Interestingly, melanoma is the most common malignancy to metastasize to the placenta or fetus. In general, the placenta is resistant to metastatic disease; therefore, case reports are extremely rare [61]. Dildly and colleagues [63] reviewed 53 reported cases of maternal cancer metastatic to either the placenta or fetus between 1866 and 1987. Despite accounting for only 8% of maternal cancers, melanoma represented 30% of the cases metastasizing to the placenta and more than 50% of the cancers metastasizing to the fetus. After delivery, the placenta should be sent for pathologic evaluation in all women who have concurrent malignancies.

## Summary

The incidence of surgical disease is the same in pregnant and nonpregnant patients. Approximately 1 in 500 pregnancies requires a nonobstetric surgical intervention. Most of the presenting symptoms of surgical diseases in pregnant women are similar to those in nonpregnant patients, but many of these symptoms may be confused with normal complaints of pregnancy, leading to delays in diagnosis. The surgical tenets of treatment remain largely unchanged. Prognosis also is largely unchanged by the pregnant state and depends more on the extent of disease at diagnosis. Consultation with maternal-fetal medicine during treatment planning is invaluable to ensure optimal outcomes for both the mother and fetus.

## References

[1] Parangi S, Levine D, Henry A, et al. Surgical gastrointestinal disorders during pregnancy. Am J Surg 2007;193:223–32.

[2] Coleman MT, Trianfo VA, Rund DA. Nonobstetric emergencies in pregnancy: trauma and surgical conditions. Am J Obstet Gynecol 1997;177(3):497–502.

[3] Gomez A, Wood MD. Acute appendicitis during pregnancy. Am J Surg 1979;137(2):180–3.

[4] McGee TM. Acute appendicitis in pregnancy. Aust N Z J Obstet Gynaecol 1989;29(4): 378–85.

[5] Mourad J, Elliott JP, Erickson L, et al. Appendicitis in pregnancy: new information that contradicts long-held clinical beliefs. Am J Obstet Gynecol 2000;182(5):1027–9.

[6] Mazze RI, Kallen B. Appendectomy during pregnancy: a Swedish registry study of 778 cases. Obstet Gynecol 1991;77(6):835–40.

[7] Babaknia A, Parsa H, Woodruff JD. Appendicitis during pregnancy. Obstet Gynecol 1977; 50(1):40–4.

[8] Al-Mulhim AA. Acute appendicitis in pregnancy: a review of 52 cases. Int Surg 1996;81(3): 295–7.

[9] Hale DA, Malloy M, Pearl RH, et al. Appendectomy: a contemporary appraisal. Ann Surg 1997;225(2):252–61.

[10] Tamir IL, Bongard FS. Acute appendicitis in the pregnant patient. Am J Surg 1990;160(6): 571–6.

[11] Epstein FB. Acute abdominal pain in pregnancy. Emerg Med Clin North Am 1994;12(1): 1511–65.

[12] Visser BC, Glasgow RE, Mulvihill KK, et al. Safety and timing of nonobstetric abdominal surgery in pregnancy. Dig Surg 2001;18(5):409–17.

[13] Affleck DG, Handrahan DL, Egger MJ, et al. The laparoscopic management of appendicitis and cholelithiasis during pregnancy. Am J Surg 1999;178(6):523–9.

[14] Firstenberg MS, Malangoni MA. Gastrointestinal surgery during pregnancy. Gastroenterol Clin North Am 1998;27(1):73–88.

[15] Kammerer WS. Nonobstetric surgery during pregnancy. Med Clin North Am 1979;63(6): 1157–64.

[16] Cohen-Kerem R, Railton C, Oren D, et al. Pregnancy outcome following non-obstetric surgical intervention. Am J Surg 2005;190(3):467–73.

[17] Baer JL, Reis RA, Arenas RA. Appendicitis in pregnancy with changes in the position and axis of the normal appendix in pregnancy. JAMA 1932;52:1359–64.

[18] Beck WW. Intestinal obstruction in pregnancy. Obstet Gynecol 1974;43(3).374–8.

[19] Nathan L, Huddleston JF. Acute abdominal pain in pregnancy. Obstet Gynecol Clin North Am 1995;22(1):55–67.

[20] Hodjati H, Kazerooni T. Location of the appendix in the gravid patient: a re-evaluation of the established concept. Int J Gynaecol Obstet 2003;81(3):245–7.

[21] Cunningham FG, McCubbin JH. Appendicitis complicating pregnancy. Obstet Gynecol 1975;45(4):415–20.

[22] Richards C, Daya S. Diagnosis of acute appendicitis in pregnancy. Can J Surg 1989;32(5): 358–60.

[23] Kilpatrick CC, Monga M. Approach to the acute abdomen in pregnancy. Obstet Gynecol Clin North Am 2007;34(3):389–402.

[24] Poortman P, Lohle PN, Schoemaker CM, et al. Comparison of CT and sonography in the diagnosis of acute appendicitis: a blinded prospective study. Am J Roentgenol 2003; 181(5):1355–9.

[25] Shellock FG, Crues JV. MR procedures: biologic effects, safety, and patient care. Radiology 2004;232(3):635–52.

[26] Malangoni MA. Gastrointestinal surgery and pregnancy. Gastroenterol Clin North Am 2003;32(1):181–200.

[27] Gurbuz HT, Peetz ME. The acute abdomen in the pregnant patient: is there a role for laparoscopy? Surg Endosc 1997;11(2):98–102.

[28] Paik PS, Towson JA, Antbone GJ, et al. Intra-abdominal abscesses following laparoscopic and open appendectomies. J Gastrointest Surg 1997;1(2).188–93.

[29] Hee P, Viktrup L. The diagnosis of appendicitis during pregnancy and maternal and fetal outcome after appendectomy. Int J Gynecol Obstet 1999;65(2):129–35.

[30] Indar AA, Beckingham IJ. Acute cholecystitis. BMJ 2002;325:639–43.

[31] Walcher T, Haenle MM, Kron M, et al. Pregnancy is not a risk factor for gallstone disease: results of a randomly selected population sample. World J Gastroenterol 2005;11(43):6800–6.

[32] Augustin G, Majerovic M. Non-obstetrical acute abdomen during pregnancy. Eur J Obstet Gynecol Reprod Bio 2007;131:4–12.

[33] Bolukbas FF, Bolukbas C, Horoz M, et al. Risk factors associated with gallstone and biliary sludge formation during pregnancy. J Gastroenterol Hepatol 2006;21(7):1150–3.

[34] Ko CW, Beresford SA, Schulte SJ, et al. Incidence, natural history, and risk factors for biliary sludge and stones during pregnancy. Hepatology 2005;41(2):359–65.

[35] Ko CW. Risk factors for gallstone-related hospitalization during pregnancy and the postpartum. Amer J Gastroenterol 2006;101:2263–8.

[36] Gilat T, Konikoff F. Pregnancy and the biliary tract. Can J Gastroenterol 2000;14(Suppl D): 55D–9D.

[37] Diettrich NA, Kaplan G. Surgical considerations in the contemporary management of biliary tract disease in the postpartum period. Am J Surg 1998;176:251–3.

[38] Stone K. Acute abdominal emergencies associated with pregnancy. Clin Obstet Gynecol 2002;45(2):553–61.

[39] Cosenza CA, Saffari B, Jabbour N, et al. Surgical management of biliary gallstone disease during pregnancy. Am J Surg 1999;178:545–8.

[40] Lu EJ, Curet MJ, El-Sayed YY, et al. Medical versus surgical management of biliary tract disease in pregnancy. Am J Surg 2004;188:755–9.

[41] Swisher S, Schmidt P, Hunt K, et al. Biliary disease during pregnancy. Am J Surg 1994;168: 576–9.

[42] Barone JE, Bears S, Chen S, et al. Outcome study of cholecystectomy during pregnancy. Am J Surg 1999;177:232–6.

[43] Bisharah M, Tulandi T. Laparoscopic surgery in pregnancy. Clin Obstet Gynecol 2003; 46(1):92–7.

[44] Graham G, Baxi L, Tharakan T. Laparoscopic cholecystectomy during pregnancy: a case series and review of the literature. Obstet Gynecol Surv 1998;53:566–74.

[45] Cappell MS. The safety and efficacy of gastrointestinal endoscopy during pregnancy. Gastroenterol Clin North Am 1998;27:37–71.

[46] Perdue PW, Johnson HW, Stafford PW. Intestinal obstruction complicating pregnancy. Am J Surg 1985;164:384–8.

[47] Lamah M, Scott HJ. Inflammatory bowel disease and pregnancy. Int J Colorectal Dis 2002; 17:216–22.

[48] Mahadevan U, Sandborn WJ, Li D, et al. Pregnancy outcomes in women with inflammatory bowel disease: a large community-based study from northern California. Gastroenterol 2007;133:1106–12.

[49] Caprilli R, Gassull A, Escher JC, et al. European evidence based consensus on the diagnosis and management of Crohn's disease: special situations. Gut 2006;55(Suppl I):i36–58.

[50] Lepisto A, Sarna S, Tiitinen A, et al. Female fertility and childbirth after ileal pouch-anal anastomosis for ulcerative colitis. Br J Surg 2007;94:478–82.

[51] Mahadevan U. Fertility and pregnancy in the patient with inflammatory bowel disease. Gut 2006;55:1198–206.

[52] Miller JP. Inflammatory disease in pregnancy: a review. J R Soc Med 1986;79:221–5.

[53] Dozois EJ, Wolff BG, Tremaine WJ, et al. Maternal and fetal outcome after colectomy for fulminant ulcerative colitis during pregnancy: case series and literature review. Dis Colon Rectum 2006;49(1):64–73.

[54] Haq AI, Sahai A, Hallwoth S, et al. Synchronous colectomy and caesarean section for fulminant ulcerative colitis: case report and review of the literature. Int J Colorectal Dis 2006;21:465–9.

[55] Nisar PJ, Scholefield JH. Managing haemorrhoids. BMJ 2003;327:847–51.

[56] Abramowitz L, Sobhani I, Benifla JL, et al. Anal fissure and thrombosed external hemorrhoids before and after delivery. Dis Colon Rectum 2002;45(5):650–5.

[57] Swenson RE, Goff BA, Koh WJ, et al. Cancer in the pregnant patient. In: Hoskins WJ, Perez CA, Young RC, et al, editors. Principles and practice of gynecologic oncology. 4th edition. Philadelphia: Lippincott Williams & Wilkins; 2005. p. 1279–311.

[58] Jemal A, Siegel R, Ward E, et al. Cancer statistics, 2007. CA Cancer J Clin 2007;57:43–66.

[59] Loibl S, von Minckwitz G, Gwyn K, et al. Breast carcinoma during pregnancy: international recommendations from an expert meeting. Cancer 2006;106(2):237–46.

[60] Lishner M. Cancer in pregnancy. Annals Oncol 2003;14(Suppl 3):iii31–6.

[61] Berman ML, Di Saia PJ, Brewster WR. Pelvic malignancies, gestational trophoblastic neoplasia, and nonpelvic malignancies. In: Creasy RK, Resnik R, editors. Maternal-fetal medicine. 4th edition. Philadelphia: WB Saunders; 1999. p. 1128–50.

[62] O'Meara AT, Cress R, Xing G, et al. Malignant melanoma in pregnancy. Cancer 2005;103: 1217–26.

[63] Dildly GA, Moise KJ, Carpenter RJ, et al. Maternal malignancy metastatic to the products of conception: a review. Obstet Gynecol Surv 1989;44(7):535–40.

SURGICAL
CLINICS OF
NORTH AMERICA

ELSEVIER
SAUNDERS

Surg Clin N Am 88 (2008) 421–440

# Trauma and Surgical Emergencies in the Obstetric Patient

Christina C. Hill, MD[a],*, Jennifer Pickinpaugh, DO[b]

[a]*Division of Maternal Fetal Medicine, Department of Obstetrics and Gynecology, Tripler Army Medical Center, 1 Jarrett White Road, Honolulu, HI 96859-5000, USA*
[b]*Department of Obstetrics and Gynecology, Tripler Army Medical Center, 1 Jarrett White Road, Honolulu, HI 96859-5000, USA*

Pregnancy always must be considered when evaluating a female trauma victim of reproductive age. When managing the pregnant trauma victim, one must optimize the well-being of two patients, but the health of the mother is of paramount importance. Rapid assessment, treatment, and transport are critical to optimizing maternal and fetal outcome. Evaluation must be performed with an understanding of the physiologic changes that occur in pregnancy. These changes alter maternal response to trauma and require adaptations to care. Management requires a multidisciplinary approach involving emergency medical technicians, trauma surgeons, anesthesiologists, emergency medicine physicians, obstetricians, maternal fetal medicine specialists, pediatricians, radiologists and nurses. The obstetrician can assess fetal status and can provide consultation regarding radiation and medication exposure as well as the indications for emergent cesarean delivery.

## General considerations

Trauma complicates 6% to 7% of all pregnancies and is the leading non-obstetric cause of maternal morbidity and mortality [1–6]. Trauma also is the leading cause of non–pregnancy-related death in women under 40 years of age in the United States, accounting for 46% of maternal deaths [7,8]. Pregnancy itself does not increase maternal mortality from trauma, because

The views expressed in this article are those of the authors and do not reflect the official policy or position of the Department of the Army, Department of Defense, or the US Government.
* Corresponding author.
*E-mail address:* christina.hill@amedd.army.mil (C.C. Hill).

mortality seems to be more a function of injury severity [9]. Because of the increasing size of the uterus and fetus, the risk of trauma to the mother and fetus increases as pregnancy progresses. Pregnancy seems to alter the pattern of injury, making the gravida more prone to abdominal trauma, particularly as gestation advances, and less vulnerable to head trauma [9]. The distribution of trauma includes motor vehicle accidents (55%), falls (22%), assaults (22%), and burns (1%) [10]. In a review by Connolly and colleagues [10], the mean maternal age at the time of trauma was 24 years, and the mean gestational age was 25.9 weeks. The average gestational age at delivery following trauma was 37 weeks.

## Physiologic changes of pregnancy

When managing the pregnant victim of trauma, appreciation of the physiologic and anatomic changes associated with pregnancy is critical [3,11]. These physiologic changes begin as early as the first trimester and can alter or mimic maternal response to trauma, thereby confounding evaluation.

The pregnant patient is physiologically prepared for the blood loss associated with delivery. Blood volume increases by 50%, and there is a 30% increase in erythrocyte volume. As such, the pregnant patient can hemorrhage up to 2000 mL of blood (or 30% to 40% of her blood volume) before manifesting changes in heart rate or blood pressure [12]. A patient's condition can deteriorate rapidly after hemorrhage approaching 2500 mL. The increase of plasma volume over red blood cell volume results in hemodilution and a physiologic anemia. Therefore, a normal pregnancy hematocrit is approximately 32% to 34%, which is lower than nonpregnant values. Cardiac output increases up to 50% beginning in the first trimester and peaks somewhere between 20 and 30 weeks' gestation. Cardiac output remains at third trimester values for the first 48 hours postpartum and then decreases gradually to nonpregnant values over the following 2 weeks. Uterine blood flow comprises about 20% of cardiac output, increases up to 600 mL/min during pregnancy, and can serve as a significant source of hemorrhage in the face of trauma. Uterine blood flow has no autoregulation and therefore is dependent on maternal mean arterial blood pressure. As such, changes in blood pressure can impact uterine blood flow negatively, thereby compromising fetal perfusion and oxygenation. By 20 weeks' gestation the enlarging uterus is capable of aortocaval compression, which can compromise venous return to the heart and reduce cardiac output. When the pregnant woman is supine, aortocaval compression reduces cardiac output by approximately 30% and can result in maternal pallor, sweating, nausea, vomiting, hypotension, tachycardia, and mental status changes.

Blood pressure is lower in pregnancy secondary to decreased systemic vascular resistance. Lower vascular resistance is the result primarily of the vasodilatory effects of progesterone and the low resistance of the placental bed. Systolic and diastolic blood pressures decrease by 5 mm Hg to 15 mm Hg, reaching a nadir at 28 weeks' gestation and gradually returning to normal at term [1]. Central venous pressure drops slowly from 9 mm Hg to about 4 mm Hg by term. Estrogen-mediated increases in myocardial alpha receptors result in heart rate increases of approximately 15 beats per minute [13].

ECG changes during pregnancy are common. Normal findings include sinus tachycardia, ectopic beats, left axis deviation, inverted or flattened T waves, and a Q wave in lead III and the augmented voltage unipolar left foot lead [1,14].

The increased metabolic demands of pregnancy increase oxygen consumption by 15% to 20% in the gravida. Minute ventilation increases by 50%, largely as a result of increased tidal volume, because respiratory rate changes minimally. The diaphragm moves approximately 4 cm upward in pregnancy, and the thoracic anteroposterior diameter increases. These anatomic alterations, in addition to the enlarging uterus, cause decreased expiratory reserve and residual lung volumes, thereby decreasing functional residual capacity. The 20% decrease in functional residual capacity coupled with increased oxygen consumption of pregnancy results in rapid maternal desaturation in the face of depressed respiration or apnea.

Normal chest radiographic findings in a pregnant patient include mild cardiomegaly, a widened mediastinum, an increased anteroposterior diameter, and prominence of the pulmonary vasculature [1,3]. The pregnant woman exists in a state of mild respiratory alkalosis. Elevated progesterone levels act on the medullary respiratory center stimulating ventilatory drive causing a decrease in $Pa_{CO_2}$ values to levels approaching 25 mm Hg to 30 mm Hg. Because values are lower in pregnancy, a $Pa_{CO_2}$ value in the nonpregnant range is concerning. There is a compensatory renal excretion of bicarbonate resulting in serum levels of 17 mEq/L to 22 mEq/L, thereby maintaining an arterial pH of 7.40 to 7.45. The increased minute ventilation results in $Pa_{O_2}$ levels that are higher than nonpregnant values, ranging between 104 mm Hg and 108 mm Hg. Maternal oxygen saturation should be maintained at 95% to maintain a $Pa_{O_2}$ greater than 70 mm Hg, optimizing oxygen diffusion across the placenta. Fetal oxygenation is maintained when maternal $Pa_{O_2}$ remains above 60 mm Hg to 70 mm Hg, and it is compromised immediately at lower levels.

The smooth muscle relaxation effects of progesterone contribute to decreased gastric tone and motility as well as reduced lower esophageal sphincter tone. These changes, in addition to the cephalad displacement of the stomach, result in an increased risk of aspiration when the trauma victim is unable to protect her airway. Normal pregnancy complaints include nausea, vomiting, and abdominal pain, symptoms that can confound the examination of a trauma patient.

Venous pooling in the lower extremities can lead to more extensive blood loss with lower extremity injuries and can predispose the patient to deep venous thrombosis. The increased engorgement of pelvic vessels associated with pregnancy also places the patient at increased risk of retroperitoneal hemorrhage and hematomas following lower abdominal and pelvic trauma [2].

It is normal to have a leukocytosis during pregnancy with a count ranging from 5000 to 25,000 per $mm^3$. Most procoagulant factors also are increased during pregnancy and may be beneficial for the patient in achieving hemostasis after injury. Fibrinogen levels normally approach 400 mg/dL. Therefore, findings of a normal or low fibrinogen level, in addition to elevated fibrin degradation products and low platelets, suggest disseminated intravascular coagulation. Increase in procoagulants, in addition to venous stasis and endothelial damage, place the gravida at risk for thromboembolic complications including pulmonary embolism. Therefore, when possible, thromboembolic prophylaxis is recommended following trauma.

## Fetal considerations

Although less than 8% of trauma injuries are life-threatening injuries, life-threatening injuries carry a 40% to 50% risk of fetal loss. Although fetal loss is much less common with mild injuries (1% to 5%) than with life-threatening trauma, mild injuries account for the majority of fetal losses because they occur so much more frequently [11]. Situations in which fetal death occurs include motor vehicle accidents (82%), gunshot wounds (6%), and falls (3%), with maternal death accounting for 11% of fetal deaths [11,15]. Predictors of fetal death include injury severity, high base deficit, high abdominal or thoracic abbreviated injury score, direct fetal or uterine injury, fetal heart rate abnormalities, uterine activity, maternal coma, and maternal death [9,11,16,17]. Fetal death may be a result of placental abruption, direct fetal injury, maternal shock, hypoxia, disseminated intravascular coagulation, or unexplained reasons [18,19].

## Diagnostic radiation

In the face of trauma, all indicated tests must be performed, including diagnostic radiologic studies. The diagnostic studies should be obtained as for similar indications in the nonpregnant patient, but studies should be limited, and the uterus should be shielded whenever possible. Radiation risk to the fetus is determined by gestational age, type of study, proximity to the uterus, use of uterine shielding, and the type of machine used [1,3]. The unshielded fetus receives approximately 30% of the radiation dose that the mother receives. Fetal risks from radiation are greatest during the period of major organogenesis, between 2 and 7 weeks postconception. The fetal central nervous system is vulnerable between 8 and 15 weeks' gestation. Radiation carries negligible fetal risk of anomalies after 20 weeks' gestation, especially if cumulative doses are less than 10 rads (100 mGy). Radiation doses of less than 1 rad (10 mGy) are believed to contribute little fetal risk. Radiation doses of less than 5 rads (50 mGy) are not associated with an increase in pregnancy loss or fetal anomalies [20]. Exposure to 15 rads (150 mGy) is associated with a 6% chance of mental retardation, a 3% chance of childhood cancer, and a 15% chance of microcephaly [3,21]. A plain-film radiograph of the pelvis exposes the fetus to 1 rad (10 mGy) of ionizing radiation. Plain radiographs of the chest and spine expose the fetus to little radiation, particularly if the uterus is shielded [3]. CT imaging is an excellent modality to evaluate for internal and intrauterine injuries and hemorrhage. A typical abdominal CT study, however, can expose the fetus to 5 to 10 rads (50–100 mGy); if possible, its use should be avoided in the first trimester with ultrasound or diagnostic peritoneal lavage used instead. Head and chest CT imaging exposes the fetus to far less radiation, particularly with uterine shielding, and may be used with little fetal exposure risk [3].

## Blunt trauma

Pregnant women are more likely than nonpregnant women to sustain abdominal trauma [3]. Blunt abdominal trauma is associated with a 3% to 38% incidence of fetal mortality. Blunt trauma may be the result of motor vehicle accidents, pedestrian automobile accidents, falls, direct abdominal trauma, and assault. Motor vehicle accidents are the leading cause of maternal blunt trauma and account for 55% to 82% of maternal trauma cases [1–3]. Although maternal death is uncommon, when it occurs it is a result of head and neck trauma, respiratory failure, or hypovolemic shock from hemorrhage. The most common cause of fetal death is maternal shock and death [3]. When the mother survives, abruption is the next leading cause of fetal mortality, followed by uterine rupture [3,22,23].

Before 13 weeks' gestation the uterus has not yet become an abdominal organ and is protected by the bony pelvis [11]. Fetal loss in the first trimester is less likely the result of direct trauma (occurring less than 1% of the time) but instead is likely to be caused by uterine hypoperfusion resulting from maternal hypotension or death [11]. As the uterus enlarges, it displaces the bowel cephalad, thereby protecting these structures, but rendering the fetus more vulnerable to injury [2]. Thinning of the uterine wall with growth and the relative decrease in amniotic fluid volume also contribute to fetal vulnerability.

The bladder is displaced cephalad by the enlarging uterus, making it susceptible to injury. As such, hematuria after injury should be evaluated aggressively [1]. Splenic injuries occur most commonly in the third trimester and may occur after even apparently mild trauma. Engorgement of the spleen renders it vulnerable to injury and excessive blood loss [1]. Injuries to the liver or spleen may result in abdominal pain, shoulder pain, and elevated transaminases [1]. Pelvic fractures commonly are associated with blunt trauma and are associated with significant retroperitoneal hemorrhage as a result of the myriad of engorged pelvic vessels. Pelvic fractures are the most common trauma resulting in direct fetal injury manifest by skull fractures and brain injury, particularly when the head is engaged in the pelvis. Fetal mortality can approach 25% in these cases [2]. Pelvic fractures commonly are associated with injuries to the bladder, urethra, and rectosigmoid colon. Pelvic radiographs must be interpreted with caution, because there is a normal widening of the sacroiliac joints and symphysis pubis with pregnancy.

Obstetric complications of blunt abdominal trauma include preterm labor, preterm delivery, preterm premature rupture of membranes, abruption, fetomaternal hemorrhage, and, rarely, uterine rupture. These topics are discussed sequentially.

## Preterm labor and delivery

Premature labor complicates 25% of trauma cases after 22 to 24 weeks' gestation [11]. Connolly and colleagues [10] found that 39% of all incidents of trauma were associated with uterine contractions of varying frequencies, although only 11.4% of cases were associated with preterm labor. Of trauma cases with preterm labor, 25% delivered preterm. The majority of these preterm deliveries occurred remote from the trauma. Preterm labor is managed using standard obstetric protocols.

## Abruption

Abruption occurs with 1% to 5% of minor injuries and 20% to 50% of major life-threatening injuries. It also occurs at a higher rate in women suffering trauma than in the general obstetric population [7,22,24–26]. Next to maternal death, abruption is the most frequent cause of fetal death from trauma [7]. Abruption occurs when acceleration-deceleration injuries result in shearing forces that separate the relatively elastic myometrium from the inelastic placenta [1,7]. Placental injury results in the release of thromboplastin into the circulation, and uterine injury releases plasminogen activator, resulting in fibrinolysis. These processes can lead to disseminated intravascular coagulation. The patient may complain of abdominal pain, bleeding, and/or back pain. Examination may demonstrate vaginal bleeding and a tender, rigid uterus. Goodwin and Breen [24] reviewed 205 cases of noncatastrophic trauma during the second half of pregnancy. They found that pregnancy-related morbidity was associated most frequently with vaginal bleeding, uterine tenderness, and/or uterine contractions. Abdominal or uterine tenderness and/or vaginal bleeding associated with direct abdominal trauma suggest placental abruption and require evaluation. The pregnant trauma patient should be admitted, and continuous fetal monitoring should be initiated if the fetus is viable. Electronic fetal monitoring is the most sensitive tool in identifying abruption. In a study by Pearlman and colleagues [25], patients experiencing uterine contractions demonstrated a 20% risk of placental abruption. Cardiotocography has demonstrated a 100% negative predictive value for adverse outcomes when monitoring was reassuring and there were no significant early clinical findings. Initial external fetal monitoring for a minimum of 4 hours is recommended for all patients of 20 weeks' gestation who have experienced any multisystem or minor abdominal trauma. Monitoring should be continued if there is evidence of persistent contractions, uterine tenderness, vaginal bleeding, significant maternal injury, rupture of membranes, or a nonreassuring fetal heart rate pattern [3]. Monitoring may be discontinued and the patient discharged if laboratory evaluation is normal, the fetal tracing is reassuring, contraction frequency is less than 1 per 10 minutes, and there is no evidence of vaginal bleeding or nonreassuring maternal status.

*Fetomaternal hemorrhage*

Fetomaternal hemorrhage occurs in 10% to 30% of pregnant trauma patients [27]. It occurs more commonly in women who suffer abdominal trauma with an anterior placenta and/or experience uterine tenderness [28]. Fetal risks of fetomaternal hemorrhage include anemia, arrhythmias, and exsanguination with resultant fetal distress and death [25]. Maternal risks include Rh sensitization. Less than 1 mL of Rh-positive fetal blood can result in sensitization in an Rh-negative woman.

The Kleihauer-Betke blood test assesses for hemorrhage of fetal cells into maternal circulation. It allows quantification of the amount of fetal red blood cells introduced into the maternal bloodstream. All Rh-negative pregnant trauma victims should receive 300 μg of Rh-immune globulin within the first 72 hours of fetomaternal hemorrhage and another 300 μg for each additional 30 mL of estimated fetal blood identified in the maternal circulation [11]. Kleihauer-Betke testing is not indicated in Rh-positive women [10].

*Uterine rupture*

A rare complication of blunt abdominal trauma is uterine rupture. Uterine rupture accounts for approximately 0.6% of all injuries during pregnancy and can result in a maternal mortality rate of up to 10% and nearly universal fetal mortality [2,7]. Uterine rupture occurs most commonly with rapid deceleration or direct compression injuries and is found most often in women who have had prior cesarean deliveries [1,3,29]. The risk for uterine rupture tends to increase with advancing gestational age and with increasing severity of direct abdominal trauma. The uterine wall separates, thereby rupturing the membranes and allowing extrusion of the umbilical cord and fetal parts into the abdomen. This rupture often is accompanied by extensive intra-abdominal hemorrhage [1]. Rupture of an unscarred uterus tends to occur posteriorly and commonly is associated with a bladder injury, presenting occasionally with blood or meconium in the urine [3,21].

Symptoms of uterine rupture include severe abdominal pain and cessation of uterine contractions. Examination is remarkable for vaginal bleeding, a rigid abdomen, rebound tenderness, and an asymmetric uterus or fetal parts palpable through the abdomen [1,3]. There may be no fetal heart rate, decreased fetal heart rate beat-to-beat variability, decelerations, or fetal tachycardia as a result of anemia or hypoxemia [30]. The diagnosis is suggested on abdominal radiograph or ultrasound and may require emergent surgical management [1]

## Seatbelts

Approximately 46% to 74% of pregnant trauma patients are restrained during motor vehicle accidents [3,11,31]. Poor compliance with restraint use may be caused by maternal concerns that seatbelt use can harm the pregnancy [11]. When trauma is the result of motor vehicle accidents, Crosby and Costiloe [23] found that among unrestrained women who were ejected, the maternal mortality rate was 33%, with a 47% fetal mortality rate. They found that although there is no evidence that seatbelt use in pregnancy decreases overall maternal mortality, there is an increase in mortality in mothers ejected from the vehicle. They therefore recommended that women wear seatbelts to prevent ejection-associated mortality. The use of restraints is associated with reduced injury severity, thereby also reducing risk of fetal demise [31]. The American College of Obstetricians and Gynecologists and the National Highway Traffic Safety Administration recommend that seatbelts be placed as low as possible over the protuberant portion of the abdomen and across the thighs. The shoulder strap should be worn to the side of the uterus, between the breasts and over the midportion of the clavicle [2,20]. An improperly placed seatbelt may result in uterine rupture and fetal demise [1,32]. The National Highway Traffic Safety Administration does not consider pregnancy as an indication to deactivate airbags, but the woman should position herself at least 10 in back from the center of the airbag cover [33].

## Penetrating trauma

Penetrating trauma is caused primarily by gunshot wounds, followed by knife wounds; the former are more lethal for the mother and fetus. Maternal mortality occurs in fewer than 5% of cases of penetrating trauma. The incidence of visceral injury with penetrating trauma in pregnancy is 16% to 38%, compared with 80% to 90% in the nonpregnant population [2,3]. Gunshot wounds to the abdomen result in fetal injury in up to 70% of cases; unfortunately, 40% to 70% of these fetuses die [11,34]. Fetal death is the result of direct fetal injury or preterm delivery [35]. Missiles such as bullets cause a transient shock wave and cavitations as they transmit their kinetic energy to the high-density tissues of the body, thereby causing more severe injury than the lower-velocity knife wounds [3]. The density of the uterus rapidly dissipates the energy of a low-velocity projectile, but high-velocity missiles are far more devastating to the mother and fetus. In early pregnancy the uterus is dense and protects the fetus and viscera. This density contributes to fairly low incidences of maternal visceral injury and improved maternal outcomes [1]. As pregnancy advances, the enlarging uterus displaces the abdominal contents cephalad and cushions against penetrating injury [2], but this displacement leaves the uterus vulnerable to penetrating trauma and renders abdominal contents vulnerable with upper abdominal wounds [1,3]. In knife wounds, the location of the injury is a critical determinant of outcome. Upper abdominal stab wounds can result in more complex bowel injury because of the upward displacement of intraperitoneal contents [11]. Therefore upper abdominal injuries are explored surgically more often [3,36].

Treatment guidelines for penetrating injuries are similar to those for nonpregnant patients [1]. Management options include immediate surgical exploration, diagnostic peritoneal lavage, laparoscopy, CT imaging, local wound exploration, and observation. Radiographic studies are helpful in localizing a bullet that has not exited. Management often is individualized and should involve a multidisciplinary team including trauma surgeons and obstetricians [3]. Laparotomy typically is performed for the management of gunshot wounds to the abdomen; however, selective observation may be considered in gravid patients who have stable vital signs and anterior and subfundal entry sites and when diagnostic imaging indicates that the missile has not exited the posterior uterine wall. Patients should receive antibiotics to cover streptococcal and clostridium infections. Management in an intensive care setting with continuous fetal monitoring and serial evaluations is recommended.

## Burns

The incidence of burns in pregnancy is relatively low and is difficult to determine. Maternal and fetal mortality are directly related to the type, location, and severity of the burn sustained, in addition to the presence of complications. Fetal outcome also is related to gestational age. The fetal loss rate is approximately 56% when patients sustain burns over 15% to 25% of the total body surface area (TBSA) [1]. Fetal mortality is as high as 63% when 25% to 50% of the TBSA is burned and approaches 100% when burns exceed 50% of TBSA [1,3,37,38]. When fetal loss occurs, it usually is within a week of the initial burn injury [3]. Maternal and fetal deaths often are a result of inadequate fluid resuscitation, prolonged hypotension, shock, hypoxia, septicemia, and hyponatremia [1]. Burn severity is determined by the depth and size of the burn. Burn depth is described as partial thickness (superficial and deep layers of skin) or full thickness. The TBSA affected is estimated using the "rule of nines" and is related directly to maternal and fetal outcome. The head, extremities, and torso are each assigned a score of 9% or a multiple thereof. Summed together, this score estimates the TBSA involved.

When caring for the pregnant burn patient, one should consider the potential for carbon monoxide poisoning. Carbon monoxide crosses the placenta and preferentially binds with fetal hemoglobin, creating fetal carboxyhemoglobin. Carboxyhemoglobin levels should be evaluated and hyperbaric oxygen therapy considered when levels are abnormal.

When burns are a result of electrocution, electrical current is the most significant predictor of pregnancy outcome. The severity of the injury depends on the strength of the voltage and the resistance and pathway through which the current traveled. The spectrum of injury ranges from an unpleasant sensation to cardiac arrest. Current most often travels from hand to hand. When voltage travels from hand to foot, it may involve the fetus. Electric current passing through the uterus often results in fetal demise [39].

Burns are managed aggressively using treatment protocols for nonpregnant victims. When trauma occurs in conjunction with burns, trauma care takes precedence [1]. Early prompt resuscitation and transport are critical [1]. Patients who have major burns over more than 20% of TBSA should be transferred to a burn center for management with care coordinated between trauma surgeons and obstetricians [3]. Resuscitation includes assessment of burn severity, assessment for other injuries, airway protection, oxygenation, aggressive fluid replacement, and pain management [3]. Oxygenation prevents maternal and fetal hypoxemia. Burn patients often have compromised airways, and early endotracheal intubation should be performed when signs of airway burn are present. Signs of potential airway compromise include facial burns, copious secretions, hoarseness, stridor, singed nasal hairs or eyebrows, soot in the nares or oropharynx, hypoxia, respiratory distress, or a history of combustion within a small area [7]. Aggressive hydration is critical [1,3]. Fluid loss and uteroplacental hypoperfusion are most likely to occur within the first 12 hours following a burn [3,40]. Hydration protocols such as the Parkland formula are used to estimate fluid replacement requirements. Volume amounting to 4 mL/kg/percent TBSA burned is replaced over the first 24 hours, with half of the fluid infused over the first 8 hours and the remainder infused over the following 16 hours [41]. Volume requirements may be greater, because protocols often are derived from nonpregnant victims. Electrolytes should be followed carefully during fluid resuscitation, as should input and output. Central hemodynamic monitoring may be indicated, particularly in the face of pulmonary or cardiac compromise or oliguria. Patients often require parenteral nutrition supplementation, and broad-spectrum systemic antibiotic therapy is administered to prevent infection and sepsis. Wound care practice is similar to that of nonpregnant patients and involves early, careful eschar débridement and cleaning of burned areas to improve healing. Sterile dressings and topical antibiotics are applied regularly. Stabilization typically occurs within 36 to 72 hours [42]. Decisions regarding delivery involve consideration of gestational age and fetal well-being. Urgent delivery has been considered the treatment of choice in term or near-term pregnant women who have suffered extensive burn injury [43].

## Falls

Falls account for 3% to 31% of injuries [1,10]. The morbidity associated with falls is modest and typically is associated with a less than 10% incidence of maternal or fetal complications [44]. Connolly and colleagues [10] found that falls occur more frequently between 20 and 30 weeks' gestation. Williams and colleagues [45] noted that more than 80% of falls occur after 32 weeks' gestation.

The gravid female has an increase in spinal lordosis that allows the shifting of her center of gravity over her legs [1]. This change in the center of gravity contributes to more falls as pregnancy progresses. As such, overly aggressive, high-impact activity should be avoided as pregnancy advances. The degree of injury is related to the distance of the fall and the specific body part involved [1]. When patients fall, they fall primarily on their buttocks, side, or onto their abdomen. The nature of injuries includes bruises, cuts, ankle sprains, strains, and fractures [1]. Associated complications include preterm labor, abruption, uterine rupture, low birth weight neonates, and stillbirths [1].

## Assault

The prevalence of domestic violence ranges from 10% to 30% and is associated with a 5% risk of fetal death [3,11,46]. Approximately 1 million women sustain nonfatal violence by an intimate partner annually [1]. Up to 60% of abused women report multiple episodes of abuse [10,47,48]. Abused pregnant women have a threefold higher risk of being victims of attempted and completed homicide than do nonabused controls [47]. Most often the abuser is the patient's boyfriend or partner. Interpersonal violence is not associated with marital status, age, race, or socioeconomic status. Pregnancy and the postpartum period may escalate the incidence and severity of the abuse, and the uterus and fetus may sustain the brunt of the force [1,27,28,47]. Common sites of abuse include the face, head, breasts, and abdomen [3]. Assault is associated with delay in prenatal care, fetal death, low fetal birth weight, low maternal weight gain, maternal infections, anemia, maternal drug and alcohol use, preterm labor, preterm premature rupture of membranes, and abruption [1,3, 47–49].

## Initial assessment

Most pregnant trauma victims should be transported to a recognized trauma center [3]. Prehospital findings of tachycardia (defined as a heart rate > 110 beats/min), chest pain, loss of consciousness, and third trimester pregnancy have been independently associated with the need for care in a trauma center [3,24]. The guidelines for Advanced Trauma Life Support and prehospital trauma care of the pregnant patient are similar to those for nonpregnant patients. Life-saving interventions, including medications and diagnostic imaging, should be undertaken irrespective of pregnancy status. Extrication procedures are similar to those used for nonpregnant victims. The physical examination is identical to that for any trauma patient with consideration given to any pregnancy-related findings [11]. Initial assessment involves the airways, breathing, and circulation and is focused on achieving maternal cardiopulmonary stability. Evaluation and management requires a multidisciplinary approach, with trauma surgeons and obstetricians collaborating with maternal-fetal medicine specialists, emergency medical technicians, emergency room physicians and nurses, anesthesiologists, and pediatricians.

### Primary survey

The initial assessment is similar to that of the nonpregnant victim and is rapid, taking no longer than 30 to 60 seconds. While inline cervical spine immobilization is maintained, the airway is assessed and rendered free from obstruction and secretions [1]. The patient's head should be maintained in a neutral position if there is concern for a cervical spine injury. Respiratory rate and effort should be assessed and pulse oximetry applied. Central and peripheral pulse quality, skin color, skin temperature, and capillary refill should be evaluated.

Disability and neurologic function should be assessed by a basic neurologic examination [1]. Eclampsia should be considered as a cause for altered mental status or seizures. The Glasgow Coma Scale is used to evaluate neurologic status. Patients who have a score of 8 or less typically require intubation and mechanical ventilation for control of the airway or intracranial pressure control [7].

While cervical spine immobilization is maintained, the patient should be exposed briefly and the extent of injuries quickly assessed. It is important to search for any gunshot entry or exit wounds.

### Secondary survey

The secondary survey is a head-to-toe comprehensive inspection with palpation and auscultation. Obtain information regarding the mechanism of injury and information regarding weapons used, use of drugs or alcohol, and use of seatbelts. It is essential to obtain a complete past medical and

obstetric history, including last menstrual period, current and past pregnancy complications, and estimated gestational age.

Fetal heart tones should be assessed as soon as possible during the secondary survey. The normal baseline fetal heart rate ranges from 120 to
160 beats per minute. Fetal heart tones can be auscultated with a stethoscope
after 20 weeks' gestation and with Doppler ultrasound at 10 to 14 weeks'
gestation. Continuous monitoring should be initiated when gestational age
is approximately 24 weeks. The fetal monitoring tracing should be evaluated
by providers skilled in interpreting heart rate tracings. Fetal compromise
may be manifest by tachycardia, bradycardia, loss of beat-to-beat variability, or recurrent decelerations. When the pregnant trauma victim experiences hemorrhage, blood is shunted to vital organs at the expense of the
uteroplacental unit and splanchnic beds. Therefore, an abnormal fetal heart
rate may be the first indication that hemodynamic instability is impending
[50]. Monitoring also can assess for uterine irritability or contractions that
may not be perceived by the patient.

It is critical to pay close attention to the abdominal component of the secondary survey, because the protuberant abdomen is more vulnerable to injury. One should check for ecchymoses and asymmetry. Gradual growth
and distention of the peritoneum as the uterus expands seem to desensitize
the pregnant patient to peritoneal injury. Therefore abdominal tenderness,
rebound, and guarding may not be present on physical examination.

One should assess uterine size to help determine gestational age and to
assess for contractions, rigidity, or tenderness. The distance of the uterine
fundus from the pubic symphysis measured in centimeters correlates with
gestational age [3]. The fetus probably is viable if the uterus can be palpated
3 to 4 cm above the level of the umbilicus.

A sterile-speculum vaginal examination is performed to assess for evidence of rupture of membranes and to evaluate vaginal bleeding. Vaginal
bleeding may indicate preterm labor, abruption, uterine rupture, or pelvic
fracture with vaginal involvement. A digital cervical examination is performed to assess for cervical dilation and effacement but should be deferred
in the presence of bleeding until the possibility of placenta previa is elimi-
nated. A rectal examination is performed to evaluate for hematomas and
blood.

Initial laboratory studies should assess hemoglobin and studies sent for
immediate packed red blood cell cross-matching. Comparison of the hematocrit with prenatally obtained levels can help determine if blood loss is present or significant. Coagulation studies and a urinalysis are also obtained.
Kleihauer-Betke testing is obtained when indicated. Arterial blood gases
with serum bicarbonate or lactate levels also may be indicated when there
is significant trauma. Toxicology testing may be indicated also, because
such tests may be positive up to 16% of the time [19].

Diagnostic studies, including cervical spine imaging, CT studies, and
chest and pelvic radiographs, should be obtained for indications similar to

those in the nonpregnant patient but should be limited, if possible. The uterus should be shielded whenever possible.

Focused abdominal sonography for trauma (FAST) is used to assess for free fluid in the pericardial and pleural cavities and in the peritoneum and retroperitoneum. This study has 85% sensitivity and 99% specificity for detecting intraperitoneal fluid and 100% sensitivity and 99% specificity for detecting pericardial fluid [1,51].

Ultrasound also may be used in the emergency room to confirm fetal heart rate, assess gestational age, evaluate for possible placenta previa or abruption, and to assess fetal well-being [1,11,52]. Using ultrasound whenever possible avoids exposing the fetus to ionizing radiation. Although the sensitivity of identifying abruption with ultrasound is poor (less than 50%), its positive predictive value is high [3,25,53].

Diagnostic peritoneal lavage (DPL) may be indicated if there are abdominal signs or symptoms suggestive of intraperitoneal bleeding, altered mental status, unexplained shock, multiple abdominal, thoracic or orthopedic injuries, or when FAST examination is equivocal [48]. Although DPL may be performed earlier in pregnancy, it becomes technically more challenging as pregnancy progresses. The supraumbilical approach is used when the uterus is palpated above the pubic symphysis and is performed using an open or mini-laparotomy technique to minimize complications such as inadvertent uterine or fetal injury.

## Management

When managing the pregnant trauma patient, it is important to consider that there are two patients. Maternal well-being and stability takes precedence, however. Evaluation of the fetus should take place only after stabilization of the mother. High-flow oxygen should be administered initially by either nasal cannula or facemask. Because of diminished maternal oxygen reserve, when assessing breathing and the airway, there should be early consideration for placement of an oral or nasal airway or performing endotracheal or nasotracheal intubation [1]. Pregnant women are at increased risk for aspiration because of decreased gastric motility and reduced lower esophageal sphincter tone. Early intubation protects the airway to prevent aspiration. When intubating a pregnant trauma patient, one should assume she has a full stomach and a cervical spine injury and therefore should lift the chin and thrust the jaw forward. Early intubation also is recommended because developing airway edema can compromise an already challenging maternal airway. Nasopharyngeal airways are not recommended if there is facial trauma. Intubation and placement of airways should be undertaken with care and caution. Airway edema, tongue enlargement, increased breast size, and the generalized weight gain of pregnancy make laryngoscopy and intubation difficult [7]. The hyperemic mucosa and oropharynx predispose to bleeding with manipulation and further compromise attempts at achieving an airway. In a patient who has a cervical spine injury, direct laryngoscopy should be avoided, and fiberoptic or awake fiberoptic intubation should be performed. Denitrogenation and preoxygenation with 100% oxygen is performed before intubation because of the maternal decreased functional residual capacity and increased oxygen consumption associated with pregnancy [1]. Intubation is accomplished with a rapid sequence induction and application of cricoid pressure. Because placental production of pseudocholinesterase increases levels in pregnancy, lower doses of succinylcholine are required [54]. Both depolarizing and nondepolarizing agents cross the placenta and may result in an initially depressed neonate. After establishing an airway, high-flow 100% oxygen is administered.

The presence of decreased breath sounds, dyspnea, subcutaneous edema, and hypotension may suggest a tension pneumothorax. A chest tube should be placed immediately at the third or fourth intercostal space. The insertion is moved one to two intercostal spaces higher than in nonpregnant individuals because of the 50% increase in substernal angle, the rising diaphragm, and the increase in anteroposterior diameter of the chest [1]. Alternatively, needle aspiration can be performed by placing a needle in the second intercostal space along the midclavicular line.

Aggressive fluid resuscitation in the pregnant trauma victim is critical and should be accomplished with placement of two large-bore intravenous lines. One to 2 L of warm crystalloid such as lactated Ringer's solution or normal saline should be infused immediately to replace volume. Fluids are given in a 3:1 ratio for the estimated blood loss. If indicated, transfusion with typed and cross-matched packed red blood cells is preferred. In emergent circumstances, however, type O Rh-negative blood is used. Because vasopressors compromise uteroplacental perfusion, it is preferable to replace volume to manage cardiac output and blood pressure [55]. Pressors may be required, however, as a life-saving intervention. Norepinephrine and epinephrine restore maternal blood pressure but compromise uterine perfusion. Ephedrine and mephentermine increase maternal blood pressure while preserving uterine blood flow. Dopamine at doses no greater than 5 μg/kg per minute also raises maternal blood pressure without compromising uterine blood flow.

The patient should be tilted on her left side by placing a wedge (towels or blankets) under her right hip or using a backboard tilted to a 15° angle. This tilting displaces the uterus laterally, thereby maximizing cardiac preload and cardiac output. Displacing the uterus laterally can increase cardiac output by 30% [1]. This increase is of particular importance in pregnancies beyond 20 weeks' gestation.

Military antishock trousers or pneumatic antishock garments may be used to control hemorrhage, but use of the abdominal compartment is contraindicated, because it may compromise uterine perfusion [1]. The lower compartments also may be used to stabilize fractures.

A Foley catheter is inserted for accurate urinary output assessment. Lack of urine output after catheter placement may be the result of misplacement, recent urination, incontinence, depleted intravascular volume with compromised renal blood flow, or bladder rupture. Placement of a nasogastric or orogastric tube may be required to evacuate gastric contents and minimize aspiration risk.

Knives and other penetrating objects should not be removed but instead should be stabilized in place with packing. Doing so allows exploration of the exact injury pathway when the patient is taken to surgery and allows control of hemorrhage, because the object provides some tamponade of bleeding [1]. When performing exploratory laparotomy with a living fetus in utero, it is imperative to handle the uterus gently and avoid applying excessive traction or twisting, which could compromise uteroplacental perfusion. Exploratory laparotomy is not an indication for cesarean delivery, which rarely is indicated unless there is fetal death or a direct perforating injury to the fetus. When performing exploratory laparotomy, appropriate antibiotic coverage should be administered to cover for streptococcus, staphylococcus, clostridium, and polymicrobial infections.

For patients who have penetrating injuries, tetanus toxoid administration is not contraindicated. Patients should receive 0.5 mL of tetanus toxoid if they have not received a booster in the past 5 years. They should receive 250 units of tetanus immunoglobulin intramuscularly in addition to the tetanus toxoid if they have not been immunized and have suffered a high-risk injury [1].

## Special considerations

### Cesarean delivery

Emergency cesarean deliveries occasionally are performed for maternal or fetal indications [1]. Emergency cesarean is indicated when the uterus interferes in trauma-related surgical interventions, cardiopulmonary resuscitation has been unsuccessful after 4 minutes, there is fetal compromise in a viable fetus with a stable mother, or there is obvious impending or recent maternal death [56]. Fetal and maternal survival rates after emergency cesarean delivery at greater than 25 weeks' gestation have been documented to be as high as 45% and 72%, respectively. There was no fetal survival when no fetal heart beat was heard before emergent delivery, whereas there was 75% survival when fetal heart tones were present and gestational age was 26 weeks or more [57]. Optimum infant survival has been described when cesarean delivery was performed within 5 minutes of maternal death [56,58]. It is recommended that cesarean delivery be performed if the patient has not responded after 4 minutes of resuscitation. Four minutes of resuscitation and 1 minute to deliver the neonate is the basis for the "5-minute rule." One may want to consider proceeding with delivery even if resuscitation efforts have extended beyond 4 minutes, because neonatal survival has been reported. In addition to optimizing fetal outcome, cesarean delivery removes aortocaval compression, resulting in a 60% to 80% increase in cardiac output and optimizing chances for maternal survival.

*Cardiac arrest*

Cardiac arrest during pregnancy is rare, occurring in approximately 1 in 30,000 pregnancies. Prompt initiation of cardiopulmonary resuscitation is critical while addressing the underlying etiology for the arrest [1]. Standard Advanced Cardiac Life Support algorithms for medications, intubation, and defibrillation are applied. Chest compressions and ventilations are performed in the usual manner; they are less effective in the latter trimesters, however, because aortocaval compression compromises cardiac output. Moving the hand position cephalad improves compressions, because the heart is displaced upward during pregnancy. Defibrillatory shocks transfer no significant current to the fetus. A decision to move toward cesarean delivery should be made quickly, with delivery of the fetus accomplished within 5 minutes of the cardiopulmonary arrest [1,20]. Katz and colleagues [56] looked at 61 infants born to women by perimortem cesarean delivery between 1900 and 1985. They found that 70% of neonates delivered within 5 minutes of maternal death survived, and all survivors were neurologically intact. When cesarean delivery was delayed for more than 5 minutes, only 13% of infants were living, and all had neurologic morbidity. The degree of neurologic handicap correlated with the time between maternal death and delivery.

**Prevention**

Of paramount importance in managing trauma in pregnancy is preventing its occurrence in the first place. Education in trauma prevention should be incorporated into prenatal care and should include instruction on the appropriate use of seatbelts, encouraging their use and addressing the misconceptions that using them may harm the fetus somehow. Outpatient visits, whether for a prenatal visit or other reasons, should incorporate screening for domestic violence. It is important to understand that pregnancy loss can occur even in patients who have minor or no injuries. Health care providers must not assume that minimal maternal injury confers no fetal risk. Therefore, all pregnant women should be advised to seek medical attention after trauma, regardless of how minor the trauma is considered to be.

**References**

[1] Tweddale CJ. Trauma during pregnancy. Crit Care Nurs Q 2006;29(1):53–67.
[2] Stone K. Trauma in the obstetric patient. Obstet Gynecol Clin North Am 1999;26(3):459–67.
[3] Shah AJ, Kilcline BA. Trauma in pregnancy. Emerg Med Clin North Am 2003;21(3):615–29.

[4] Fildes J, Reed L, Jones N, et al. Trauma: the leading cause of nonobstetric maternal death. J Trauma 1992;32(5):643–5.

[5] El-Kady D, Gilbert WM, Anderson J, et al. Trauma during pregnancy: an analysis of maternal and fetal outcomes in a large population. Am J Obstet Gynecol 2004;190(6):1661–8.

[6] Rosenfeld JA. Abdominal trauma in pregnancy: when is fetal monitoring necessary? Postgrad Med 1990;88(6):89–91, 94.

[7] Kuczkowski KM. Trauma in the pregnant patient. Curr Opin Anaesthesiol 2004;17(2): 145–50.

[8] Baker BW. Trauma. In: Chestnut DH, editor. Obstetric anesthesia: principles and practice. 1st edition. St Louis (MO): Mosby; 1999. p. 1041–50.

[9] Shah KH, Simons RK, Holbrook T, et al. Trauma in pregnancy: maternal and fetal outcomes. J Trauma 1998;45(1):83–6.

[10] Connolly AM, Katz VL, Bash KL, et al. Trauma and pregnancy. Am J Perinatol 1997;14(6): 331–5

[11] Mattox KL, Goetzl L. Trauma in pregnancy. Crit Care Med 2005;33(10):S385–9.

[12] Greiss FC Jr. Uterine vascular response to hemorrhage during pregnancy, with observations on therapy. Obstet Gynecol 1966;27(4):549–54.

[13] Norwitz ER, Robinson JN, Malone FD, et al. Critical care obstetrics. In: Clark SL, Cotton DB, Hankins GDV, editors. Critical care obstetrics. 4th edition. Malden (MA): Blackwell Scientific; 2004. p. 19–42.

[14] Anderson RN. Trauma and pregnancy: prehospital concerns. Emerg Med Serv 2002;31(7): 71–5, 79.

[15] Weiss HB, Songer TJ, Fabio A. Fetal deaths related to maternal injury. JAMA 2001;286(15): 1863–8.

[16] Rogers FB, Rozycki GS, Osler T, et al. Multi-institutional study of factors associated with fetal death in injured pregnant patients. Arch Surg 1999;134(11):1274–7.

[17] Sperry JL, Casey BM, McIntire DD, et al. Long-term fetal outcomes in pregnant trauma patients. Am J Surg 2006;192(6):715–21.

[18] Ali J, Yeo A, Gana T, et al. Predictors of fetal mortality in pregnant trauma patients. J Trauma 1997;42(5):782–5.

[19] Esposito TJ, Gens DR, Smith LG, et al. Evaluation of blunt abdominal trauma occurring during pregnancy. J Trauma 1989;29(12):1628–32.

[20] Guidelines for Diagnostic Imaging During Pregnancy. ACOG Committee Opinion Number 299. American College of Obstetricians and Gynecologist 2004;104(3):647–51.

[21] Neufeld J, Moore E, Mars J, et al. Trauma in pregnancy. Emerg Med Clin North Am 1987; 5(3):623–40.

[22] Rothenberger D, Quattlebaum F, Perry J, et al. Blunt maternal trauma: a review of 103 cases. J Trauma 1978;18(3):173–9.

[23] Crosby WM, Costiloe JP. Safety of lap-belt restraint for pregnant victims of automobile collisions. N Engl J Med 1971;284(12):632–6.

[24] Goodwin T, Breen M. Pregnancy outcome and fetomaternal hemorrhage after noncatastrophic trauma. Am J Obstet Gynecol 1990;162(3):665–71.

[25] Pearlman M, Tintinalli J, Lorenz R. A prospective controlled study of outcome after trauma during pregnancy. Am J Obstet Gynecol 1990;162(6):1502–10.

[26] Drost TF, Rosemurgy AS, Sherman HF, et al. Major trauma in pregnant women: maternal/ fetal outcome. J Trauma 1990;30(5):574–8.

[27] Hull SB, Bennett S. The pregnant trauma patient: assessment and anesthetic management. Int Anesthesiol Clin 2007;45(3):1–18.

[28] Rose PG, Strohm PL, Zuspan FP. Fetomaternal hemorrhage following trauma. Am J Obstet Gynecol 1985;153(8):844–7.

[29] Pearlman M, Tintinalli J. Evaluation and treatment of the gravida and fetus following trauma during pregnancy. Obstet Gynecol Clin North Am 1991,18(2):371–80.

[30] Pak LL, Reece EA, Chan L. Is adverse pregnancy outcome predictable after blunt abdominal trauma? Am J Obstet Gynecol 1998;179(5):1140–4.

[31] Curet M, Schermer C, Demarest G. Predictors of outcome in trauma during pregnancy: identification of patients who can be monitored for less than 6 hours. J Trauma 2000; 49(1):18–25.

[32] Astarita D, Feldman B. Seat belt placement resulting in uterine rupture. J Trauma 1997; 42(4):738–40.

[33] Metz TD, Torri D, Abbott JT, et al. Uterine trauma in pregnancy after motor vehicle crashes with airbag deployment: a 30-case series. J Trauma 2006;61(3):658–61.

[34] Sandy EA, Koemer M. Self inflicted gunshot wound to the pregnant abdomen: report of a case and review of the literature. Am J Perinatol 1989;6(1):30–1.

[35] Buchsbaum H. Penetrating injury of the abdomen. In: Buchsbaum H, editor. Trauma in pregnancy. Philadelphia: WB Saunders; 1979. p. 82–100.

[36] Awwad J, Azar G, Seoud M, et al. High velocity penetrating wounds of the gravid uterus: review of 16 years of civil war. Obstet Gynecol 1994;83(2):259–64.

[37] Polko L, McMahon M. Burns in pregnancy. Obstet Gynecol Surv 1997;53(1):50–6.

[38] Schmitz J. Pregnant patients with burns. Am J Obstet Gynecol 1971;110(1):57.

[39] Fish R. Electric shock. Part I: physics and pathophysiology. J Emerg Med 1993;11(3): 309–12.

[40] Lavery J, Staten-McCormick M. Management of moderate to severe trauma in pregnancy. Obstet Gynecol Clin North Am 1995;22(1):69–90.

[41] Reiss G. Thermal injuries. In: Lopez-Viego MA, editor. The Parkland trauma handbook. St. Louis (MO): Mosby; 1994. p. 389–412.

[42] Mabrouk A, El-Feky A. Burns during pregnancy: a gloomy outcome. Burns 1997;23(7/8): 596–600.

[43] Kuczkowski KM, Fernandez CL. Thermal injury in pregnancy: anesthetic considerations. Anesthesia 2003;58:931–2.

[44] Fort A, Harlin R. Pregnancy outcome after noncatastrophic maternal trauma during pregnancy. Obstet Gynecol 1970;35(6):912–5.

[45] Williams JK, McClain L, Rosemurgy AS, et al. Evaluation of blunt abdominal trauma in the third trimester of pregnancy: maternal and fetal considerations. Obstet Gynecol 1990;75(1): 33–7.

[46] Guth AA, Pachter HL. Domestic violence and the trauma surgeon. Am J Surg 2000;179(2): 134–40.

[47] McFarlane J, Campbell JC, Sharps P, et al. Abuse during pregnancy and femicide: urgent implications for women's health. Obstet Gynecol 2002;100(1):27–36.

[48] Poole G, Martin J, Perry K, et al. Trauma in pregnancy: the role of interpersonal violence. Am J Obstet Gynecol 1996;174(6):1873–6.

[49] Parker B, McFarlane J, Soeken K. Abuse during pregnancy: effects on maternal complications and birth weight in adults and teenage women. Obstet Gynecol 1994;84(3):323–8.

[50] Baerga-Varela Y, Zietlow SP, Bannon MP, et al. Trauma in pregnancy. Mayo Clin Proc 2000;75(12):1243–8.

[51] Ma OJ, Mateer J, Ogata M, et al. Prospective analysis of a rapid trauma ultrasound examination performed by emergency physicians. J Trauma 1995;38(6):879–85.

[52] Goodwin H, Holmes JF, Wisner DH. Abdominal ultrasound examination in pregnant blunt trauma patients. J Trauma 2001;50(4):689–93 [discussion: 694].

[53] Dahmus M, Sibai B. Blunt abdominal trauma: are there any predictive factors for abruptio placentae or maternal-fetal distress? Am J Obstet Gynecol 1993;169(4):1054–9.

[54] Schneider R. Muscle relaxants. In: Walls R, editor. Emergency airway management. Philadelphia: Lippincott Williams & Wilkins; 2000. p. 121–8.

[55] Baker BW. Trauma. In: Chestnut DH, editor. Obstetric anesthesia: principles and practice. 3rd edition. Philadelphia: Elsevier Mosby; 2004. p. 942–50.

[56] Katz VL, Dotters DJ, Droegemueller W. Perimortem cesarean delivery. Obstet Gynecol 1986;68(4):571–6.
[57] Morris JA, Rosenbower TJ, Jurkovich GJ, et al. Infant survival after cesarean section for trauma. Ann Surg 1996;223(95):481–8 [discussion: 488–91].
[58] Katz VL, Balderston K, Defreest M. Perimortem cesarean delivery: were our assumptions correct? Am J Obstet Gynecol 2005;192(6):1916–20 [discussion: 1920–1].

ELSEVIER
SAUNDERS

Surg Clin N Am 88 (2008) 441–450

SURGICAL
CLINICS OF
NORTH AMERICA

# Index

*Note:* Page numbers of article titles are in **boldface** type.

## A

Abdominal wall injury, gynecologic surgery and, imaging of, 386

Abnormal uterine bleeding. *See* Gynecologic emergencies.

Abscesses
    tubo-ovarian. *See* Gynecologic emergencies.
    vaginal cuff, gynecologic surgery and, 352

Adhesions, postoperative, and bowel obstruction, 350

Adnexal masses, benign. *See* Benign gynecologic conditions.

Adnexal torsion. *See* Gynecologic emergencies.

Airway compromise, in pregnant burn victim, 430

Antibiotics
    for appendicitis, in pregnancy, 407
    for infections, after gynecologic surgery, 351
    for pelvic inflammatory disease, 262
    for tubo-ovarian abscesses, 275

Appendicitis, in pregnancy. *See* Pregnancy.

Arterial embolization, for vascular injuries, after gynecologic surgery, 347

Aspiration, of gastric contents, in pregnancy, 396–397, 434

Assault, in pregnancy, 431

Autotransfusion, in pregnancy, 393

## B

Benign gynecologic conditions, **245–264**
    adnexal masses, 245–249
        clinical features of, 247–248
        diagnosis of, 248
        etiology of, 245–247

endometriomas, 246
functional ovarian cysts, 245–246
neoplasms, 247
pelvic inflammatory disease, 246
imaging of, 368–371
laparoscopic surgery for, 327–330
management of, 248–249
endometriosis, 254–259
    clinical features of, 255–256
    diagnosis of, 256–257
        laparoscopic surgery in, 327
    etiology of, 254–255
    management of, 257–259
leiomyomas, 249–254
    clinical features of, 250–251
    diagnosis of, 251–252
    etiology of, 250
    management of, 252–254
pelvic inflammatory disease, 246, 259–262
    clinical features of, 260–261
    diagnosis of, 261
        laparoscopic surgery in, 327
    etiology of, 260
    management of, 262

Beta-human chorionic gonadotropin, in ectopic pregnancy, 267–268

Bevacizumab, for advanced epithelial ovarian cancer, 293

Biologic therapy, for advanced epithelial ovarian cancer, 293

Bladder, female, anatomy of, 229

Bladder injury, gynecologic surgery and, 344–345
    imaging of, 385

Bleeding, abnormal uterine. *See* Gynecologic emergencies.

Blood loss, in pregnant trauma victim, 422

Blood pressure changes, in pregnancy, 393, 422–423

doi:10.1016/S0039-6109(08)00030-3                    *surgical.theclinics.com*